Nursing care in eye, ear, nose, and throat disorders

Nursing care in eye, ear, nose, and throat disorders

WILLIAM H. HAVENER, B.A., M.S. (Ophth.), M.D.

*Professor and Chairman, Department of Ophthalmology, The Ohio State University
College of Medicine; Member, Attending Staff, University Hospitals;
Member, Consulting Staff, Children's Hospital and
Mt. Carmel Hospital, Columbus, Ohio*

WILLIAM H. SAUNDERS, B.A., M.D.

*Professor and Chairman, Department of Otolaryngology, The Ohio State
University College of Medicine, Columbus, Ohio*

CAROL FAIR KEITH, R.N., B.S.N., M.S.

*Assistant Professor in Medical-Surgical Nursing, The Ohio State University
School of Nursing, Columbus, Ohio*

ARDRA W. PRESCOTT, R.N.

Head Nurse, Eye Clinic, The Ohio State University Hospital, Columbus, Ohio

Third edition

With 357 illustrations

The C. V. Mosby Company

Saint Louis / 1974

Library of Congress Cataloging in Publication Data

Main entry under title:
  Nursing care in eye, ear, nose, and throat disorders.

  First ed. by W. H. Havener, W. H. Saunders, and
B. S. Bergersen.
  1. Ophthalmic nursing. 2. Otolaryngological
nursing. I. Havener, William H. II. Havener,
William H. Nursing care in eye, ear, nose, and
throat disorders. [DNLM: 1. Eye diseases—Nursing.
2. Otorhinolaryngologic diseases—Nursing.
WY158 N974 1974]
RE88.N8 1974   610.73'6   73-12693
ISBN 0-8016-2101-1

VH/VH/VH 9 8 7 6 5 4 3 2 1

Preface

This book is designed to assist the nurse in her expanding role in the health care system, including outpatient, inpatient, and homegoing preparation situations.

We hope this text will assist the nurse in her assessment role and in her development of a plan of care based upon a better understanding of the pathophysiology, the treatment, and the related problems of patients with disorders of the eye, ear, nose, and throat.

In assisting with the chapters concerning the nursing care of patients with eye disorders thanks go to Miss Sallie Gloeckner, Mr. Vincent McGuire, and Mrs. Ruth Davis for their invaluable assistance.

Preparation of the chapters regarding nursing care of patients with problems of the mouth, nose, ear, and throat was greatly facilitated by the able assistance of Mrs. Gretchen Meske.

William H. Havener

William H. Saunders

Carol Fair Keith

Ardra W. Prescott

Contents

Glossary

The patient with eye disorders

CHAPTER ONE

Structure and function

The eye (Figs. 1-1 to 1-3) is made of three layers (sclera, choroid, retina) of tissue, which enclose a fluid-filled center. The outer layer, which provides strength, is called sclera posteriorly and cornea anteriorly. Both the sclera and cornea are very strong and resistant to stretching and tearing; however, they are quite flexible and not at all rigid like an eggshell. The firmness of the eye results from its fluid contents, which are normally under a pressure of 15 to 20 mm. Hg. Hence the structure of the eye is similar to that of an inflated basketball. If the sclera or cornea is cut, the fluid contents may escape, permitting the structure of the eye to collapse like a flat tire.

The cornea is normally completely transparent and invisible. It focuses and transmits light to the interior of the eye. Its surface must be moist at all times, or it will lose its transparency and may even develop permanent scarring. A film of tear fluid is spread upon the cornea with each blink of the lids. Failure of the lids to close properly (as may happen in an unconscious patient) may result in drying of the cornea, unless the lids are adequately closed by the nurse. The physician's order for protective eye ointment should be obtained.

The surface of the cornea is covered with a thin layer of epithelial cells. These cells are much more resistant to infection than are the deeper layers of the cornea; hence an abraded cornea is quite susceptible to infection. Fortunately damage to the corneal epithelium is easily recognized because of pain. The cornea has many more pain-recognizing nerve fibers than does any other part of the eye.

The back of the cornea is covered by a layer of endothelial cells. Their function is to remove excess water from the cornea. If the endothelial cells are diseased, the cornea becomes swollen and opaque.

The sclera is directly continuous with the edge of the cornea and encircles the eye completely, except where it joins the emerging optic nerve. Numerous arteries, veins, and nerves penetrate the sclera. The tendons of the extraocular muscles (which rotate the eye) attach to the sclera. The sclera is white and nontransparent and is responsible for the color of the white portion of the eye.

The middle layer of the eye is called the uveal tract. It is divided into three portions—iris, ciliary body, and choroid.

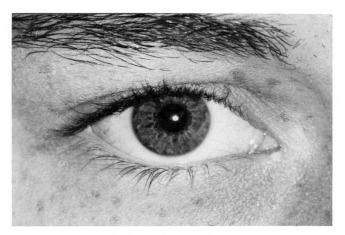

Fig. 1-1. External view of human eye.

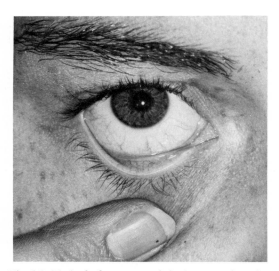

Fig. 1-2. Method of exposure of the lower conjunctiva.

The iris is the doughnut-shaped structure that gives the eye its blue, gray, or brown color. It surrounds the pupil, which appears black because no light can be seen to emerge from the eye. (The pupil is **not** a black structure but is simply a hole in the center of the iris.) Two muscles in the iris change the size of the pupil. The iris sphincter encircles the pupil, and its contraction decreases the pupil diameter. This iris dilator runs radially from the pupil to the iris periphery, and its contraction enlarges the pupil. The sphincter is supplied by the parasympathetic nervous system,

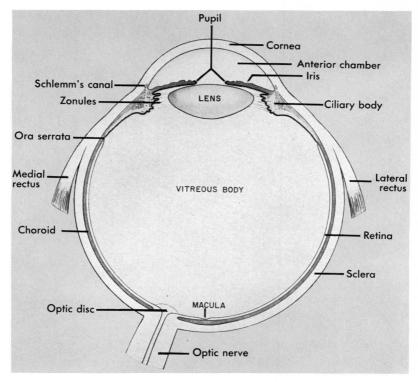

Fig. 1-3. Diagrammatic cross section of the eye.

may be activated by such drugs as pilocarpine or echothiophate (Phospho-line), and is paralyzed by drugs such as atropine or cyclopentolate (Cyclo-gyl). The dilator is sympathetically innervated and may be activated by drugs such as phenylephrine (Neo-Synephrine) or epinephrine (Adrenalin). The function of the iris is to adjust the pupil size appropriately to adapt the eye to the existing brightness of light. As is well known, the pupil becomes large in the dark and small in bright light.

The ciliary body (Fig. 1-4) cannot be seen by the nurse as she observes the patient's eye, but it encircles the eye just behind the iris. The ciliary body has both muscular function and secretory function. The circular por-tion of the ciliary muscle lies upon its inner surface and by its contraction relaxes the tension of the zonular fibers. (These fibers are attached to the lens and will be described with it.) The longitudinal portion of the ciliary muscle lies upon its outer surface and by its contraction opens the trabecular spaces through which the aqueous fluid escapes from the eye. The ciliary processes lie just behind the peripheral iris and produce the aqueous fluid, which fills the anterior portion of the eye.

The choroid is a richly vascular layer and supplies the nutrition of the outer half of the retina. The outer layer of the choroid is composed of large

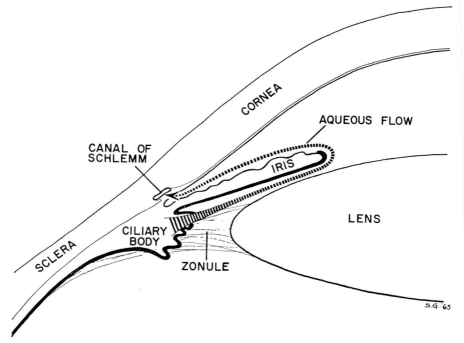

Fig. 1-4. Diagrammatic section of the anterior eye and the aqueous circulation.

vessels; the inner layer is composed of fine capillaries. If the retina falls away from its normal position (retinal detachment), it no longer receives its nourishment from the choroid and hence loses vision. The choroid lines the entire posterior portion of the eye and extends from the ciliary body to the optic nerve.

The innermost layer of the eye, the retina, is the part that perceives light. The retina is an enormously complex and precise network of nerve cells and fibers. Each retina contains more than 125 million nerve cells, which are able to "see" light. Many millions of additional nerve cells co-ordinate and transmit the impulses from the seeing cells to the optic nerve. The optical portion of the eye (cornea and lens) focuses the details of the outside world into a tiny image upon the retina. The pattern of this retinal image is detected by the multimillions of retinal cells and is relayed via the optic nerve to the brain.

The visual cells are more compactly arranged in the center of the retina, which is called the macula. The very center of the macula is called the fovea centralis. Because of the arrangement of visual cells, the central retina, which sees straight ahead, has a considerably better visual acuity than the peripheral retina, which sees to the side.

The optic nerve leaves the eye about 3 mm. nasal to the fovea centralis. The nerve exit creates an oval retinal defect, measuring about 1.5 mm.

across. This defect is responsible for the physiologic blind spot, which is present in every eye, about 15 degrees to the side, and is 5 to 8 degrees across.

The retina has two types of visual cells, called rods and cones. The rods are very sensitive cells that are used for vision in dim light. The cones are used for daylight vision. Colors are recognized by cones but not by rods. The ingenious combination of these different types of visual cells permits the human eye to see usefully through a wide range of illumination—from the intense light of noonday to the dimness of a starlit night.

Within the eye and just behind the iris is the lens. This transparent structure consists of a very thick gelatinous mass of fibers encased in an elastic capsule. Attached at about the equator of the lens are a number of delicate ligaments—the zonular fibers, which suspend the lens in proper position behind the pupil. The zonular fibers are attached to the ciliary body, and their tension may be varied by contraction or relaxation of the circular portion of the ciliary muscle. The shape of the lens changes, depending upon the tension of the zonular fibers. The function of the lens is to focus light upon the retina, which it does automatically in younger persons. With age the lens structure becomes rigid, and the eye loses its ability to change focus (accommodate). Sometimes an older lens loses its transparency; this condition is called cataract.

Most of the space inside the eye is behind the lens. This area is filled with a viscous fluid of a consistency somewhat resembling gelatin. This vitreous gel is formed only during the growth of the eye, remains relatively inert during life, and is never regenerated if lost. The vitreous framework often disintegrates and becomes watery in older persons. Fragments of embryonic blood vessels or of partially disintegrated vitreous framework are often suspended within the vitreous and cast visible shadows (floaters) upon the retina. Loss of vitreous as the result of injury or as an operative complication is serious because the tension exerted by the framework of the remaining vitreous may distort the internal ocular structures.

The anterior chamber is the space between the iris and cornea; the posterior chamber is the space between the iris and lens. Both anterior and posterior chambers are filled with the aqueous. Aqueous is a crystal clear, watery solution of nutrients that is formed by the ciliary body; it bathes and feeds the lens, circulates anteriorly through the pupil, and flows out of the eye through a circular meshwork situated just peripherally to the cornea. This meshwork (trabecular spaces) may be considered as an extremely fine sieve, the apertures of which can be varied somewhat by contraction or relaxation of the longitudinal muscle of the ciliary body. This sieve is so fine that it creates a resistance to the outflow of aqueous, thereby causing a rise in pressure as the aqueous flow is held back. The normal intraocular pressure is regulated by means of the trabecular meshwork. In about 2% of older persons the trabecular meshwork becomes sclerotic and obstructed; aqueous cannot escape at the proper rate, and the intraocular pressure rises to abnormal heights. This elevated intraocular pressure is called glaucoma.

Beyond the trabecular meshwork is a circular channel called the canal of Schlemm. This canal conveys the aqueous to scleral veins, through which it returns to the bloodstream.

The eyes are suspended in the orbits (Fig. 1-5) by means of muscles, ligaments, vessels, nerves, and a cushion of fat.

Six extraocular muscles are attached to each eye. Four of these muscles are attached just in front of the equator of the eye, to the top, bottom, and inner and outer sides. These four muscles extend straight back to the apex of the orbit and are therefore called the rectus (straight) muscles. According to their position in the eye, they are designated as the superior rectus, inferior rectus, medial rectus, or lateral rectus muscle. The remaining two muscles insert on the back of the eye (top and bottom) and extend obliquely forward and medially to their origin from the orbital wall. Hence they are called oblique muscles and are designated the superior oblique muscle and the inferior oblique muscle.

The extraocular muscles of the eyes are remarkably coordinated so that they automatically aim the two eyes at exactly the same point in space, regardless of whether it is near or far, high or low, right or left. The extraocular muscles are innervated by the third, fourth, and sixth cranial nerves; therefore, brain diseases that damage these nerves may be recognized because of the corresponding muscle paralysis.

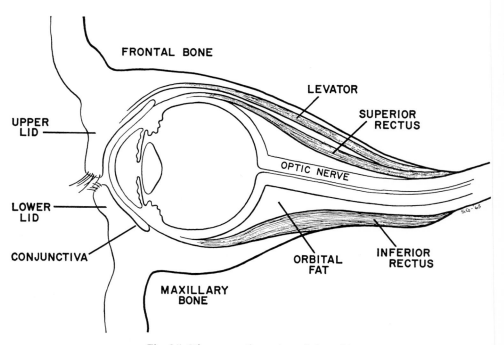

Fig. 1-5. Diagrammatic section of the orbit.

Ligaments and sheets of connective tissue ensheath the extraocular muscles, the optic nerve, and the posterior part of the eye and help to support the eye by means of their attachments to the bony orbital walls.

Much of the posterior orbit is filled with semifluid orbital fat, which acts as a soft cushion supporting the eye. Loss of this fat by injury results in an unsightly sunken appearance of the eye.

Assorted vessels and nerves are also contained within the orbit. Most of the arterial circulation of the eye originates from the ciliary arteries. About a dozen posterior ciliary arteries enter the back of the eye by passing through the sclera. Six or seven anterior ciliary arteries run within the rectus muscles and enter the eye at their insertions. Blood leaves the eye through four or more large vortex veins that emerge from the posterior sclera and also through the conjunctival veins anteriorly. The inner part of the retina has a separate circulation that enters through the optic nerve and is entirely independent of the circulation of the rest of the eye. These vessels are called the central retinal artery and the central retinal vein. Because of this vascular anatomy, occlusion of the central retinal artery can result in death of the retina and blindness, although the appearance of the eye as a whole is unchanged.

The space contained within the rectus muscles is called the muscle cone. The third, fifth, and sixth nerves pass through the superior orbital fissure to enter the muscle cone. Because of this anatomic fact, retrobulbar injection of an anesthetic into the muscle cone will block movement of the lateral rectus (sixth nerve); superior, medial, and inferior rectus (third nerve); and orbital pain sensation (fifth nerve). Such an anesthetic is commonly used in cataract surgery. Being outside the muscle cone, the fourth nerve (superior oblique muscle) is not blocked by a retrobulbar injection. The seventh cranial nerve (innervates facial muscles, including the orbicularis muscle, which closes the lids) runs forward from just below the ear, is not within the orbit, and is not blocked by a retrobulbar injection.

The bony cavity surrounding the eye and its supporting structures is known as the orbit (Fig. 1-6). Anteriorly the orbital walls are quite sturdy and provide considerable protection for the eye against injury. In the orbital apex two large openings, the superior orbital fissure and the optic foramen, transmit nerves and vessels to and from the brain. This is the least well-protected part of the brain, for a sharp wire or icepick could easily penetrate through the orbit and superior orbital fissure and then deeply into vital brain tissue.

The medial wall of the orbit is extremely thin, as is implied by its name, the lamina papyracea (paper layer). The ethmoid sinuses lie just medial to the orbit. Ethmoid infections are particularly dangerous because they may easily spread through this thin bone to invade the eye socket.

The lacrimal apparatus (Fig. 1-7), which supplies and drains the tears, consists of the lacrimal gland, lacrimal puncta and canaliculi, lacrimal sac, and nasolacrimal duct. The lacrimal gland, situated in the upper outer part of the orbit, produces the tears, which drain down and inward across

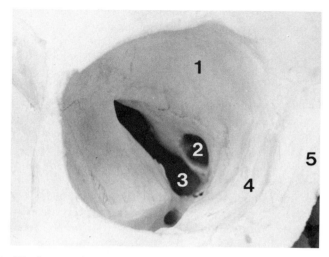

Fig. 1-6. Orbit. The bony orbital cavity, **1**, communicates with the brain via the optic foramen, **2**, which transmits the optic nerve, and the superior orbital fissure, **3**, which transmits most of the other nerves and vessels entering the orbit. The lacrimal fossa, **4**, contains the lacrimal sac. **5** is the nasal bone.

the eye. Regular blinking of the lids helps to spread the tears evenly in a lubricating and protective film across the cornea. The tears drain into the lacrimal puncta, at the inner part of the upper and lower lids, and are carried by the canaliculi into the lacrimal sac. The lacrimal sac is a small pouch located in the corner of the orbit nearest the nose. From the sac the nasolacrimal duct drains into the nose. Obviously the running nose associated with crying is caused by drainage of tears into the nose.

The function of the tears is to bathe and lubricate the eye. Tears perform this function far better and more safely than any eyewash. Contrary to popular belief, the eye itself does **not** need to be washed—indeed, routine irrigation of the eye with proprietary eyewashes is far more likely to irritate and infect the delicate ocular membranes than to help them.

The eyelids are remarkably adaptive, flexible, protective coverings. They are closed by the orbicularis muscle of the eye, which lies just beneath the thin lid skin and completely encircles the opening between the lids. The orbicularis muscle is innervated by the facial (seventh cranial) nerve. The upper lid is opened by the levator muscle, which pulls the lid up into the orbit. The levator muscle lies just above the superior rectus muscle and is innervated by the third cranial nerve.

The shape of the lids is maintained by a tough sheet of connective tissue called the tarsal plate. The tarsal plate and orbicularis muscle hold the lids in proper position against the eye. Should the lower lid sag away from the eye, tears will run annoyingly down the cheek. If the lid margins turn abnormally inward, the eyelashes will painfully abrade the cornea.

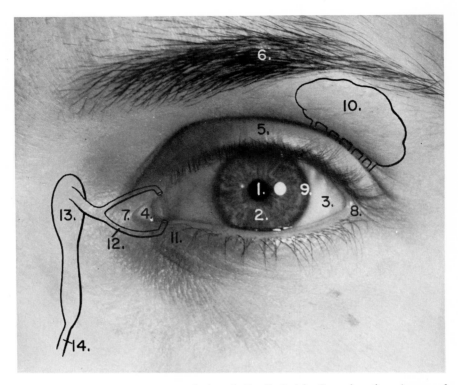

Fig. 1-7. Lacrimal apparatus, external view. **1,** Pupil; **2,** iris; **3,** conjunctiva; **4,** caruncle; **5,** upper lid; **6,** brow; **7,** inner canthus; **8,** outer canthus; **9,** limbus; **10,** lacrimal gland; **11,** near lower lacrimal punctum; **12,** lower lacrimal canaliculus; **13,** lacrimal sac; **14,** naso-lacrimal duct.

Many small glands are located along the lid margin. Their oily secretion prevents the tears from overflowing upon the skin. Infection of these glands is a fairly common cause of local discharge and irritation (sty).

A delicate mucous membrane, the conjunctiva, lines the back surface of the eyelids and the front surface of the eyeball (except for the cornea). The conjunctiva is semitransparent and therefore assumes the color of the underlying tissue (white sclera or reddish eyelid). Naturally the conjunctiva contains blood vessels, just as do almost all other living tissues. Surprisingly often a patient notices the presence of these conjunctival vessels and erroneously thinks that they are abnormal. The common "pink eye" of childhood represents infection of the conjunctiva.

The visual messages are transmitted back to the brain (Fig. 1-8) via the optic nerves. Within the orbit the optic nerves are sinuous and about 1 cm. longer than necessary in order to permit free movement of the eyes. The meningeal sheaths encircling the optic nerves are directly continuous with the meninges of the brain. This permits increased intracranial pressure

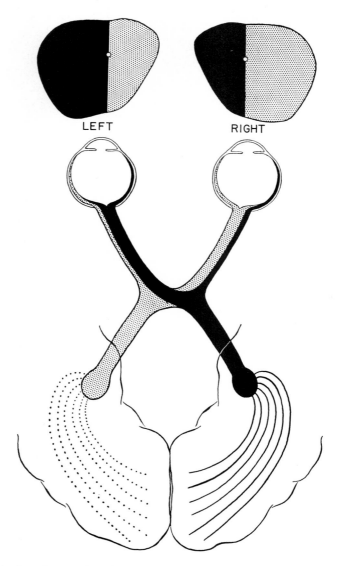

Fig. 1-8. Visual pathway. The left half of the visual field is seen by the right half of both eyes. As drawn, the nerve fibers seeing the left visual field all travel to the right side of the brain and vice versa. Because of the changing anatomic arrangement of the visual fibers as they travel backward within the brain, measurement of the visual field is helpful in localizing the position of brain tumors or other lesions affecting the visual pathway. (From Havener, William H.: Eyes. In Prior, John A., and Silberstein, Jack S.: Physical diagnosis, ed. 4, St. Louis, 1973, The C. V. Mosby Co.)

(as from brain tumor) to be carried forward to the eye, where it causes ophthalmoscopically visible swelling of the optic disk (papilledema).

Just behind the orbits, overlying the pituitary gland, the optic nerves join to form the optic chiasm. Within the chiasm the fibers from the medial half of each optic nerve cross over to run to the opposite side of the brain. Since this crossing causes a marked difference in arrangement of nerve fibers before, at, and after the chiasm, it is possible to diagnose the location of visual pathway disease by study of the visual field.

Extending backward from the chiasm, the optic tract and radiation carry the visual impulses to the occipital lobes at the very back of the brain. Here we first become aware of what the eyes see. Nearby are cortical areas for visual interpretation and memory.

In *summary*, the eye is composed of a seeing retina, a nourishing choroid, and a protective sclera. The front part of the eye focuses the light. The lids and tears protect the cornea. Eye movements are coordinated by the extraocular muscles. The optic nerves carry the message to the brain. The whole seeing apparatus is encased in the bony orbit and skull for protection.

SUGGESTED READINGS

Moses, Robert A.: Adler's physiology of the eye, ed. 5, St. Louis, 1970, The C. V. Mosby Co.

Wolff, Eugene: The anatomy of the eye and orbit, ed. 5, New York, 1961, McGraw-Hill Book Co.

CHAPTER TWO

Clinical examination

Since the human eye is located upon the surface of the body and is largely composed of transparent substance, it can be examined easily and precisely. The presence or absence of disease and the type of disease are much more readily determined than if an internal organ were affected. Indeed, a number of general diseases cause such characteristic ocular changes that diagnosis may be made upon the appearance of the eye alone. Examples of such diseases include diabetes, hypertension, and brain tumor.

MEASUREMENT OF VISUAL ACUITY

Determination of visual acuity is often the responsibility of the office or clinic nurse. The ease and speed with which visual acuity may be measured tends to mislead lay persons into underestimating the value of this test. As a matter of fact, **the most rewarding single test of ocular function is the evaluation of visual acuity.** Reduced acuity will betray the presence of a great variety of eye diseases as well as the need for refractive correction. Determination of visual acuity should be a part of every complete physical examination and is mandatory when the patient complains of blurred vision or other ocular symptoms or when the eye has been injured.

Distance acuity is measured with the aid of a wall chart (Fig. 2-1) 20 feet from the patient. Visual acuity is recorded as a fraction; the numerator indicates the distance to the chart, and the denominator is the distance at which a normal eye could read the line. Thus, 20/30 means that the patient is 20 feet from the chart and can read the line which a normal eye should see at 30 feet. By 20/200 is meant that he can read only the largest letter at the top of the chart, ordinarily legible to a normal eye at 200 feet. Lesser visual acuity than this may be recorded as hand movements (H. M.) or light perception (L. P.). An eye is not termed "blind" unless it cannot even perceive light. (Some confusion is caused by the term "legal blindness," which is defined as less than 20/200 or less than a 20-degree field of vision and which entitles the individual to an additional income tax exemption.)

The acuity of each eye is measured separately. The other eye should be occluded with an opaque card (Fig. 2-2). Always be alert for failure to cover the eye completely or for head turning, which permits the patient to peek around the card. Such "cheating" may be an involuntary attempt to see with the only good eye or may be a deliberate fraud. **Never** allow a patient to cover his eye with his fingers because of the ease with which he may

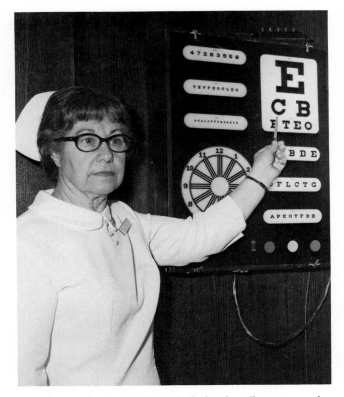

Fig. 2-1. Visual acuity may be measured routinely by the office nurse and recorded upon the chart before the patient is seen by the doctor.

look between them. Glasses (Fig. 2-3) should be worn if the patient customarily uses them for distance. Reading glasses will often blur distant vision.

The patient should be asked to read the smallest line he can see. Reading the whole chart from top down is an unnecessary waste of your time. Always coax the patient with apparently reduced visual acuity to try to read another line. Surprisingly often he can! If the patient reads correctly the majority of letters in a given line, he is credited with this line of vision, even though he may miss one or two letters. The number of missed letters may be designated by a minus sign, for example, 20/20—2.

Illiterate patients may say they "can't see it" rather than admit their ignorance. Charts composed of E letters of various sizes and positions are useful for such patients, who can then indicate the direction the E is pointing. E charts or an E block (Fig. 2-4) enable the nurse to measure visual acuity of cooperative children as early as $3\frac{1}{2}$ to 4 years of age.

Is it a waste of time to measure the acuity of children because they are "too young to have eye trouble"? **No!** At least 5% of children will be found to have defects in eyesight that require medical attention. Many of these

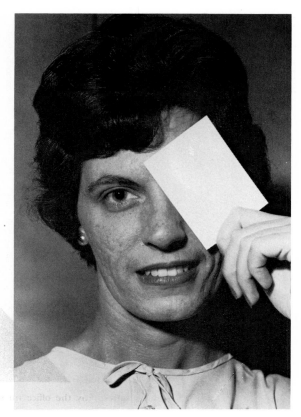

Fig. 2-2. During measurement of visual acuity the other eye should be completely covered.

faults will be refractive errors, which can easily be corrected—with great benefit to the child's schoolwork and general pleasure. Measurement of visual acuity is also one of the best ways to detect suppression amblyopia at 4 to 5 years of age, when it can be corrected by proper treatment. Suppression amblyopia (discussed in more detail on pp. 100-101) is a serious and common loss of vision in one eye in children, usually caused by crossing of the eyes. Visual loss because of suppression is irreversible unless treated before the age of 6 years.

Measurement of near vision is relatively unimportant as a routine procedure except for patients complaining specifically of reading difficulty or in persons over 40 years of age. After the age of 40 years the lens of the eye becomes sufficiently inflexible to interfere with clear focusing upon near objects. This condition is termed *presbyopia*. Most patients who cannot read newspaper print at a 1-foot distance will benefit from an ophthalmologic examination and prescription of glasses.

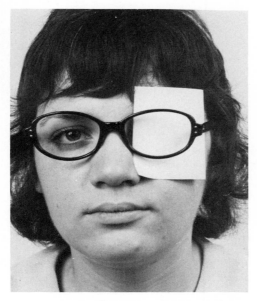

Fig. 2-3. When eyeglasses are worn, the eye not being tested may conveniently be occluded by positioning a card behind the frame of the glasses.

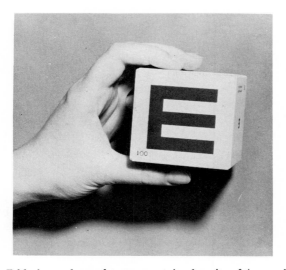

Fig. 2-4. An E block may be used to measure visual acuity of 4-year-old children.

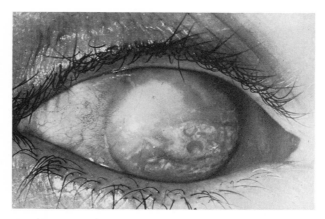

Fig. 2-5. Exposure damage to the cornea results if the lids do not properly close. Adequacy of closure of the lids should be checked during the physical examination. (From Havener, William H.: Synopsis of ophthalmology, ed. 3, St. Louis, 1971, The C. V. Mosby Co.)

INSPECTION OF THE LIDS

Lid examination has three objectives: (1) to see if the lids adequately cover the eyes, (2) to seek signs that betray systemic disease, and (3) to detect local disease.

Do the lids close completely? This question should be answered in all patients and particularly in those with abnormally prominent eyes or facial paralysis. Potentially serious damage may be sustained through drying of the cornea if the lids do not close properly (as in unconsciousness resulting from disease, injury, or anesthesia or if the lid defects are present) (Fig. 2-5).

Systemic disease may cause characteristic lid changes such as edema, abnormal prominence of the eyes, or ptosis. Excess fluid collects more readily in the thin lid skin than elsewhere in the body and is responsible for the puffy lids (Fig. 2-6) so characteristic of nephrosis or hypothyroidism. Undoubtedly the most common cause of forward protrusion of the eye from the orbit (exophthalmos) is thyroid disease (Fig. 2-7). Exophthalmos may be so severe as to cause exposure damage to the cornea unless it is properly protected, as by lubricants. Ptosis (drooping of the upper lid) may be an early sign of third nerve damage from any cause. Congenital defects rank high among causes of ptosis.

Local infections of the lids are quite common. (More detailed discussion will be found in Chapter 8.) The characteristic signs of lid infection are discharge and redness. Such infections are caused by potentially contagious organisms, which may be transmitted to other patients or to the nurse herself. The nurse should always wash her hands between examinations of patients, whether or not evidences of infection are present.

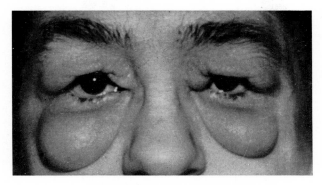

Fig. 2-6. Because the lid skin is thin and loosely adherent to underlying tissue, it more easily becomes swollen than skin elsewhere. Such lid edema may result from nonocular disease, e.g., kidney disorder. (From Havener, William H.: Synopsis of ophthalmology, ed. 3, St. Louis, 1971, The C. V. Mosby Co.)

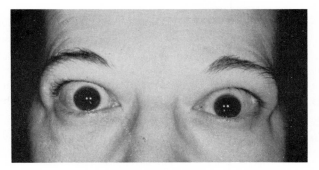

Fig. 2-7. Retraction of the upper lids so that the upper sclera is exposed to view is almost pathognomonic of thyroid disease.

Great care must be taken in examining an injured eye. **Never** press upon the eye when trying to separate the lids, since this may destroy the eye. This must not be forgotten when the nurse opens an injured eye for inspection. She should always limit pressure to the portions of the lids overlying the bony orbital rims. The upper eyelid may be gently elevated by lifting upward over the brow, and the lower lid may be retracted by pulling down the skin overlying the cheek bone (Fig. 2-8). If at any time during examination of an injured eye it is evident that the eye has been penetrated (obvious laceration, protruding iris or vitreous, blood within the eye, etc.), the examination should be stopped immediately to avoid the possibility of further damage.

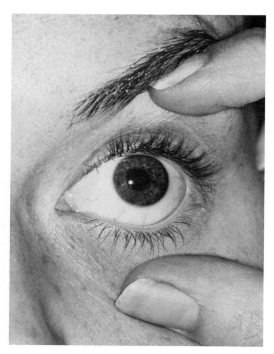

Fig. 2-8. Proper lid separation, with no pressure directed upon the eyeball.

INSPECTION OF THE CONJUNCTIVA

The conjunctiva is a delicate, transparent mucous membrane that lines the back surface of the lids (this part is called the *palpebral conjunctiva*) and covers the front of the eye (this part is called the *bulbar conjunctiva*) from its equator to the *limbus* (junction of cornea and sclera). The bulbar conjunctiva is readily examined by separating the lids widely as the patient looks up, down, and to each side. It is normally quite transparent, permitting the white color of the sclera to show through. In heavily pigmented individuals yellow discoloration of the conjunctiva may be the only visible sign of liver disease. Many small blood vessels are normally visible in the conjunctiva. Dilation of these vessels is responsible for the various patterns of redness characteristic of many types of eye disease.

A small fleshy elevation known as the caruncle is situated in the nasal corner of the bulbar conjunctiva. Fine hairs and tiny yellowish spots (sebaceous glands) are normally seen in the caruncle, especially in older persons. Just lateral to the caruncle is a flat fold called the plica semilunaris, which is the remnant of the third eyelid found in lower animals.

The palpebral conjunctiva overlies the fleshy lid tissue and therefore appears much redder than the bulbar conjunctiva. Vertical yellowish striations are commonly seen in the palpebral conjunctiva and represent the

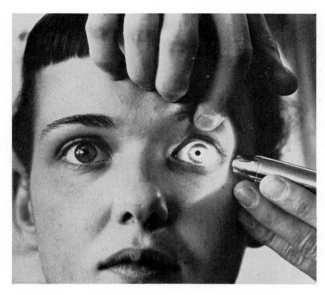

Fig. 2-9. Use of oblique moving illumination is best for examination of the cornea. (From Havener, William H.: Synopsis of ophthalmology, ed. 3, St. Louis, 1971, The C. V. Mosby Co.)

sebaceous glands of the eyelids. The lymph follicles of the palpebral conjunctiva often enlarge, causing a finely nodular appearance, which is best seen with flashlight illumination from the side in a semidarkened room.

The palpebral conjunctiva cannot be seen until the lids are everted. The lower lid is easily everted by pulling down the skin overlying the lower orbital rim. (See Fig. 7-8.) More of the conjunctiva will be exposed if the patient simultaneously looks upward. The inferior conjunctival folds are the commonest location of superficial foreign bodies. Foreign bodies on the conjunctival surface may safely be removed by the nurse, as described in Chapter 7.

The technique of everting the upper lid is described on p. 84. This permits examination of the upper palpebral conjunctiva. Foreign bodies embedded here are exceptionally annoying because they abrade the highly sensitive cornea with each blink of the lid.

Almost all inexperienced persons are much too rough during examination of the eyes. All manipulations, including lid eversion, must be performed *gently*. Move your hands slowly and carefully and you will retain the patient's confidence.

EXAMINATION OF THE CORNEA

The cornea is the most important and delicate part of the surface of the eye and therefore deserves careful examination. Good vision requires a perfectly smooth and transparent cornea, which is normally invisible except for surface reflections. Oblique moving illumination (Fig. 2-9) with a small flashlight is particularly effective in demonstrating corneal abnormalities. Two of the most common abnormalities of the cornea are abrasions and opacities. Superficial irregularities are best detected by noting the defects appearing in the light reflections of the normal surface (Fig. 2-10). Occasionally an opaque defect casts shadows on the iris, which may be more readily visible than the corneal lesion producing the shadow.

INSPECTION OF THE PUPIL

Particularly during the care of patients with diseases of the central nervous system the nurse will observe pupil signs. Normal pupils are perfectly round, equal in size, and constrict visibly to light and during accommodation. The *direct reaction to light* refers to the constriction of the pupil receiving increased illumination. Constriction of the opposite pupil (even though no light increase strikes this opposite eye) is termed the *consensual* pupil reaction. Stimulation of either optic nerve will cause both pupils to constrict. Therefore, in monocular blindness, as with a severed optic nerve, the affected eye will have no direct pupil response but will react consensually to stimulation of the opposite eye. Illumination of the blind eye, however, will not cause constriction of either pupil.

The nurse should not check the light reflex with a flashlight approaching from straight ahead, since the patient will accommodate on the light source. This induces the accommodation pupil reflex, which may be misleading. The nurse should bring the light in from the side, which is also the best position for inspection of the eye. Stray light from the flashlight should not be permitted to strike the opposite eye during evaluation of the pupil signs. Absence of the light reflex should not be reported unless the examination has been done with a bright light source used in a darkened room.

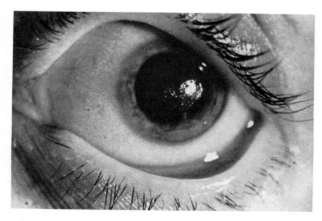

Fig. 2-10. Note the conspicuous reflections seen when a corneal abrasion is illuminated obliquely. Study of the cornea with an obliquely directed, moving, bright flashlight is the best way to locate irregularities of the corneal surface. Fluorescein staining is unnecessary if the lesion can be demonstrated in this fashion. (From Havener, William H.: Synopsis of ophthalmology, ed. 3, St. Louis, 1971, The C. V. Mosby Co.)

Pupils are normally smaller in infancy and old age. A readily observable difference in pupil size occurs in 5% of apparently normal persons. Unless the patient knows of the previous existence of such a pupil unequality, it should be regarded as a possible indicator of serious neurologic or ocular disease. Since mydriatics and miotics are frequently used medications, inquiry as to the use of drops is pertinent when pupil abnormalities are found.

Enlargement of the pupil may be caused by eye injury (recent or old), acute glaucoma, systemic poisoning by parasympatholytic drugs, or local use of dilating drops. Constriction of the pupil is seen in iris inflammation, in glaucoma patients treated with pilocarpine, as an effect of morphine or heroin, and physiologically in sleep. Irregularity of pupil contour is *invariably* abnormal, occurring in iritis, central nervous system syphilis, injury, and congenital defects, for example.

INSPECTION OF THE ORBIT

The position of the eye in its bony socket may be altered by tumor, inflammation, injury, thyroid disease, or developmental defect. Forward displacement is termed *exophthalmos;* backward displacement is *enophthalmos.* Although abnormal prominence of the eye is recognizable by inspection, the false impression of exophthalmos may be produced by widely open lids, and enophthalmos may be simulated by a drooping upper lid.

Undoubtedly the most common cause of forward protrusion of the eye from the orbit is thyroid disease (Fig. 2-7). Exophthalmos may be so severe as to cause exposure damage to the cornea unless it is properly protected by lubricants.

VISUAL FIELD MEASUREMENT

The pathways whereby visual sensations pass from the retina to the brain are well defined and constant (Fig. 1-8). Considerable separation occurs along these nerve pathways into the brain—for instance, the right half of the retina of each eye sends fibers only to the right half of the brain. Similarly the upper half of each retina sends its fibers through the upper part of the parietal lobe, whereas the lower half of each retina sends fibers through the inferiorly located temporal lobe. The central retina is connected to the most posterior tip of the brain, whereas peripheral retinal fibers connect to the anterior part of the calcarine fissure. Because of these anatomic facts, brain tumors or other intracranial diseases will cause typical visual field defects, which can be diagnosed by perimetry. A perimeter (Fig. 2-11) is a semicircular instrument, marked in degrees, with which an accurate map can be made of the extent of the patient's side vision. Visual field defects may also be caused by diseases of the retina and optic nerve.

Perimetry is useful in the examination of patients with suspected intracranial disorders. It has the great advantage of being completely safe and painless, in contrast to neurosurgical diagnostic procedures. However, perimetry will not detect brain defects that do not involve the visual pathways.

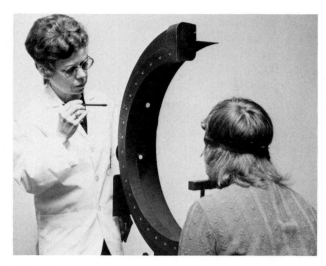

Fig. 2-11. Vision in the peripheral field is measured with a perimeter.

REFRACTION

Refraction is the clinical measurement of the optical faults of the non-accommodated eye. Refraction is done when patients complain of blurred vision or of symptoms (such as headache or rapid fatigue) related to use of the eyes. One of the most convenient methods of refraction employs a refractor (Fig. 2-12), which is an instrument containing a large number of lenses mounted in rotating wheels. A great variety of lens combinations can be dialed very quickly into the refractor eyepiece.

Determination of which lenses to use is aided by the retinoscope. A retinoscope (Fig. 2-12) is a source of focused light with which the eye is examined at a distance of about 2 feet. Since the focus of light is characteristically distorted by a given refractive error, the ophthalmologist using a retinoscope can quickly and precisely determine the refractive error of an eye. Since retinoscopy is an objective measurement, it permits accurate refraction of young infants, who cannot select lenses that improve vision.

The accuracy of a refraction may be enhanced by use of cycloplegic eye drops, which may be used only by physicians.

OPHTHALMOSCOPY

The tiny blood vessels, nerves, and other structures in the back of the eye can be seen with the aid of an ophthalmoscope (Fig. 2-13). The magnification of an ophthalmoscope view is so great that details as small as several times the diameter of a single cell can be identified (Fig. 2-14). The optic nerve and the center part of the retina can usually be seen with the ophthalmoscope through an undilated pupil. Most of the peripheral retina is normally hidden from clear view by the iris, but it can easily be seen if the pupil is dilated with an eye drop.

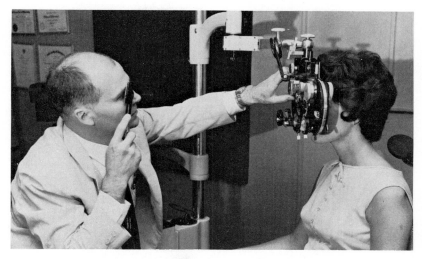

Fig. 2-12. Observation of the light reflex with a retinoscope helps to determine the patient's refractive error.

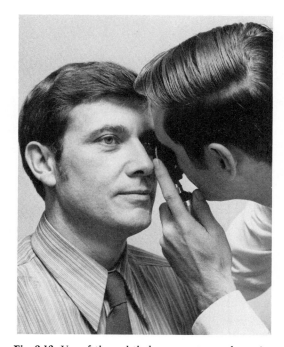

Fig. 2-13. Use of the ophthalmoscope to see the retina.

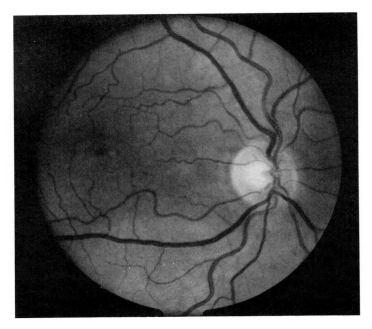

Fig. 2-14. The optic nerve and retinal blood vessels are easily seen in the living eye with an ophthalmoscope.

Ophthalmoscopy through a dilated pupil is a very important part of the medical examination of every patient with an eye complaint.

BIOMICROSCOPY

Just as the interior of the eye is examined with an ophthalmoscope, so also the anterior part of the eye can be inspected in great detail with the biomicroscope (slit-lamp microscope) (Fig. 2-15). Such abnormalities as tiny abrasions of the transparent corneal surface, inflammation of the iris, or early cataract are readily recognized.

PRESSURE MEASUREMENT

Eyes as well as automobile tires perform best at certain internal pressures. Excessive pressures may develop within an eye—this condition is called *glaucoma*. The instrument used to measure intraocular pressure is a *tonometer* (Fig. 2-16). A number of different types of tonometers are in use. The most accurate is the applanation tonometer (Fig. 2-17), which is applied to the cornea during observation with the biomicroscope. When placed upon the cornea, a tonometer causes corneal indentation, the amount of which depends upon intraocular pressure. Anesthetic eye drops are used before tonometric measurement. Since the anesthetic effect lasts for ten to fifteen minutes, a patient should be cautioned not to rub his eyes for this period of time after tonometry, lest he scratch his own eye without realizing it.

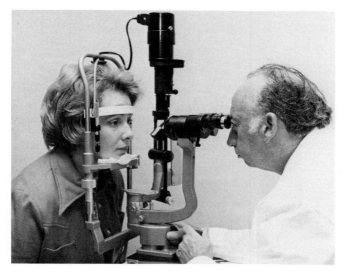

Fig. 2-15. Biomicroscopic examination of the eye is a routine clinical procedure whereby the earliest signs of disease may be detected.

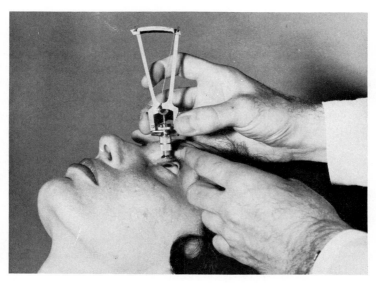

Fig. 2-16. The Schiøtz tonometer is positioned vertically upon the anesthetized cornea to measure intraocular pressure.

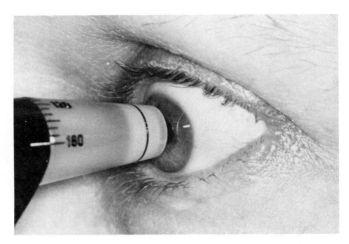

Fig. 2-17. More precise measurements of intraocular pressure may be obtained by use of an applanation tonometer.

Early detection of glaucoma by tonometry is of great importance because glaucoma is common (2% of persons over 40 years of age), it slowly and painlessly leads to blindness (12% of blind persons in the United States have glaucoma), and blindness can usually be prevented simply by the daily use of eye drops if started during the early stages of this disease. Here is an area of patient teaching for the alert nurse. She should encourage older persons to have regular ophthalmologic examinations, which always include pressure measurement.

ORTHOPTIC EXAMINATION

The way in which the eyes work together may be evaluated with stereoscope-like instruments (Fig. 2-18). Such a stereoscope presents a slightly different picture to each eye and thereby permits determination of whether these two pictures are combined to a single picture by the brain (normal fusion), seen as two separate pictures (double vision; diplopia), or whether the brain simply ignores the picture from one eye (suppression). Since these stereoscopes can be adjusted to different angles, they may also be used to measure the amount by which eyes cross. Also, certain types of defective binocular function may benefit from stereoscopic training.

EXAMINATION OF A CHILD

When ophthalmology or other ocular examination must be performed on an uncooperative child, some type of restraint is necessary. (Distraction with lollypops is better, but it will not always work.) "Mummying" the child by wrapping him snugly in a sheet is a common method of holding him quiet. A quicker and simpler way of simultaneous immobilization of

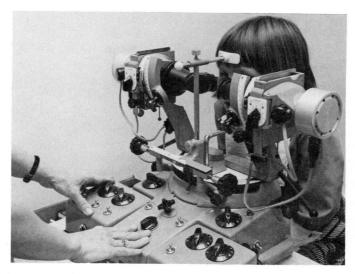

Fig. 2-18. Orthoptic measurement of binocular function.

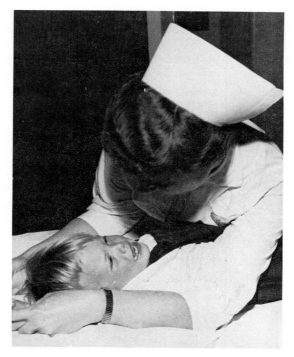

Fig. 2-19. An uncooperative child may be held for eye examination by pressing his arms firmly on each side of his head. (From Havener, William H.: Synopsis of ophthalmology, ed. 3, St. Louis, 1971, The C. V. Mosby Co.)

head and arms is to lay the child upon a cot, take hold of both his elbows, and press his arms firmly against his ears (Fig. 2-19). The nurse can greatly assist an eye examination by holding the child securely in this fashion. If the child moves his body and legs enough to disturb the eye examination, the nurse may lean gently upon the child's body.

OTHER EXAMINATIONS

Although a skilled nurse is most helpful in the use of a great number of other eye examining devices and techniques, they are too specialized to warrant detailed description and will be learned by individual nurses who enter the field of eye care.

SUMMARY

Nursing duties related to ocular examination will frequently include measurement of visual acuity, instillation of appropriate drops (dilating drops before ophthalmoscopy and refraction, constricting drops afterward, or anesthetic drops before pressure measurement), maintenance of instruments (e.g., tonometer sterilization), positioning and holding of patients, and assorted technical functions. While performing these important but mechanical tasks, the nurse should not forget that her personality, if warm and friendly, will greatly reassure the patient. Remember that the patient has sought medical care because he is concerned and uncertain about his eyes. Perhaps he fears blindness or brain tumor or is apprehensive that the examination will be painful. Your kindness and understanding can be of greater importance to a worried patient than you ordinarily realize. Also, let us not forget the many opportunities available for patient teaching, which may be tremendously important in the prevention of blindness.

SUGGESTED READINGS

Ballantyne, Arthur J., and Michaelson, Isaac C.: Textbook of the fundus of the eye, Baltimore, 1962, The Williams & Wilkins Co.

Berliner, Milton: Biomicroscopy of the eye, 2 vols., New York 1943, Paul B. Hoeber, Inc., Medical Book Division, Harper & Row, Publishers.

Prior, John A., and Silberstein, Jack S.: Physical diagnosis, ed. 4, St. Louis, 1973, The C. V. Mosby Co.

CHAPTER THREE # Meaning of eye symptoms

Knowledge of the causes of common eye symptoms is important to the nurse because these symptoms are the way in which an eye seeks help. Some symptoms are very dangerous and require prompt evaluation; others are benign but annoying. Since the nurse is often the first person the patient encounters, she should be able to evaluate accurately the importance of his symptoms.

FOREIGN BODY SENSATION

If the foreign body sensation began suddenly, and particularly if the patient is reasonably sure that something entered or struck the eye, by far the most likely cause is the presence of the foreign particle somewhere upon the surface of the eye. Removal of such a particle, discussed on p. 82, may be done by the properly trained nurse if the foreign body can be found upon the conjunctiva. Foreign bodies embedded in the cornea should be removed by a physician.

A foreign body sensation following injury can result from an abrasion of the cornea, which may feel exactly as if a foreign particle were present. Because tiny particles can easily be overlooked and because corneal abrasions require prophylactic antibiotic treatment, a physician should be consulted for care of such a painful eye after possible injury.

Eyelashes rather frequently loosen and drop upon the eye. This causes a brief stinging sensation, which rapidly subsides. Spontaneous blinking and tearing usually move the lash away from the eye, or the lash may be easily removed with a clean tissue. Sometimes eyelashes are misdirected backward and scratch the cornea with lid movement. The offending lash may be too fine to be seen easily, but if recognized, epilation of the lash will relieve the foreign body sensation.

Acute infection of the corneal surface is another common cause of foreign body sensation. This is caused by inflammatory damage to the sensitive corneal surface. If of bacterial etiology, such inflammations will be helped by administration of antibiotics.

31

PAIN

Mild pain in the general region of an eye is an extremely nonspecific symptom that may result from eye disorder, psychosomatic difficulty, or referred pain from sinus, tooth, or brain diseases. If transient and unaccompanied by other symptoms, mild ocular pain is usually of no significance and can be ignored with reasonable safety.

Severe and persistent ocular pain ordinarily indicates serious disease (Fig. 3-1), urgently requiring attention. If other ocular symptoms (such as decreased vision, photophobia, etc.) are present, the eye itself is probably at fault. If other ocular symptoms are absent, the pain probably originates elsewhere in the orbit, sinuses, or along the intracranial course of the fifth nerve. Severe pain may be caused by inflammations within the eye or by increased intraocular pressure.

Although some pain can be expected after eye surgery, the analgesics ordered by the ophthalmologist will ordinarily relieve such discomfort. Should the patient continue to complain of more than usual pain after the ordered medications have been given, the nurse should notify the physician. This will enable him to prescribe stronger drugs to relieve the patient or to recognize a complication of surgery. Unless specifically authorized, the nurse should **never** remove the bandage to inspect a recently operated eye, regardless of any complaints of pain and discomfort.

HEADACHE

One of the most common and annoying symptoms encountered in medical practice is headache. Each patient with this complaint presents a serious problem to his physician, who must determine with reasonable accuracy the cause of the pain. The problem is complicated by the great frequency of functional headaches, each of which forces the conscientious physician to

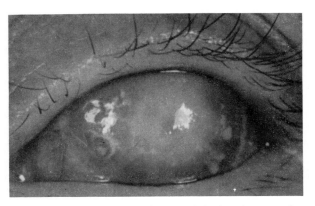

Fig. 3-1. Pain resulting from a corneal injury or infection is an early warning signal that should lead to treatment of the disease before the transparency of the cornea is destroyed by scarring.

decide how much diagnostic effort and expense is justified to rule out organic disease.

The possibility of eye origin of unexplained headaches should be considered. Ocular headaches may be situated anywhere—orbital, frontal, temporal, vertex, or occipital. Eye-induced pains may vary from the dull headache associated with use of eyes with uncorrected refractive error to the severe and almost intolerable pain of acute glaucoma. The pain of eye inflammation, glaucoma, or injury may start rather abruptly. Such pains are usually correctly identified as affecting the eye, although they often radiate to adjacent parts of the head. Acute eye diseases causing headache are rather easily identified by a physician.

Since refractive errors or muscle imbalance do not begin suddenly, a need for glasses is not indicated by headaches of abrupt, recent onset. Refractive errors cause chronic, persistent, mild headaches, which characteristically become *worse with use of the eyes*. Chronic headaches definitely related to the use of the eyes for detailed work of any kind (reading, sewing, driving, television, occupational tasks) certainly warrant refraction and will often be relieved by a prescription of proper glasses. Headaches *unrelated* to use of the eyes are seldom caused by a need for glasses. Other symptoms associated with refractive errors may include reduced visual acuity, burning and irritation of the eyes, rapid ocular fatigue, and dislike of reading.

It must be emphasized that many headaches referred specifically to the eyes are of functional origin. Thorough examination is, of course, necessary to rule out eye disease, but if the physician finds no visible eye disorder and if the symptoms are not related to use of the eyes, it is very unlikely that the eyes are the source of the discomfort.

Of course everyone is aware that headaches may be caused by general or cerebral diseases, such as high blood pressure or brain tumor.

BURNING AND IRRITATION

Although burning and irritation of the eyes are very annoying complaints, these two symptoms are not characteristic of serious eye disease. Chronic infection of the lid margin or conjunctiva is a frequent cause of burning and irritation. Excessive exposure to smoke, dust, or wind may be responsible. Another cause is deficiency of tears, particularly common in middle-aged women with arthritis. Prolonged use of the eyes and fatigue may cause mild irritation. Cold compresses will usually relieve burning and irritation quite rapidly. Such treatment is preferable to self- medication with the types of eye drops available without a prescription.

ITCHING

The classic sign of ocular allergy is itching. Chronic lid infection is more likely to cause irritation than itching.

FATIGUE

Falling asleep after supper is commonly and erroneously blamed upon refractive error—it simply means the patient is tired. So, also, the reading of homework assignments or other uninteresting subject matter may rapidly bore a student, particularly if distracting thoughts or emotions compete for attention. After prolonged use even the healthiest eye and mind will ultimately fatigue.

Certainly the added strain of poor lighting or need for eyeglasses will hasten fatigue, and eye examination is appropriate in the evaluation of unduly rapid fatigue with eye use. However, the symptom of fatigue does not indicate presence of serious eye disease; nor does prolonged use of eyes, even under adverse circumstances, induce eye disease.

TEARING

Watering of the eye (epiphora) is usually caused by excessive tear production. Crying from emotional causes is familiar to everyone. The irritation of a cinder or other foreign body in the eye causes a flow of tears intended by nature to wash away the offending particle. The watery eye and running nose associated with the common cold and allergy are well known.

Failure of the tears to flow into the nose will also result in tearing. This may occur if the lower lid sags (because of age, disease, or injury) so that the lacrimal punctum no longer is in contact with the tear film. The lacrimal canaliculi, sac, or nasolacrimal duct (Fig. 1-7) may become blocked by disease, with resultant tearing. Blockage of the nasolacrimal duct predisposes the eye and lacrimal sac to the development of surface infections.

PHOTOPHOBIA

Sensitivity to light is a nonspecific symptom accompanying many types of ocular irritation and inflammation. Since serious conditions such as iritis cause photophobia, the abrupt appearance of severe and persistent intolerance to light should cause suspicion of eye disease.

People vary considerably in their tolerance of bright sunlight. This is more likely a personality characteristic than an ocular condition.

Dark glasses effectively shield sensitive eyes from excess light. Contrary to popular opinion, the wearing of dark glasses is not harmful to the eyes. Commercially available sunglasses are ordinarily of adequate quality and are considerably less expensive than prescription glasses. Of course if a person has sufficient refractive error to require the wearing of corrective lenses, he will also require a prescription correction in his dark glasses. Dark glasses may be used freely and safely as desired for comfort.

DIPLOPIA

Double vision almost always indicates that both eyes are not pointing at the same object (see Chapter 9). Since this indicates a disorder of the extraocular muscles or their innervation, persistent diplopia requires medical evaluation for the possibility of serious disease.

Transient double vision that promptly disappears with effort to see clearly is usually of no consequence and simply indicates a temporary relaxation of the fusion mechanism that maintains ocular straightness.

"FLOATERS"

"Floaters," small moving spots that seem to drift about in front of the eye, are very common causes of complaint. Such spots represent shadows cast upon the retina by vitreous debris. Although most floaters are either benign or untreatable, they may indicate presence of several very serious diseases that can be greatly helped by early care. Any patient complaining of a sudden onset of floaters must be evaluated by careful ophthalmoscopic examination through a well-dilated pupil. Any other management of such a case is as inexcusable as failure to examine the interior of a rectum that is the source of bright red bleeding.

Floaters may be caused by developmental remnants, hemorrhage, inflammation, or degenerations.

Developmental remnants. Before birth the vitreous cavity of the eye contains a network of blood vessels, which atrophy and almost completely disappear when the eye is fully formed. When looking at a uniform, brightly lighted background such as a ceiling, almost everyone can see moving spots and irregular lines, which represent remnants of this embryonic vascular network. Such floaters are nonprogressive and harmless but sometimes cause considerable alarm when first discovered. Accidental discovery of these harmless remnants is by far the commonest cause of floaters in a young person; nevertheless, the serious nature of many of the other causes indicates performance of an adequate medical eye examination for such complaints.

Hemorrhage. Vitreous hemorrhage may cause a multitude of small and large floaters, the extent of which varies with the severity of the hemorrhage. Often a reddish discoloration of vision is reported. The cause is obvious if there is history or evidence of recent injury. Traumatic intraocular hemorrhage ordinarily requires ophthalmologic consultation for evaluation of the extent of injury and for proper care. Spontaneous intraocular hemorrhage most frequently is caused by systemic disorders such as diabetes, hypertension, blood dyscrasia, or increased intracranial pressure. Even if the vitreous hemorrhage completely obscures the retina, diagnosis of these conditions can easily be made by examining the other eye.

Purely ocular disease may cause spontaneous vitreous hemorrhage. Examples include occlusion of the retinal veins, cancer, retinal detachment, and inflammation.

Inflammation. Chorioretinitis is the result of infection of the inner coats of the eye by a variety of microorganisms. Quite commonly inflammatory cells enter the vitreous, where they are perceived as floaters. Inflammatory debris adherent to the vitreous framework forms netlike masses, which greatly disturb the patient's vision. Inasmuch as intensive corticosteroid therapy is often most valuable in preventing loss of vision, prompt recognition of chorioretinitis is very important.

Degenerations. Retinal detachment is the most important degenerative disease causing floaters. When the retina tears, a shower of pigment or red cells suddenly appears in the vitreous, causing the floaters. Flashes of light, somewhat resembling distant lightning, are often seen during the early stages of retinal detachment. When a portion of the retina has fallen out of position, a corresponding part of the visual field is lost. Proper surgery for detached retinas gives good results if done early; hence the recognition of this cause of floaters indicates emergency care.

VISUAL FIELD DEFECTS

Visual defects that move exactly with the eye are readily differentiated by history from vitreous floaters. These fixed defects are caused by damage of the retina or visual pathways. Common causes include chorioretinitis, injury, macular degeneration, glaucoma, and occlusion of vessels of the eye or brain. Loss of a noticeable portion of the visual field certainly deserves adequate medical evaluation.

SUDDEN LOSS OF VISION

Surprisingly, one of the commonest explanations of supposedly "sudden" loss of vision is the recognition by the patient of a slowly progressive disease. Rather commonly, patients with gradual visual loss in one eye will be unaware of this condition.

Closure of the central retinal artery causes instantaneous complete blindness of the eye. It is painless and almost always permanent. Cerebral artery occlusions may cause sudden loss of extensive portions of the visual field.

Intraocular hemorrhages may occur abruptly or slowly. Vision will be obscured in the area of hemorrhage. A considerable variety of eye and general disorders (diabetes, hypertension, blood dyscrasia, chorioretinitis, macular degeneration, retinal detachment, etc.) can cause intraocular hemorrhage.

Corneal edema, as from infection, abrasion, or acute glaucoma, will cause severe blurring of vision. The possibility of injury must be considered whenever sudden visual loss has occurred. Intraocular penetration of a tiny foreign body may be almost painless, yet may severely impair vision by causing corneal edema, cataract, or hemorrhage.

Retinal detachment is a rare cause of rapidly progressive visual loss. It is usually preceded by showers of floating spots and the sensation of lightning flashes. As the detachment progresses, a dark shadow is seen to move across the field of vision. Most commonly affected are myopes, elderly persons, or persons with previously injured eyes.

Poisons such as wood alcohol may selectively destroy the retina. Drinking of denatured alcohol or of alcohol substitutes (such as chemical solvents) is extremely hazardous.

GRADUAL LOSS OF VISION

Gradual reduction of vision in old age is very common and often is accepted uncomplainingly as a natural accompaniment of age. It must be emphasized that a healthy eye sees clearly even in extreme old age and that decreased vision (uncorrectable with glasses) indicates disease—often of a type responding to treatment.

Cataract is one of the commonest causes of this gradual, painless visual loss, and it may be years before the patient can no longer read. It is well known that operation is indicated only for advanced cataract, at such time that the patient no longer has satisfactory vision. Often an elderly patient is erroneously advised not to see an ophthalmologist until his vision is gone. Obviously this advice leads to tragedy should he have glaucoma rather than cataract (or in addition to cataract).

Glaucomatous visual loss (Fig. 3-2) is usually insidious, gradual, painless, and not readily differentiated by history from cataract. Glaucomatous loss of

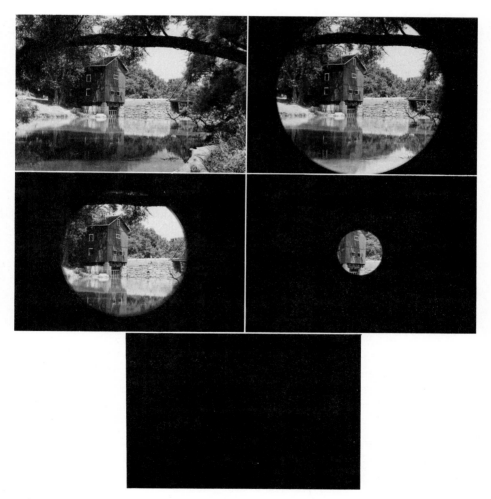

Fig. 3-2. The gradual loss of sight from glaucoma so insidiously destroys vision that the patient is unaware of impending blindness until extensive and irreversible damage is already present.

vision is, however, *irreversible* and, most important, *preventable* by proper early treatment. Twelve percent of all blindness is caused by glaucoma. Invariably the patient fails to recognize his difficulty until a far-advanced stage of the disease is reached. Hence it is the duty of his physician to diagnose glaucoma by routine tonometer measurement of intraocular pressure before a late stage of glaucoma is reached.

Senile macular degeneration causes gradual bilateral loss of central vision. Although no treatment is effective, comfort is usually derived from knowledge that peripheral vision is never affected by this degeneration.

Optic atrophy is another cause of gradual visual loss that may mimic the history of cataract. Treatment depends upon the cause and may be dramatically effective, as in the case of early neurosyphilis or early brain tumor.

Diabetes, hypertension, and blood dyscrasias may cause gradual or sudden visual loss. The course of diabetic retinopathy is affected very little by medical treatment. There are many instances of dramatic improvement of hypertensive or leukemic retinopathy through proper systemic treatment.

The average older person believes all painless and gradual loss of vision indicates only a need for a change of glasses. Frequently he really does need new glasses, but he may also have early symptoms of a serious eye disease. Prescription of glasses only may permit insidious irreversible visual loss. For this reason the nurse should advise older patients with eye symptoms to obtain regular medical eye care from their ophthalmologist.

REDNESS

Redness of the eye is a warning signal common to many diseases; most frequent are the relatively insignificant, superficial allergies and minor conjunctival infections. There is a danger that the frequency of these minor causes of red eye may result in a serious red eye being overlooked. Fortunately it is unnecessary to learn the characteristics of a multitude of diseases in order to exclude a serious cause of eye redness. The following five easily recognized findings may be used as a checklist:

1. Reduced vision
2. Pain
3. Visible loss of transparency of the normally clear parts of the eye
4. Irregularity or unequal size of the pupils
5. Location of the redness as a definite circular pattern immediately surrounding the cornea

A really serious red eye will almost always show not only one but usually several of these associated findings.

SUMMARY

Eye symptoms requiring immediate medical attention include rapid loss of vision (whether straight ahead or to the side), persistent severe pain or foreign body sensation, and sudden onset of many floaters.

Less urgent are symptoms such as gradual visual loss, double vision, photophobia, headache, and redness. However, these symptoms do require medical evaluation, which should not be unduly delayed.

Itching, burning, irritation, and fatigue of the eyes, as well as tearing and redness, are annoying symptoms but are unlikely to indicate serious disease (unless accompanied by the other symptoms just mentioned). The nurse should encourage the patient with any eye complaint to seek prompt medical attention, which will often relieve his symptoms.

Knowledge of the relative importance of these symptoms will be of value in the triage function of a busy emergency room nurse. Also, the nurse entrusted with making office appointments must be able to differentiate the patient with an urgent problem from one needing a routine refraction.

SUGGESTED READING

Havener, William H.: Synopsis of ophthalmology, ed. 3, St. Louis, 1971, The C. V. Mosby Co.

CHAPTER FOUR

Medical therapy

Being located on the surface of the body, the eyelids and the anterior portion of the eye can be treated effectively with medications applied directly. Local application of medications is desirable because high concentrations can quickly be achieved and because systemic side effects can be minimized. Furthermore, the lesser quantities of medication required are cheaper.

Because the technique of instilling a drop into the eye is so simple and since a drop of fluid appears so small and harmless, a nurse may be unaware of the great potency of some types of eye drops. Atropine is a good example of a commonly used, highly toxic eye medication. A single drop of 1% atropine solution contains almost 1 mg. of drug. This is an amount equivalent to the atropine premedication given before general anesthesia. An effective demonstration of the potency of 1% ophthalmic atropine is provided by putting 1 drop (only 1!) on your tongue. Rapid systemic absorption will cause several hours of unpleasant dryness of the mouth. The profuse nasal drainage of a fresh cold can be likewise stopped almost completely with 1 drop of 1% atropine.

A child, being much smaller than an adult, will be much more susceptible to the effect of a given amount of atropine absorbed from the eye. For this reason atropine should not be instilled repeatedly at very short intervals. Any excess fluid should be wiped from the eye rather than being permitted to drain through the tear duct to the nose and stomach. The accurate refraction of a cross-eyed child requires atropinization, usually achieved by instilling a small amount of 1% atropine ointment in each eye three times a day for three days before refraction. Recognition of atropine toxicity, which rarely occurs, is important so that misdiagnosis of some other disease can be avoided and the further administration of atropine can be stopped during the period of toxicity. The effects of atropine upon a child may include fever, dry skin, irritability, and delirium; of course the pupils will be widely dilated and nonreactive.

Isoflurophate is an even more toxic eye medication, used in only 0.025% concentration for treatment of crossed eyes. This drug is one of the "nerve gases" developed during World War II. Similar chemicals are used as insecticides. Isoflurophate is helpful in treatment of about one third of children with crossed eyes and is usually instilled upon the eye several times weekly. It incidentally causes the pupil to become very small.

Obviously atropine and isoflurophate, as well as other potent eye medications, must be kept safely out of reach of children. Even a tiny 5 ml. eye bottle holds a fatal dose of these drugs.

Eye drops are used for many different purposes, some of which are exactly the opposite of others. For instance, in treatment of acute glaucoma the pupil must be made very small in order to pull the iris away from the aqueous drainage channels at the iris periphery. If the pupil is dilated, the iris blocks the aqueous outflow and the intraocular pressure rapidly rises high enough to destroy the retina and optic nerve. In contrast, treatment of acute iritis requires dilation of the pupil. If iritis causes a small pupil, inflammatory adhesions may grow across the small opening, destroying sight.

Acute glaucoma is treated with pilocarpine, which constricts the pupil. Acute iritis is treated with atropine, which dilates the pupil. If the glaucoma or iritis is severe, accidental interchanging of these two drugs could easily lead to blindness. Do **not** conclude that because they all come in little bottles, eye drops are all the same. **Do** read the labels carefully and double-check for accuracy before putting drops into a patient's eye. Pilocarpine and Paredrine may sound alike, but pilocarpine constricts the pupil, whereas Paredrine dilates. Atropine may dilate the pupil for a week, but homatropine only lasts for a day.

Not only the identity but also the concentration of the drug must be verified. The most dramatic example of this is the 1% silver nitrate that is routinely instilled into the eyes of a newborn infant to prevent blindness from gonococcal infection. If 10% silver nitrate is used, the delicate infant cornea will be burned and a permanent blinding scar may result. A number of such tragedies have actually happened.

A not uncommon practice is the exchange of eye drops between patients, apparently based upon the assumption that a "good eye drop" has universal value. Certainly a given antibiotic drop might be useful against infection in several different eyes (although bacterial sensitivity to antibiotics does vary considerably). Unfortunately the symptoms and appearance of an allergic eye somewhat resemble those of an infected eye. The corticosteroid drops prescribed for allergy reduce resistance to infection and may predispose to permanent corneal scarring if used during certain virus infections. Clearly the use of another person's eye drops without knowledge of the type of drop or the nature of the eye disease is a practice to be severely condemned.

Proper frequency of instillation may be very important. Just as the diabetic must take insulin regularly, so also the patient with glaucoma must faithfully follow his schedule of eye drops if the intraocular pressure is to be maintained within normal limits. Neither a joyful vacation nor an unexpected hospitalization should interfere with the regular antiglaucoma eye drops. The nurse should consider it important that the hospitalized patient follow his usual eye-drop routine. Control of an acute corneal ulcer may require day-and-night antibiotic instillation. Proper preoperative dilation of a pupil may contribute to the success or failure of a cataract extraction. In a patient with faulty lid closure, forgetting to instill ointment at bedtime may permit corneal exposure and ulceration to develop by morning. Excessively frequent instillation of isoflurophate in a cross-eyed child may cause painful spasms of accommodation, redness of the eye, and photophobia, and sometimes results in growth of iris cysts. Instructions followed inaccurately are worthless, possibly dangerous.

Unfortunately, drugs and eye drops are often not labeled by name when dispensed to patients. This may lead to dangerous confusion when multiple drugs are mixed up in the medicine cabinet. Old, unidentified medications should be disposed of beyond the reach of children (e.g., flushed down the toilet). Some medications (particularly antibiotic solutions) lose potency with age. Contamination of eye drops may occur in old bottles, especially if the eyedropper is touched to the eyelid and then returned to the bottle. Occasionally bacteriologic study uncovers an old bottle of eye drops that is teeming with germs. Unlike pills, eye drops should be sterile. A diseased eye, even more than a healthy one, may be quite susceptible to infection introduced via contaminated eye drops. The practice of using an eye cup should therefore be strongly discouraged, since the solution washes germs from the skin into the eye.

Commonly used eye medications may be grouped in the following general categories: anesthetics, antibiotics, astringents, constricting drops, corticosteroids, diagnostic stains, dilating drops, and lubricants. Our intent is to present the general principles of drug action that will be of value to the nurse and to avoid excessive detail.

ANESTHETICS

Local anesthesia of the eye may be achieved quickly and easily with eye drops. These drops cause a brief stinging, followed within less than a minute by a "stiff" or numb sensation of the eye and eyelids. Repeated instillation of anesthetic drops will produce more profound and deeper anesthesia, but 1 or 2 drops usually suffice for minor procedures such as removal of a superficially embedded corneal foreign body or measurement of intraocular pressure with the tonometer. These procedures can be performed as quickly as one minute after instilling the anesthetic drop. Depending upon the amount of anesthetic used, ocular sensation will return in about fifteen minutes to a half hour. During this period of anesthesia a patient could abrade his own cornea without pain should he wipe his eye while it is open. Since tearing is common when irritating drops are instilled and minor ocular procedures are performed, it is almost certain that each patient will, indeed, wipe his anesthetized eye. Hence the patient must always be cautioned to be sure the lids are completely closed before wiping his eye during the duration of anesthesia. He should be provided with absorbent tissue or clean cotton for such wiping.

Because the superficially injured (sunlamp burn, corneal scratch, etc.) eye is immediately relieved of pain by an anesthetic drop, the patient is likely to request the drop for home use. The dispensary nurse must not provide eye anesthetics for home use because they inhibit the healing of corneal epithelium and destroy the protective corneal reflex that closes the eye and guards against injury. An anesthetic acts by reversibly poisoning nerve cells; it also poisons epithelial cells, which completely cease to grow while anesthetized. If constantly anesthetized, a corneal abrasion will never heal; indeed, prolonged anesthesia will destroy normal corneal epithelium.

Commonly used eye anesthetics are 0.5% tetracaine and 0.5% proparacaine (Ophthaine). Cocaine, in concentrations to 4%, was formerly popular, but it is relatively more toxic to corneal epithelium. Furthermore, federal narcotic regulations make the use of cocaine a nuisance. Less commonly used topical eye anesthetics are butacaine (Butyn) and piperocaine (Metycaine). The anesthetic agents effective upon topical application are quite toxic and ordinarily should not be used as injection anesthetics. Conversely, procaine and lidocaine (Xylocaine), the common injectable anesthetics, are relatively ineffective when dropped into the eye.

ANTIBIOTICS

Infections of the lids and surface of the eye are treated with topically applied antibiotics. Systemic administration is usually reserved for infections that threaten sight or involve the deeper parts of the eye and orbit. Before each antibiotic application it is desirable to clean away the bacteria-laden crusts that accumulate on the lid margins during the course of an eye infection; hot moist compresses will help to soften and remove these adherent crusts. This material is infectious and should be disposed of in a sanitary fashion.

Topical antibiotics are also used prophylactically to prevent infection of corneal abrasions. Many ophthalmologists order antibiotic instillation before intraocular surgery to help prevent wound infection.

Although ophthalmic preparations of almost all antibiotics are available, those antibiotics that are commonly used systemically (e.g., penicillin, oxytetracycline [Terramycin], chlortetracycline [Aureomycin]) are infrequently used for ocular instillation. Instead, ophthalmologists prefer to use the antibiotics that are toxic on systemic administration (e.g., bacitracin, neomycin, polymyxin B, nitrofurazone [Furacin]). This usage is preferred because bacteria are less likely to be resistant to an uncommon antibiotic than to the commonly used drugs such as penicillin. Also, penicillin causes ocular allergy in about 5% of adult patients.

Indiscriminate dispensing of antibiotics for treatment of red eyes is unwise. The red eye of allergy, iritis, acute glaucoma, embedded foreign body, and other diseases may be mistaken for infection. Antibacterial therapy instituted on the basis of an erroneous diagnosis delays proper treatment and may permit serious, permanent ocular damage to develop. Dispensary nurses should resist the temptation to give out antibiotics to a red-eyed patient.

ASTRINGENTS

Used as a nonspecific astringent, 0.25% zinc sulfate reduces redness and swelling and soothes itching and irritation. It is often prescribed in combination with 0.125% Neo-Synephrine, which is an effective vasoconstrictor. Although these medications cure no disease, they whiten an irritated eye and make it more comfortable. Annoying ocular irritation may result from many causes (fatigue, dust or smoke, minor infections of low virulence, chronic allergy, wearing of contact lenses). As would be expected, eye drops of this kind are popular and relatively harmless and may be purchased without prescription under a variety of proprietary names. Equal relief can usually be derived from a cold pack (an ordinary washcloth moistened with cold water and applied to the eyelids for several minutes), which is preferable to the use of drops, if effective.

CONSTRICTING DROPS (MIOTICS)

Constriction and dilation of the pupil result from the autonomic innervation of the eye, briefly outlined in Fig. 4-1. Miotic drops cause the pupil to become small (Fig. 4-2). Commonly used drugs of this type are

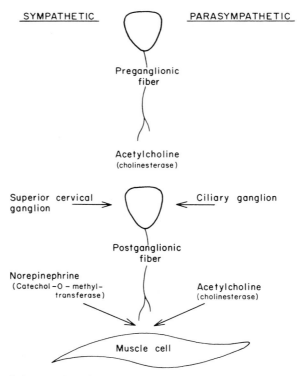

Fig. 4-1. Autonomic innervation of the eye. (From Havener, William H.: Ocular pharmacology, ed. 2, St. Louis, 1970, The C. V. Mosby Co.)

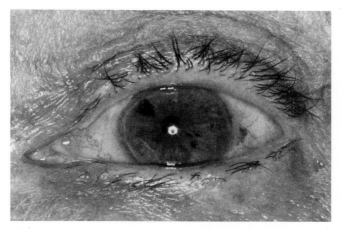

Fig. 4-2. A miotic pupil, resulting from pilocarpine treatment of aphakic glaucoma.

pilocarpine 1 to 4%, eserine 0.25%, carbachol 0.75%, and echothiophate 0.06%. The most valuable use of miotics is in the treatment of glaucoma. They improve the ease with which the aqueous fluid escapes from the eye and thereby decrease intraocular pressure. The frequency of miotic instillation is determined in each patient's eye by clinical trial. A sufficient strength and frequency of instillation is used to maintain intraocular pressure within normal limits, as measured by the tonometer. Once the eye is regulated, the same dosage will usually maintain pressure control; therefore routine tonometer pressure checks may be made as infrequently as every two to three months. Should these routine tonometer measurements detect increased pressure, the patient's miotic dosage is appropriately increased. Sometimes a patient will continue to use his drops as prescribed but will fail to visit his ophthalmologist for a year or more. Safe glaucoma control requires more frequent examinations. The nurse should remember that the pressure elevation of chronic simple glaucoma causes no pain or discomfort and that visual loss is so insidious and slow the patient is unaware of progressive ocular damage. Glaucoma is not adequately controlled just because the patient's eyes "feel fine."

One type of cross-eyed child is helped by echothiophate. The same type of crossed eye is also helped by wearing glasses. Often surgery can be avoided by proper use of glasses and/or echothiophate.

Miotic drops may also be used by physicians to return pupils to normal size at the completion of an eye examination during which the pupils have been dilated in order to permit thorough visualization of the interior of the eye.

CORTICOSTEROIDS

Therapy with cortisone and its derivatives is of great value in allergic eye conditions and for a variety of chronic inflammations. Corticosteroid therapy does not cure disease but merely suppresses the inflammation. In most cases, therefore, prolonged treatment is necessary—sometimes for months. Dosage is determined by ocular response. A great number of corticosteroid preparations exist, and there is very little difference in their effect when used locally in the eye.

Unfortunately corticosteroid therapy reduces the resistance of the eye to invasion by microorganisms. Bacteria, viruses, and fungi have all been proved to cause considerably more damage to a corticosteroid-treated eye than to an untreated eye. Clinical evidence of active infection is therefore an important contraindication to corticosteroid treatment.

Long-continued use of corticosteroids may increase intraocular pressure or cause cataract. As many as one third of the population carry a genetic tendency to develop glaucoma in response to long-term topical use of corticosteroid eye drops. Prolonged unsupervised use of such eye drops may result in loss of sight from glaucoma and must not be allowed.

DIAGNOSTIC STAINS

Visualization of surface defects is aided by selective staining. Fluorescein 0.5% will stain corneal epithelial defects a bright green. The staining is transient, washing off within a few minutes. Fluorescein is most useful in determining the extent of a corneal abrasion or ulcer. As long as a stainable defect persists, antibiotic treatment should continue.

Fluorescein is also commonly used to study the fit of a contact lens. These lenses are supposed to float upon a thin tear film and do not touch the cornea if the fit is proper. Fluorescein stains the tear film so that a thin green space may be seen everywhere between the cornea and a perfectly fitted contact lens.

Although all eye drops should be sterile and protected from contamination, this precaution is especially important with fluorescein because it is used diagnostically in injured eyes, which are especially vulnerable to infection.

Argyrol 10% is instilled into eyes as part of the routine preparation immediately before surgery. Its purpose is to stain mucus strands and surface debris so that all such matter may be recognized and removed completely before surgery. Argyrol also has a mild antiseptic action, but this is of negligible value for the few minutes it remains in the eye.

DILATING DROPS (MYDRIATICS AND CYCLOPLEGICS)

Dilating drops serve at least three important purposes. The first and most obvious reason for dilating a pupil is to improve the physician's view of the interior of an eye. The view of a retina through a small pupil or through a dilated pupil may be compared with the view of a room through the keyhole or with the door open! Through a dilated pupil details of the inner eye are observed with ease and can be studied much more accurately. Through a small pupil it is absolutely impossible to see the peripheral half of the retina, and posterior details are often considerably

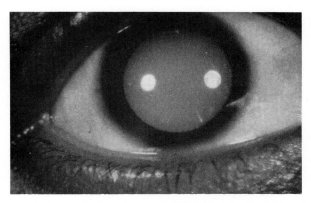

Fig. 4-3. Dilation of the pupil is a most valuable aid to eye examination. Commonly used dilating drops are Neo-Synephrine, Cyclogyl, and homatropine. This patient has a dense cataract.

harder to evaluate. Examination of the eye through a well-dilated pupil is particularly important if a patient has visual complaints of any type (Fig. 4-3).

Mydriatics are drugs that dilate the pupil but do not block accommodation (focusing of the eye). Commonly used mydriatics are Neo-Synephrine 10% and Paredrine 1%. These drops do not interfere with reading ability.

The second important use for dilating drops is to aid in refraction. A cycloplegic drug not only dilates the pupil but also blocks accommodation. The greatest obstacle to accurate determination of refractive error is the ability of the eye to change its strength by accommodation. Although nonmedical methods to relax accommodation in adults usually give accurate findings, they are more time-consuming in younger patients with active accommodation. Precise refraction in young children is impossible without the aid of cycloplegic drops. If a child has crossed eyes, cycloplegic refraction is mandatory. Difficult refractions in adults (high astigmatic errors, accommodative spasms, severe hyperopia, or refractive errors unequal in the two eyes) are corrected with greater accuracy and hence with more comfort to the patient with the aid of cycloplegics. Nonmedical refractionists are greatly handicapped by their legal inability to use dilating drops.

The commonly used cycloplegics are cyclopentolate (Cyclogyl) 1%, bistropamide (Mydriacyl) 1%, homatropine 2%, and atropine 1%. Atropine is especially long lasting and is reserved for refraction of cross-eyed children, who have exceptionally great accommodative ability.

Cycloplegic refraction has the disadvantage of causing blurring of near vision, which lasts for some hours after dilation. The duration and amount of cycloplegia vary with pigmentation, being longer and greater for blondes and shorter and less marked for darkly pigmented individuals. The importance of thorough examination of the interior of the patient's eye and accurate determination of his refractive error far outweighs the temporary inconvenience caused by dilating drugs.

The third use of dilating drops is in the treatment of inflammation of the iris. These inflammations cause shrinkage of the pupil, which becomes very small and may even be occluded by inflammatory membranes. Wide dilation of the pupil is the most important step in the treatment of iritis and is achieved by intensive use of atropine and Neo-Synephrine or other combinations of dilating drops. Proper dilation prevents blindness from pupil block, hastens healing, and relieves pain.

LUBRICANTS

Deficient tearing and inadequate protection by the lids are two common causes of corneal discomfort and damage. Tear deficiency may be caused by lacrimal gland disease, or it may occur spontaneously with age—often at the time of menopause and in association with arthritis. Faulty lid closure may result from paralysis of the facial nerve, sagging muscles of age, unusual prominence of the eye caused by thyroid disease or tumor of the orbit, unconsciousness, etc. Corneal drying from any of these causes is irritating and may result in blurred vision. Use of lubricating drops or ointments will protect the cornea.

Methylcellulose 0.5% is one of the best lubricants, since it is viscous but water soluble and therefore not greasy. This is an excellent "artificial tear" for use in dry eyes. If corneal exposure is more severe, ophthalmic ointments are required to cover the cornea. Boric acid 5% ointment is commonly used because it is quite inexpensive.

Protection of the cornea of all unconscious patients is one of the important responsibilities of the nurse. Often a nurse is the only person who will see the glazed, half-open eye of a comatose patient. Within hours the dried cornea will develop surface necrosis and permanent scarring—if the vigilant nurse does not close the lids and protect the cornea with a lubricant as necessary.

OBSOLETE MEDICATIONS

Before the development of antibiotics, bacterial infections of the eye were commonly treated with chemicals such as boric acid, yellow oxide of mercury, and Argyrol. In comparison with modern drugs these medications are relatively ineffective. However, since they may be obtained without prescription, they are still widely used by patients carrying on the traditions of their grandmothers.

Boric acid, used as an eyewash, has been considered safe because it is relatively insoluble, and a saturated solution is not strong enough to cause eye damage. Actually, when used with an eye cup, this solution (just as any other) washes bacteria from the skin into the eye. Furthermore, toxic amounts of boric acid may be absorbed if large areas of skin are soaked with this solution, especially if the skin is injured or diseased. Death of infants has been recorded as a result of absorption of boric acid powder sprinkled into the diaper. Finally, if use of boric acid delays effective treatment, ocular damage may result from the disease. Ordinary tap water is as effective for any cleaning purpose as is boric acid solution.

OSMOTIC AGENTS

Intraocular pressure may be reduced by the systemic use of osmotic agents (urea, mannitol, or glycerol), which increase the osmotic pressure of the plasma relative to that of aqueous and vitreous. Such osmotherapy is very effective for a brief period of time and is therefore useful as an emergency measure for the control of acute glaucoma or to reduce intraocular pressure during eye surgery. Osmotherapy has no place in the prolonged treatment of chronic eye disease.

The mechanism of action of osmotherapy is entirely different from that of the miotic drugs or the secretory inhibitors. The interior of the eye is separated from the bloodstream by semipermeable membranes. Since osmotic agents do not readily cross these membranes, they cause a withdrawal of intraocular water into the blood vessels, thereby decreasing intraocular pressure within a half hour of administration of an effective dose.

The dosage of urea is 1 Gm. per kilogram of body weight, given intravenously as 30% solution within a thirty- to sixty-minute period. Because of rapid decomposition, urea solutions must be freshly prepared. Accidental extravasation of the urea solution will cause necrosis and sloughing of the infiltrated area. To avoid this very serious complication the patient must be watched attentively during the period of urea infusion.

The dosage of mannitol is 2 Gm. per kilogram of body weight, given intravenously as 20% solution within a thirty- to sixty-minute period. Mannitol extravasation does not cause tissue necrosis, hence it is used more commonly than is urea.

The dosage of glycerol is 1.5 Gm. per kilogram of body weight, taken by mouth. Addition of lemon flavoring and refrigeration makes the medication more palatable. Nausea commonly is troublesome.

All osmotic agents cause severe thirst. Drinking of fluids will completely nullify the hypotensive effect and must **not** be permitted. Severe diuresis will result, and the anesthetized patient must have an indwelling catheter. Cerebral dehydration causes severe headache comparable to that after spinal puncture. A recumbent position minimizes this headache. Mental confusion is a danger sign requiring less rapid intravenous infusion. Excessive cerebral dehydration can cause convulsions, cerebral hemorrhage, and even death.

SECRETORY INHIBITORS

When the improved aqueous outflow resulting from miotic therapy is insufficient to control glaucoma, the ophthalmologist usually resorts to medications that reduce aqueous secretion. These must be given orally, since they act by inactivating an enzyme, carbonic anhydrase, in the bloodstream; this enzyme is necessary for the secretion of aqueous humor.

The most commonly used secretory inhibitor is acetazolamide (Diamox); dosage is 250 mg. or more one to four times daily. Other similar drugs are methazolamide (Neptazane), 50 to 100 mg.; dichlorphenamide (Daranide), 50 mg.; and ethoxzolamide (Cardrase), 125 mg.

The most annoying side effect of the carbonic anhydrase inhibitors is gastrointestinal upset, which may be intolerably severe. Numbness and tingling of extremities and lips bother many patients. Some become drowsy and confused after prolonged treatment. These drugs are sulfonamide derivatives and may be toxic to patients who are allergic to sulfonamides. Urinary calculi may form.

SURGICAL DRUGS

Hyaluronidase is commonly mixed with the anesthetic solution used for local injection preceding eye surgery. This enzyme increases the diffusion of the anesthetic through tissue, thereby improving the effectiveness of the anesthetic nerve block. When used in the retrobulbar injection, as for cataract surgery, hyaluronidase also helps to reduce intraocular pressure, which decreases the possibility of serious complications such as vitreous loss during surgery. The standard vial of hyaluronidase, containing 150 units, is usually mixed with the 30 ml. standard bottle of anesthetic solution; however the enzyme is nontoxic and effective over a wide range of concentrations.

Alpha-chymotrypsin helps to extract cataracts because it dissolves the zonular fibers that suspend the cartaract within the eye. If used for only a few minutes in 1:10,000 concentration, this enzyme does not significantly damage other parts of the eye. Since young persons have stronger zonular fibers than do elderly patients, alpha-chymotrypsin is used mostly for patients between 20 and 50 years of age. Persons under 20 years of age usually have their cataracts removed by a different surgical method, which does not completely remove the lens capsule; hence the enzyme is not used for very young patients.

Epinephrine in 1:1,000 concentration may be applied topically to mucous membranes such as the conjunctiva to decrease bleeding. When combined with injectable anesthetics to prolong anesthetic duration, the concentration of epinephrine is only 1:50,000. If epinephrine 1:1,000 is mistakenly injected by the surgeon, thinking the solution is a local anesthetic, the patient will immediately die of a heart attack.

Obviously drug solutions used during surgery must be accurately identified, with no possibility of confusion.

SYSTEMIC MEDICATIONS

Since drops do not penetrate to the posterior part of the eye, diseases here must be treated by medicines given by mouth or by injection. Indications for such treatment are very much the same as for diseases elsewhere in the body, for example, antibiotics for infection, corticosteroids for allergy, and sedatives and narcotics for pain. Vasodilators are often prescribed for degenerative eye changes, but they usually accomplish little.

SUMMARY

Eye drops contain the highly potent drugs that are necessary for the healing of diseased eyes. The nurse who instills these drops must be absolutely certain of the identity and concentration of the drug and of the frequency with which treatment is necessary, and she must know *which eye* is to be treated. Many eye drops are very poisonous and must not be kept within reach of children.

SUGGESTED READING

Havener, William H.: Ocular pharmacology, ed. 3, St. Louis, 1974, The C. V. Mosby Co.

CHAPTER FIVE # Nursing philosophy, care, and assessment of the patient with visual disability

PHILOSOPHY AND ASSESSMENT

The most important factor in ophthalmic nursing is the ability of the nurse to identify with her patients. She must, of necessity, have a good understanding of medical, surgical, pediatric, and psychiatric nursing to handle the challenging and demanding aspects of caring for the patient with visual impairment. The demands of ophthalmic nursing are not as dramatic or exciting as emergency room or intensive care service, but the rewards of caring for a patient whose vision will be improved or restored cannot quite be duplicated in any other area.

Imagine, if you will, what the loss of vision might mean to you. What other single sense can convey emotion and feeling between individuals as can the momentary, penetrating expression of the eye? What vistas of natural beauty are lost forever to those who once had sight and lost it, or perhaps **never** have been able to see? What aspects of simple daily living that we take for granted become frustrating impossibilities for the blind or visually limited person?

An important aspect of nursing those with visual impairment is the quiet manner and gentleness with which the patient must be physically and emotionally handled. Of course, *all* nursing should be done in a gentle dexterous manner but to the unsighted, who can only imagine your approach, any unusual or hurried motion, bumping of beds, or startling sounds can be most distressing. Therefore, ophthalmic nursing may be said to be "gentle" nursing.

In order to identify patient needs, to plan and implement nursing care, a nursing assessment should be carried out for each patient. This assessment should include information about the patient as a person, his social and physical limitations, the members of his family, and his physical surroundings at home. The nurse also needs knowledge pertinent to the patient's eye disorder, and skill in applying it to the related medical and/or surgical therapy. In gathering information about the patient the nurse uses all the resources at her disposal—the patient, the family, the chart, and other members of the health team. She uses all her interviewing and observational skills. This total patient assessment not only will help the nurse with her nursing care plan, but will also ensure that the patient will have the advantage of having an individual care plan *especially* tailored for him. A patient with a correctable eye disorder enters the hospital with hope of improved vision. Although he may have received basic information from his ophthalmologist about his scheduled surgery and the expected results, the patient may have ambivalent feelings about his hospitalization. Even with thorough briefing, patients bring with them many fears, such as fears of permanent blindness, fear of pain, fear of the unknown, and fear of the anesthetic. There is something unusually terrifying to the average patient about eye surgery and this unwarranted alarm is often caused by completely erroneous misconceptions on the part of the patient and his friends and relatives, because of "old wives' tales." Also, every person is influenced by past experiences such as previous hospitalizations. All these factors must be taken into consideration by the nurse as she forms the nursing care plan. The nursing care plan can be only as effective as the nurse's knowledge of the factors that will influence the patient's attitude and response to his therapy.

The first nursing contact with the patient is usually at the time of admission. The importance of interpersonal relationships at this time is critical if the nurse is to be effective in alleviating fear, orienting the patient to his environment, evaluating his understanding of why he is in the hospital, and clarifying misconceptions.

The nurse's responsibility for this care begins as soon as the patient enters his hospital room (Fig. 5-1). Both psychologic and physical needs may *not* be immediately apparent in the patient. The manifestations of these needs will be as individual as the patient himself.

These needs may be obvious and readily recognized or they may be hidden beneath a calm, quiet exterior. Particular situations will precipitate the emergence of some needs more than others, and the way in which they are met by capable nursing personnel conveys concern for the individuality of the patient. For example, the 70-year-old man who has gradually been losing his sight during the past ten years because of cataracts now enters the hospital for cataract extraction. His hope is to be independent again, to read his newspaper, to obtain glasses, to really *see* again. Will he find adjustment to the hospital routine difficult because he is older and his patterns of daily living are firmly established? Contrast this patient to a young man who has just returned from emergency surgery for removal of an intraocular foreign body. He lies there quietly, never verbalizing any concern, and speaking only when spoken to. However, one cannot help noticing his rigid, tense body position and the way he continually fidgets with his hands. These two patients need equal understanding and care. Whether young or old, we fear for our eyesight. After all, everyone knows that eye surgery is delicate and potentially dangerous, and the spec-

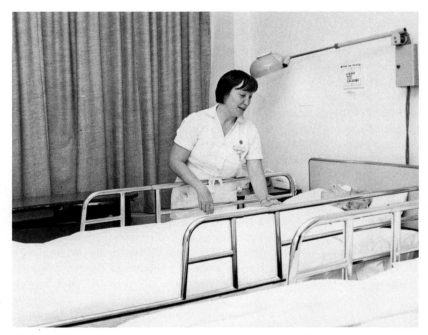

Fig. 5-1. The non-seeing patient is in particular need of a friendly and reassuring greeting.

ter of blindness is always on the patient's mind. This fear cannot be totally banished except by the successful completion of surgery and the convalescent period. Until then, the nurse must understand these anxieties and try to encourage the patient.

Close your eyes for a moment and imagine your problems if the lids would never open again. Even if you are in a room fairly familiar to you, try to find your way around and locate things with your hands. Where is the door, the chair? How many steps will it take to cross the room without bumping into things? What if this were an *unfamiliar* hospital room with unusual pieces of furniture (bed, tables, footstools, bell cords, etc.)? Where is the bathroom? What are those strange noises? Who will help you? Is anybody there?

To really feel the anxiety of the unsighted patient think of your *future* with closed lids. What am I going to do the rest of my life? Who is going to help me? Will my family still love me, and who will take care of them? These unpleasant and *real* fears affect *every* unsighted or visually handicapped person whether he communicates them to you or not. The nurse must be aware of these problems.

NURSING CARE OF THE NON-SEEING PATIENT

When you first enter the room of a non-seeing patient greet him in a relaxed, courteous, *natural* manner. Tell him your name and that you are a nurse. Address him by name so that he will know you are talking to him. Tell him your purpose for coming. Never touch a non-seeing patient without first telling him you are there, as it will surely startle him. Be sure to teach members of the patient's family these techniques, if they are unfamiliar with the patient in an unsighted condition. After all, he does not know who is walking around his bed. It could be an intruder seeking his wallet or a window-washer passing through his room to invade his privacy while he is bathing.

The most important aspect in caring for the non-seeing patient is communication. After the nurse has introduced herself to the patient she should first acquaint him with his physical surroundings. Physical contact here is extremely helpful. Gently take the patient's hand and show him where the button of his call bell is located and tell him it will always be in this specific place. Allow him to then find it and operate it himself several times so he will know he will always have this means of communication when he is alone. Next, slowly lead the patient around the room, helping him to locate with his hands the bed, the chair, the table, etc. Help him to place his personal possessions in his bedside table so he will know exactly where his toothbrush, soap, and toilet articles are. The patient who can care for himself should be guided to the sink and to the bathroom and allowed to locate the soap, towels, toilet paper, and water faucets with his hands.

If the patient is unable to go to the bathroom, the nurse should bring the wash basin to the bedside and allow the patient to feel the temperature of the bath water. Have him touch the washcloth, soap, and towels so he will be able to locate them. Be sure the area is clear enough so he will not accidentally knock over a water pitcher or a vase of flowers, for instance. Such accidents serve to frustrate and embarrass a patient who is already insecure in unfamiliar surroundings. Draw his bedside curtains and tell him you have done so, assuring that he is certain of his privacy.

Guiding and walking with the non-seeing person is the thing most commonly done wrong by well-intentioned people trying to help. Never push the patient ahead of you. He will be the first to bump into any obstacle this way. Instead, place the person's hand in the crook of your elbow (Fig. 5-2). Walk at a normal unhurried pace about one foot ahead of the patient. If he is experienced at being guided in this fashion he will adjust very quickly to your step. If he is not, he will soon find how much easier this method is than are other ways of travel. Always warn the patient when you are about to go through a door or any narrow passage. It usually helps if you carry on a descriptive conversation with him such as, "We are going down a long corridor now, Mr. Smith. Now we are entering the sunroom, where we have some comfortable chairs." Always guide the patient to the chair, allowing him to feel the front of it with his knee, and helping feel the seat and arms with his hand. Then he will feel safe sitting down, knowing which chair height he will be aiming for.

One of the most serious hazards in the area of safety for the unattended

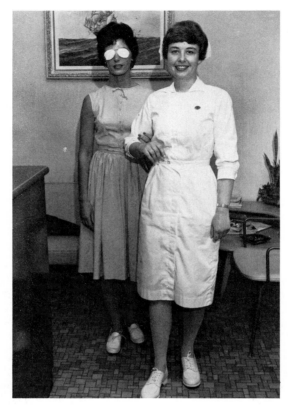

Fig. 5-2. The patient who cannot see is best guided by holding the nurse's elbow. Do not push a blind patient ahead of you.

non-seeing patient is smoking in bed. This should *never* be allowed, no matter how busy the nurse is. If the patient insists on smoking, she or someone else *must* remain at bedside until the cigarette is safely extinguished.

Patients who are non-seeing for the first time due to bilateral patching should always have siderails on their bed in the up position. Many patients experiencing sensory deprivation for the first time become disoriented within their surroundings and can easily fall and hurt themselves.

Mealtime is a very important nursing care area for the non-seeing patient. When one is deprived of the visual stimulation of even the best prepared food, it is difficult to have much appetite. Add to this the fact that the independence of self-feeding is often missing and you understand the nurse's role in encouraging good nutrition for the non-seeing individual. The nurse should exert every effort to make mealtime a pleasant event. Help the patient to select his menu by reading it to him, and when his tray arrives help him by arranging it so that he knows where things are located. Even the temporarily non-seeing patient should be encouraged to help himself, but the nurse should be on hand to assist. It is usually helpful to arrange his food on the plate in such a way that he can compare it to a clock, such as meat at six o'clock, vegetables at ten o'clock, potato at 2 o'clock. Try to be consistent and have his dessert, salad, and beverage in the same position each time. Take time to describe what is on the tray and to cut up the meat, butter the bread, pour the coffee, and generally get things started so the patient will be better able to assist himself. Mealtime is also a time to get to know your patient better. You have time for periods of conversation about many things such as the patient's family, outside interests, and problems. Many times a nurse can help allay fears during these informal talks. After meals the nurse should check the patient's tray to be sure he is getting adequate caloric intake. She should particularly note his fluid intake, as dehydration could be a problem during his short period of bed confinement.

When administering medications to the non-seeing patient, always communicate adequately with him. Be sure he knows whether a pill or liquid is in the cup. Be sure to tell him how many pills there are and assist him with a glass of water to swallow them. Always be sure a patient takes his medicine in your presence, as he may be embarrassed or reluctant to tell you if he accidentally dropped it on the floor or spilled it after you left. If an injection is ordered, always tell the patient before it is administered. Nothing is more startling than getting an unexpected "shot."

Remember that time hangs heavily on people who cannot see. Television, books, and even the passing scene in the hospital are denied the non-seeing patient. A few moments are well spent by the nurses who makes it her business to drop in several times during her tour of duty just to say "Hello" or chat a minute. These diversions help pass time which must seem endless to those whose only contacts with the world are unfamiliar sounds and voices.

PREOPERATIVE NURSING CARE

Although the ophthalmologist will have explained the surgery to the patient before he goes to the operating room, it is often the nurse who will be the target of many questions from the patient. Patients seemingly forget what they have been told by the doctor, and five minutes later will be asking the same questions of the nurse. The nurse should always be on "firm ground" when answering a patient's questions about his surgery. She should accompany the surgeon on his rounds when he talks with the patient so that she knows what the patient has been told and *should only* answer questions in those areas covered or those with which she is entirely familiar. If she does not know the answer to a question, she should say so and tell the patient she will try to find out the answer and then do so. Many patients have undue anxieties over things that those familiar with hospitals would find insignificant, such as time of surgery, how long it will take, will the family be there when they get back to their room, etc.

Routine preoperative procedures such as removal of dentures and jewelry should be explained. Always be *sure* the patient has voided before he goes to the operating room. Most eye surgery requires preoperative medication to sedate the patient and also usually includes the administration of certain eye drops, depending on the particular surgical procedure. It is the nurse's responsibility to see that the ordered preoperative medications are properly administered, thereby enhancing the possibility of successful surgery.

If the operation requires a local anesthetic the patient should know that he will be awake but feel no pain. If the surgery under local anesthesia is scheduled for late in the morning, breakfast ordinarily need not be omitted.

Surgery requiring a general anesthetic, of course, requires omission of food and fluid usually from midnight on the night before. The patient should always be informed of this and also be told that he will spend some time in the recovery room before returning to his own bed.

Transporting the patient to the operating room requires positive identification of the patient before he leaves the unit. Most hospitals have a wrist band identification system which should be checked by those responsible for the proper identity *before* he is moved.

Because a patient will be quite heavily sedated, the safety belts should always be attached during the trip to the operating room and particularly while he is on the narrow operating table. Those patients whose surgery will be done under a local anesthetic may become apprehensive about being restrained. If this occurs, the safety reasons for restraint should be explained.

POSTOPERATIVE NURSING CARE

Postoperative nursing care of the patient after eye surgery depends on the type of eye surgery performed, the anesthetic used, and specific orders of the patient's ophthalmologist. Postoperative instructions vary greatly from patient to patient as well as between different surgeons. Hence, no generalizations can be made except to say that whatever restrictions or methods of care ordered are deemed important by that particular surgeon to ensure the best healing of the eye.

Special awareness of safety and protection permeates all aspects of care for the patient after eye surgery. Generally, the time at which a patient is allowed out of bed varies from immediately to several days postoperatively. Prolonged bed rest weakens the patient and predisposes to thromboembolic and other complications. The elderly and infirm patient is particularly susceptible to the ill effects of bed rest, and it is in this older age group that a high incidence of eye pathology occurs. Being encouraged to be up and about seems to improve problems of cerebral arteriosclerosis. Getting up to go to the toilet also eliminates most of the problems of urinary retention and constipation.

Since the operated eye will be patched the nurse *must* know how much vision the patient has in his unpatched eye before expecting him to get about on his own. She may also explain the difficulty with depth perception he will experience with one eye patched. It is only when she knows how much vision the patient has that she can begin her postoperative nursing care plan for the ambulatory patient.

For patients who are to be bedfast for any period of time, many ophthalmologists recommend isometric exercises that do not jerk or shake the head. These exercises consist of pushing or pulling the arms or legs against resistance. These can easily be performed by the patient against the siderails of his bed after he has been taught by the nurse. Generally they are done at quite frequent intervals; specific instructions should be given if they are part of the medical plan of care. As with all patients who have been on bed rest for a time, care should be taken when the patient is first allowed out of bed. He should first sit on the side of the bed and be encouraged to dangle his legs for five or ten minutes. Some of these patients may feel faint or in danger of falling, so the nurse should be sure that the patient is helped when he leaves the bed for the first few times until she is certain he is adequately steady and strong.

Patients receiving a local anesthetic are permitted a regular diet immediately. Those patients who receive a general anesthetic are placed on a liquid diet postoperatively, progressing gradually to a regular diet. Many surgeons prescribe antiemetic drugs to relieve postanesthetic nausea and vomiting, not only for the comfort of the patient but because the strain of vomiting may increase intraocular pressure. The nurse should be aware that these drugs may cause postural hypotension and thereby induce fainting when the patient arises from bed. Since food and fluid worsen nausea, chewing on ice chips, sipping small amounts of carbonated beverages, or eating crackers may be helpful.

The elimination habits of the postoperative eye patient are also important. For example, a patient who always uses cathartics should be permitted to continue his routine. After intraocular surgery many ophthalmologists do not want their patients to cough or to strain, as in defecation, because of increased intraocular pressure.

Generally speaking, the most important nursing care after intraocular surgery is protection of the operated eye. This is almost universally achieved by the use of a metal shield (Fig. 5-3). An operated eye can be destroyed by inadvertent pressure upon it. The nurse should be aware of her responsibility to be sure that the shield is securely in place at all times, particularly at night. Occasionally a patient will dislodge his shield in his sleep. When this mishap is discovered, the shield and pad under it should be gently but securely put back in place. The nurse should be sure that the patient himself understands the importance of protecting his eye with the metal shield.

Usually the eye surgeon prefers to carry out all dressing changes and treatments himself. An eye bandage should *not* be changed because the eye hurts or for any other reason unless this action is approved by the surgeon. Most patients do not experience much physical pain after eye surgery. When severe pain is manifested it may indicate hemorrhage or other complications and the ophthalmologist should be notified. Most patients do have postoperative orders for mild analgesics to relieve minor discomfort.

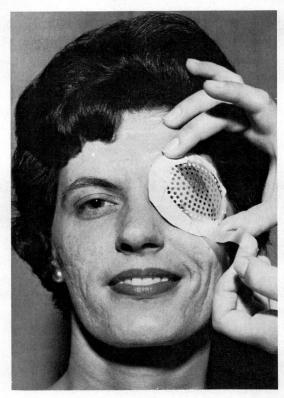

Fig. 5-3. A metal shield should protect an eye with a recent penetrating wound, whether from surgery or injury.

HOME-GOING PREPARATION

Instructions for the patient's home regimen are prescribed by the physician. It is the nurse's responsibility to go over these instructions step by step and find out how well the patient understands them. Although many doctors give detailed printed instructions to the patient, studies have shown errors in care occur because of inadequate reading or lack of comprehension of the instructions. The nurse should go over the material with the patient and include the family if possible. Since instillation of eye drops or ointment is frequently continued after discharge, instructing the patient and his family in the correct method is a part of the nursing responsibilities. It is most helpful after showing the patient how to instill the drops to have him return the demonstration to the nurse so she may correct any flaws in technique at once. She should also show the patient how to change his eye pad and shield and tape it securely in place. It is also the nurse's responsibility to find out how the patient lives. Is he living alone? Will he need assistance with care at home? Who will do the shopping, cooking, and cleaning? Does he have other medical problems which require care such as insulin injections or special diet teaching? This is the area in which a public health nursing referral can be of great importance. In addition to giving skilled nursing care, the public health nurse is in the best position through her home visits to assess the patient's living conditions and accuracy of self-care. She can also be instrumental in assisting the patient through various community resources to find meaningful diversions and in renewing contacts, such as church or community social groups.

SUGGESTED NURSING CARE PLANS

The following nursing care plans should be used only as *guides*. Again, let it be emphasized that these recommendations *cannot* be used by the nurse for all patients. There is still a great deal of diversity of opinion among eye surgeons regarding patient care. Therefore, the nurse should be sure she is following the physician's orders as prescribed.

Cataract

Prevention of infection is extremely important with cataract extraction and is the reason for preoperative instillation of antibiotic drops. Preoperative dilation of the eye is helpful in cataract extractions, since the cataract is removed through the pupil. The preoperative narcotics and sedatives are given to alleviate pain and to reduce anxiety during surgery, which is usually performed under local anesthesia.

Postoperative shielding of the operated eye with a metal shield is of greatest importance. The cataract incision encircles the entire upper half of the cornea and can be disrupted by pressing upon or bumping the eye. Rupture of the cataract incision will almost always seriously impair eye function and commonly will blind the eye permanently. Involuntary self-rubbing of an operated eye is to be expected, especially when the patient is asleep. Securely taping the metal shield over the eye virtually eliminates the danger of wound rupture. The postoperative cataract patient should be up and about as usual; being up will not harm the eye. He is allowed a soft diet immediately. Reading is not harmful. All postoperative dressings of the eye will ordinarily be performed by the surgeon. Generally there are no restrictions placed on self-care after discharge.

Corneal transplant

The hospital care for patients with corneal transplant is almost identical to that for cataract surgery, except that the operation is usually performed under general anesthesia. Preoperatively the pupil is constricted (rather than dilated, as for cataract extraction) in order to cover the lens as much as possible with the iris. This helps to protect the lens against accidental injury during surgery. Since a 6- to 8-mm. disk is cut out of the center of the cornea and replaced with a transplant which is sewn into place with many delicate sutures, the eye is extremely vulnerable to injury and must be carefully shielded.

Strabismus

Most extraocular muscle surgery is performed under general anesthesia, therefore these patients should be given no food or fluid since the preceding night. Since many muscle surgery patients are children, it may be less traumatic for them to be admitted on the morning of surgery. It is the responsibility of the physician and/or his office nurse to inform the family not to allow the child to eat or drink anything since midnight before admission. It is annoying to everyone concerned to cancel surgery because the patient has eaten, but the danger from aspiration complications precludes general anesthesia on a full stomach.

Strabismus surgery does not penetrate into the eye so there are literally no postoperative ocular rupture hazards. The patient is not restricted in any way other than the usual recovery from general anesthesia. An eye pad is generally kept on the operated eye for the first day but only to absorb blood and secretions. This bandage should be firmly applied as it will help reduce postoperative swelling. The patient usually is discharged home the day after surgery. Antibiotic drops and warm compresses three or four times daily may be ordered for home care.

Enucleation

Although removal of an eye would seem to be the most extensive and complicated eye operation possible, it is probably the procedure most free from postoperative complications. Nothing more can happen to the eye. The procedure is done under general anesthesia so the usual nursing care before and after a general anesthetic is appropriate. There is no restriction of activity. A clear plastic shell called a conformer is placed in the socket after surgery and is usually left in place until the patient is fitted with an artificial eye. Patients should be advised not to be alarmed if the conformer falls out, since this is of no consequence. It need not be replaced. The purpose of the conformer is to hold the shape of the tissues of the socket while it is healing prior to the insertion of the prosthesis.

The patient is usually discharged within two days. Antibiotic drops and warm compresses may be ordered three or four times a day. An eye pad is worn for cosmetic reasons until the prosthetic eye is fitted a month after surgery.

Retinal detachment

The most important nursing care principle to observe in caring for the patient with retinal detachment is to maintain the retinal hole down. This means to position the patient's head in such a position as to keep the retinal hole inferior with respect to the rest of the eye. Before surgery this positioning helps prevent further progression of the detachment; after surgery, this positioning maintains proper apposition of the retina. The nurse should check the patient's chart or with the surgeon before she positions and instructs the patient so that the specific instructions may be carried out. Since the patient will be on strict bed rest, good nursing care is essential. Isometric exercises and range of motion exercises that do not shake the head should be encouraged.

Since most retinal detachment surgery is done under general anesthesia, proper precautions should be taken to assure that the patient is not allowed to eat or drink anything for at least eight hours prior to surgery. Since most patients are on strict bed rest before and after surgery for one or two days, they are more likely to feel faint when allowed to first sit upright. They should be assisted to sit on the edge of the bed and dangle their legs for five or ten minutes before being allowed to stand upright and walk.

Both eyes are patched to prevent quick eye movements. Since both eyes move equally rather than independently, the unoperated eye is also patched but is uncovered as soon as possible. Activities that produce rapid eye movement (such as reading) are contraindicated for several weeks after discharge. However, television, which involves a straight ahead gaze, or radio can help pass the time. The patient is usually discharged on the third day after surgery. Dilating drops and warm compresses may be ordered for home care. An eye pad may be worn for comfort but is not absolutely necessary after discharge.

NURSING PROCEDURES
Instillation of eye drops

When the nurse gives eye drops she must be absolutely sure of three things: the correct patient, the correct eye, and the correct drop. Medication errors with eye drops can be extremely serious.

With the patient in a sitting position eye drops are most easily instilled by observing the following steps (Fig. 5-4).

1. Have the patient tilt his head back.
2. Have the patient roll his eyes up and ask him to fix at a point toward the top of his head.
3. With the forefinger, gently pull down on the tissue below the lower lid until the conjunctiva is exposed, forming a small pocket.
4. With the other hand, drop one drop of the medication directly on the conjunctiva (or lining of the lid), being careful not to touch the tip of the dropper to the eye. If the drop is properly instilled on the conjunctiva and not on the cornea the patient will tolerate it quite comfortably. The cornea is very sensitive, and properly so, as it is the body's natural warning mechanism when a foreign body is in the eye.
5. Allow the patient to blot his eye with a tissue but ask him not to rub his eye.

When giving drops to children, it is sometimes difficult to get them to hold their eyes open. Many times a simple game can be placed to get the eye drops in without frightening the child or getting into a struggle. Have the child tip his head back, tell him he can close his eye gently, then drop one drop of medication on the innermost point of the lower canthus. Tell the child the drop is in and he can now open his eye. The child will open his eye and the drop will roll in.

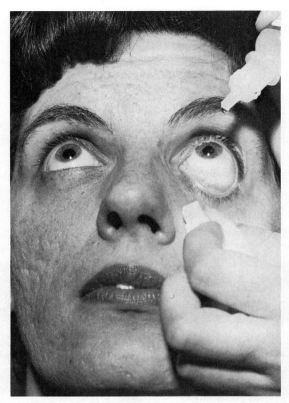

Fig. 5-4. The patient should tilt her face upward to receive an eye drop. Use an absorbent tissue to prevent excess drops and tears from flowing down the patient's face.

The natural blinking of the lids spreads the medication over the eye surface, regardless of where the drop is given. One drop at a time of the prescribed drug is sufficient.

Eye drops are sterile and should be handled in a way to prevent contamination. The tip of the dropper or squeeze bottle should never touch the eye or be touched by the nurse's finger. Always be careful when reinserting the dropper or cap not to touch it on the bottle or, in the case of a squeeze bottle, the edge of the cap. Contaminated drops should be discarded.

Eye ointments

Eye ointments are administered in exactly the same manner as eye drops (Fig. 5-5). Some nurses have been taught to put a ribbon of ointment along the entire length of the conjunctiva of the lower lid. This amount of ointment is unnecessary. Only the smallest possible amount need be placed at the same point as the eye drop is placed. Natural blinking and body temperature will distribute and melt the ointment over the eye surface.

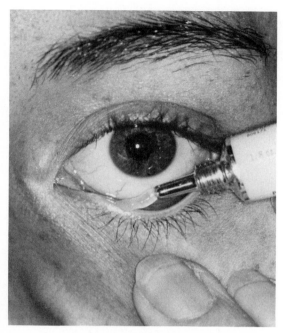

Fig. 5-5. To instill ointment, pull down the lower lid as the patient looks upward. Squeeze the ointment into the lower conjunctival sac. Avoid touching the tube to the eye or lid.

Eye pads

The purpose of the eye pad is to absorb secretions or blood, and to promote comfort (Fig. 5-6). Eye pads are *not* worn to prevent infection. Indeed, they are contraindicated in eye infections as they give bacteria a nice warm, dark, moist place to multiply! They are generally worn after eye surgery to promote comfort by preventing excessive eye motion.

In cases of corneal abrasion two pads tightly applied may be used as a pressure bandage. This helps to relieve pain.

Some patients wear an eye patch to eliminate diplopia or for cosmetic reasons.

When applying an eye pad have the patient close *both* eyes (one eye cannot be comfortably closed alone by most people). Gently place the pad on the eye without touching its inner surface.

Two diagonally placed pieces of tape stretching from the center forehead to center cheek are sufficient to keep an eye pad in place. When applying a pressure patch with two eye pads, as in treating corneal abrasions, several pieces of tape should be applied in such a manner as to hold the cheek tightly pulled up beneath the eye, thereby ensuring that the patient cannot open the affected eye.

A word should be said here about tape. Regular adhesive tape sticks

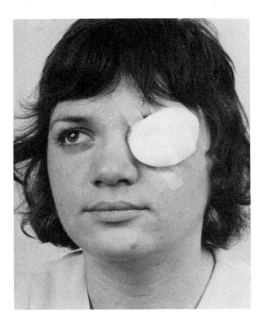

Fig. 5-6. Note the proper diagonal application of tape to secure the eye pad in position.

well but is messy, difficult, and painful to remove. Plastic tape is stretchy, sticks well, and is easily removed. There are always a few patients who will have allergic skin reactions to plastic tape, and paper tape may be used for these patients.

Hot compresses

Hot compresses are often used in the treatment of surface infections of the cornea, conjunctiva, or eyelids. They are also often prescribed for home use after eye surgery. Many patients find that the moist heat is soothing as well as cleansing for the operated eye. The easiest and most practical way of applying a hot compress to the eye is to use an ordinary wash cloth wrung out in hot water (Fig. 5-7). When the patient is discharged from the hospital the nurse should teach him to soak the wash cloth in hot water, then wring it out and fold it into a flat shape. He should allow the cloth to remain in place until it cools and repeat the process for ten to fifteen minutes. Care should be taken not to put too hot a compress on the eye; water comfortably hot to the hand sometimes needs a little cooling before it is applied to the face.

There is no need to observe any complicated ritual with sterile gauze, sterile forceps, and sterile solutions when applying hot compresses. The skin of the face and eyelids is not sterile, and of course the eye is closed and protected by the eyelids during the procedure. Hot compresses should not be used on an eye with an open penetrating laceration because of the danger of mechanically injuring the eye.

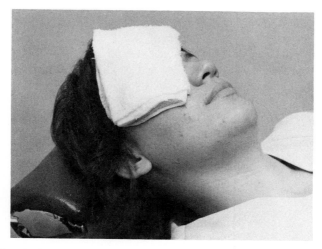

Fig. 5-7. An effective method of applying a warm compress to the eye.

Cleaning of eyelids

The application of hot compresses is probably the best method the nurse can use to soften crusts and matter adherent to eyelids. After softening with the compresses, a moist piece of cotton or a cotton-tipped applicator can then be used to remove the matter mechanically. Caution should be observed, however, if recent intraocular surgery has been done, as the eye is still vulnerable to pressure.

The cornea and conjunctiva do not need washing or irrigation. Nature takes care of this function very nicely with the normal tear secretion and blinking mechanism. The only exception to this is when the cornea and conjunctiva are irrigated immediately after a chemical burn. The eye cup, which is still seen on druggists' shelves, should be relegated to the antique shop. Its use is to be condemned for it only serves to wash organisms from the lid skin onto the delicate surface of the eye.

Cold compresses

Cold compresses are useful to relieve ocular itching, irritation, swelling, fatigue, or pain. They are prepared in exactly the same manner as hot compresses, simply substituting ice water for hot water. Small ice bags or an ice cube wrapped in a wash cloth are useful in reducing tissue edema following strabismus surgery and lid bruises. Ice should not be applied directly to the lids. Cold compresses are not used in eye infections.

Prevention of exposure damage to the eye

The cornea is very sensitive to drying and can be damaged by failure of the lids to close for even a short time. Faulty lid closure may result from

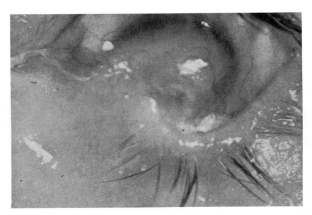

Fig. 5-8. Faulty lid closure permits severe corneal scarring to develop. The nurse must always be certain her unconscious patient's eyelids are closed.

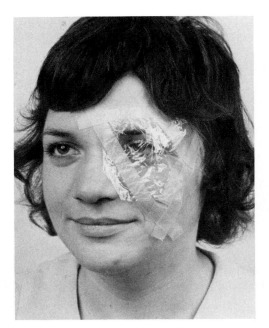

Fig. 5-9. Thin plastic, such as Saran Wrap, may be taped over an exposed eye to prevent drying.

unconsciousness from any cause, paralysis, injury to the lids, or abnormal prominence of the eyes. Lifetime scarring of a cornea may result from overnight exposure (Fig. 5-8). The alert nurse should be the first to recognize the threat of exposure damage to the cornea and can prevent scarring by closing the lids of an unconscious patient. Eye ointments, methylcellulose eye drops, and barriers of Saran Wrap (Fig. 5-9) are some of the methods used to ensure corneal protection.

Instrument care

Instruments used for eye surgery are considerably more delicate and expensive than other surgical instruments. These small, sharp instruments should receive special care, since they can easily be damaged by dropping them or using them irresponsibly. Nothing is quite so frustrating as trying to remove a 10-0 corneal suture with a fine forcep that has been misused and has its teeth malaligned.

Sterility of all equipment is necessary, of course, just as for all other surgery. The penalty for using contaminated equipment could be the loss of the eye through infection. Faulty technique observed by the nurse in the operating room should be reported immediately. The embarrassment of admitting to such a mistake should be forgotten when you know that a concealed error could cause the loss of someone's eye.

CHAPTER SIX   # Errors of refraction

Every person has some minor defects in the focusing and alignment of his eyes. Most of these defects are so small that their correction by glasses would be purely nuisance and expense to the patient. The purpose of refractive correction with glasses is to relieve symptoms. Glasses do not improve the health of an eye.

SYMPTOMS

Only two symptoms are caused by refractive errors. These are *reduced visual acuity* and *discomfort resulting from use of the eyes*. No other symptoms or problems are likely to be corrected by glasses.

Patients often do not realize they have poor eyesight. Children, especially, may endure very poor vision without any complaint. Adults are often unaware of slowly developing visual loss, especially if only one eye is affected. Measurement of vision with a reading chart is an easy, quick test that is routinely used in most schools to detect students in need of eye care.

Headaches caused by refractive error may affect the eyes, the back of the head, the forehead, the temples—almost any part of the head. Ocular fatigue, burning, and irritation (commonly called "eyestrain") may be caused by refractive errors. Since refractive errors do not develop quickly, they do not cause symptoms that appear within a short time. An exception to this might be symptoms appearing simultaneously with greatly intensified use of the eyes, such as preceding an examination. Discomfort not related to use of the eyes is very unlikely to be caused by refractive error.

Reduced acuity and ocular discomfort are **not** symptoms caused by refractive error only. Serious ocular, general, or brain disorders often cause such complaints. Other common causes are fatigue and nervous tension. Rather frequently, ophthalmologists see patients with these symptoms, which have persisted despite prescription of glasses elsewhere. Often this delay in seeking medical care is detrimental to the patient.

CAUSE

Almost all refractive errors are inherited. The parts of the eye that determine its focus are the corneal curvature, the strength of the lens, and the length of the eye. Faulty combinations of these parts result in inaccurate focusing of light upon the retina.

Disease and injury may also cause refractive errors. Uncontrolled diabetes may cause quite rapid changes in refraction, so that disabling nearsightedness may develop within a few days. Fortunately medical control of the diabetes usually corrects this. One type of senile cataract causes slowly increased nearsightedness. Often this can be corrected with glasses for several years before surgery becomes necessary. Many of the tranquilizing and antihypertensive drugs blur near vision. If this is sufficiently annoying, the drug must be given in lower dosage or discontinued. Scars resulting from injury may distort the cornea. Contact lenses sometimes improve this type of optical distortion.

TYPES

Refractive errors include nearsightedness (myopia), farsightedness (hyperopia), unequal focus of the two eyes (anisometropia), asymmetrical focus (astigmatism), and inability to change focus (presbyopia). It is easier to understand these refractive errors if we discuss accommodation first.

Accommodation is the increase in refractive power used to focus the eye upon near objects. This greater power results when the curvature of the lens is increased by contraction of the ciliary muscle. When the ciliary muscle is completely relaxed, the refractive power of an eye is at its lowest possible strength and cannot be further decreased. When the ciliary muscle is maximally contracted, the refractive power of an eye is at its greatest strength. Between these two strengths, of farthest and nearest clear vision, respectively, the eye automatically adjusts its power for best vision at any given distance.

The amount of accommodation possessed by a person gradually decreases with age, until after 40 years of age it becomes annoyingly inadequate for comfortable close work. By the age of 60 years the lens has become so inelastic that no changes in its strength are possible. This loss of accommodation because of age is called *presbyopia*. Since a presbyopic person cannot change his focus from far to near, this must be done with glasses. This correction requires a bifocal, with a different strength for lens top and bottom for far and near vision, respectively. Presbyopia does not change a preexisting refractive error (such as nearsightedness) but progressively reduces the ability to accommodate for near work.

Emmetropia. The refractive error of an eye is measured when accommodation is completely relaxed, that is, when the ciliary muscle is not working. A normal eye that, without accommodation, is focused perfectly for distance is termed emmetropic (Fig. 6-1). Such an eye sees clearly in the distance without effort and may focus upon close objects with the aid of accommodation. Emmetropia causes no symptoms, although of course even the most perfect eye will tire with prolonged use and general bodily fatigue.

Myopia. A myopic (nearsighted) eye has excessive refractive strength

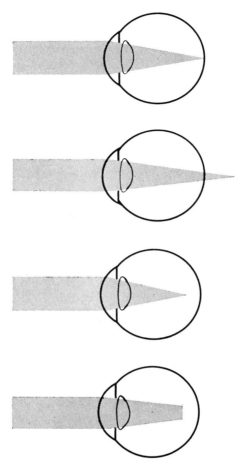

Fig. 6-1. Light is focused accurately upon the retina in an emmetropic eye, behind the retina in an uncorrected hyperopic eye, in front of the retina in an uncorrected myopic eye, and comes to a distorted linear focus in astigmatism.

and focuses light from distant objects in front of the retina. Since the eye cannot reduce this excessive power in any way, the myopic person is unable to see clearly in the distance. Near vision requires greater refractive strength than does distant vision; therefore the myope will be in focus at some near point (depending upon the amount of myopia) without the aid of accommodation. He may also accommodate, thereby focusing yet closer than would be possible with a normal eye.

The only symptom caused by myopia is decreased distance vision (without glasses). Myopia does not produce ocular discomfort, headache, fatigue with use of eyes, etc.

As children grow, their eyes tend to become less farsighted (or more nearsighted). Myopia usually first becomes evident in the early years of school and progresses at a rate requiring new glasses every year or two. After adolescence, when the child stops growing, the myopia usually becomes stationary. Use or nonuse of the eyes does not affect the rate of development of myopia. Diets, vitamins, hormones, eye exercises, or any other methods of treatment have never been proved to alter the progress of myopia. Myopia is not a valid medical reason for limiting physical, intellectual, or ocular activity.

About 1% of myopes have retinal degenerations that may lead to retinal detachment or other serious eye problems. Thorough ophthalmoscopic examination can identify these degenerative changes before they cause retinal detachment. Degenerative myopes predisposed to retinal detachment should avoid rough physical activity.

Hyperopia. A hyperopic (farsighted) eye has insufficient refractive power to focus light upon the retina, whether the light originates from far or near objects. Without the aid of accommodation, a farsighted eye is unable to see clearly at any distance. Since accommodation will supply additional focusing power, most young hyperopes are able to see clearly at distance or near—at the price of greater accommodative effort than is required by an emmetrope. If the hyperopic refractive error is large enough, the constantly required excessive accommodation will cause ocular discomfort and fatigue related to use of the eyes, especially for near work. Very high amounts of hyperopia may be greater than the accommodation available for proper focusing—such patients have reduced vision. As his accommodation gradually decreases in the late 30's and early 40's, a hyperope is forced to wear reading glasses sooner than would an emmetrope.

Anisometropia. Anisometropia refers to a different focus of the two eyes. Refractive errors are usually symmetrical, so that almost the same focus exists in each eye. Rarely, the two eyes differ considerably. Because accommodation changes both eyes by the same amount, the anisometropic patient is unable to compensate for this difference in focus. Hence he can never see clearly with both eyes at the same time (unless wearing glasses). Anisometropia commonly causes ocular discomfort and fatigue. If one eye is very much out of focus from early life, it may actually suffer loss of visual acuity from disuse.

Astigmatism. Optical surfaces in cameras, telescopes, or other precision instruments have spherical curves that are exactly equal in all meridians. Unfortunately the human cornea usually lacks this precision and is more curved in one direction than another. This unequal curvature is called astigmatism (*a,* without; *stigma,* point) because it distorts the focus of light rays so that they are not clear at any point. Hyperopia or myopia may coexist with astigmatism. Astigmatism cannot be eliminated by accommodation or by any other effort of the patient. The common, inherited form of astigmatism can be effectively corrected by glasses ground to neutralize the unequal curvature.

The symptoms of astigmatism are blurred vision and discomfort with use of the eyes.

MEASUREMENT

Refraction is the clinical measurement of the focus of a nonaccommo-dated eye. A very close objective estimate of the focus of an eye may be made with retinoscopy. Retinoscopy is the observation of the movement of focused light emerging from the patient's eye. Myopia, hyperopia, and astig-matism each have a characteristic pattern of light movement. With the aid of retinoscopy the proper corrective lenses can rapidly and accurately be determined. Hence the refractive error of even the youngest infant can be measured precisely.

Subjective refraction measures the refractive error by permitting the patient to choose the best of a series of lenses. In practice, retinoscopy is used to determine the approximately correct lens strength, and the sub-jective check is used for final confirmation.

Cycloplegics. The technique of refraction is really quite simple. The main source of error is the unknown and possibly variable amount of ac-commodation exerted by the patient during examination. Special optical techniques have been devised to reduce the possibility of error because of accommodation. In general these techniques work quite well in most adults, although they are time-consuming. Hyperopic patients, being constantly used to excessive accommodation, frequently are unsuitable candidates for these optical techniques, particularly if they are younger than 25 years of age. Accurate refraction of hyperopic children is impossible by these meth-ods. Particularly in the case of a cross-eyed child, accurate determination of the entire amount of hyperopia is vitally important.

Cycloplegic drugs (atropine, homatropine, Cyclogyl, Mydriacyl) greatly enhance the accuracy of refraction of hyperopic patients and are essential for proper refraction of children. Cycloplegics block accommodation and dilate the pupil. Aided in this way, an expert retinoscopist can easily de-termine the average uncomplicated refractive error in less than a half minute.

Performance of a refraction only is an incomplete and potentially dan-gerous examination. Symptoms of disease mimic those of refractive error. Any patient with eye symptoms sufficient to bring him for examination requires careful fundus examination through an adequately dilated pupil.

CORRECTION

Often patients with a relatively slight refractive error are happier with-out glasses, since their disadvantages (weight, reflections, dirty lenses, and expense) outweigh the benefits. Association of a significant refractive error with appropriate symptoms, in the absence of other cause for the symp-toms, indicates prescription of glasses.

Many persons believe glasses must be changed at periodic intervals, just as oil in a car. This is not true. The indications for change are the same as those for the original prescription, namely, reduced visual acuity or dis-comfort from use of the eyes—despite wearing of the existing glasses.

CONTACT LENSES

Development of strong, optically perfect plastics and of methods of precise machining and polishing to form extremely thin lenses has resulted in the modern contact lens boom. Corneal contact lenses are tiny disks about half the diameter of a cornea, precisely contoured to fit the anterior cornea, with the patient's optical correction ground in their front surface. They float freely upon the precorneal tear film. After a period of adaptation a high proportion of patients can wear accurately fitted contact lenses with minimal or no discomfort. The new "soft" lenses are especially free of discomfort, but they have some optical disadvantages and require more care.

The optical quality of visual correction by contact lenses is good. High myopes or hyperopes (especially patients after cataract extraction) are particularly benefited by the better field of vision and the absence of peripheral distortions attained through contact lenses. The annoyance of frames and dirty glasses is eliminated. Contact lenses may be worn during athletic activity. However, the desire to look more attractive is the reason for the purchase of most contact lenses.

Disadvantages of contact lenses are many. Considerable training in their insertion and removal is necessary. Definite and prolonged minor discomfort must be endured during the development of corneal tolerance. Occasional acutely painful corneal abrasions or erosions are almost inevitable. Very rarely, permanent corneal scarring may result from some misfortune connected with contact lenses (such as bacterial contamination of the lens storage case). (Patients must be cautioned against using saliva for moistening lens, since saliva has a high bacterial count, predisposing to corneal infection.) They are very expensive—the cost of a pair of contact lenses approaches that of strabismus surgery. A lens is easily dropped—and not easily found. Bifocal contact lenses are not satisfactory. Finally, not everyone can wear contact lenses successfully. Because of the potential hazards of contact lenses, they should be fitted only under medical supervision. The sudden onset of new eye symptoms should **not** be attributed to the wearing of contact lenses. The patient should seek a medical explanation for such problems, which might, for instance, be caused by retinal detachment in a myopic patient.

SUNGLASSES

Excessively bright light or abnormally light-sensitive eyes cause discomfort that can be relieved by the wearing of sunglasses. Everyone is familiar with the comfort of sunglasses at the beach or on a bright snowy day. Similarly, when eyes are abnormally light sensitive because of disease or dilation by eye drops, dark glasses help greatly to make the patient comfortable. A tinted lens may help to conceal a cosmetically disfigured eye or eyelid.

Different color shades have no merits, other than to satisfy personal preferences. The important factor is the amount of light blocked by the sunglass. A good glass for outdoor use may transmit as little as 10% of light. For indoor use some tints may transmit as much as 95% of light. The choice depends on the individual patient's comfort and preference. Polaroid glasses are especially valuable, since they selectively eliminate most reflected light, which is one of the most annoying sources of glare. A word of caution is important—some drivers wear sunglasses at night to block glare from on-coming headlights. This is an extremely dangerous practice, since it ob-scures roadside details, including signs and people.

Colored glasses have no therapeutic benefit and are not used as a treat-ment for any eye disease.

Prescription sunglasses are helpful if the patient's refractive error is sufficiently great to require constant wearing of glasses and to justify the added expense. Clip-on sunglasses are very useful and inexpensive but have the inconvenience of added weight and may scratch the front surface of the spectacle lens.

CHAPTER SEVEN   **Injuries**

In many cases of serious eye injury prompt care may restore useful vision. In contrast, rough handling or poor management may irretrievably destroy the injured eye. Because the eye has very thin walls, major damage results from small injuries that would be insignificant elsewhere on the body. Specifically, a laceration 1 mm. deep is a serious penetrating wound of the eye, although on a finger it might not even require a bandage.

Do not forget the significance of future blindness after eye injury. What residual damage would most affect **your** life one year after an accident involving the upper face? Certainly blindness of one or both eyes would handicap the majority of nurses far more than would any other scars.

HISTORY OF INJURY

Except when the patient is very young he will almost always realize that an eye injury has occurred and will remember the circumstances. Since minor bumps and bruises are so common as to prohibit seeking medical attention for every such accident, it is important for the nurse to know how to differentiate potentially serious eye injuries.

Decreased vision after injury is truly an alarming sign and definitely indicates that the eye has been damaged. If blurred vision persists for an hour or more after injury, prompt medical consultation is in order.

Pain subsequent to eye trauma indicates at least some degree of injury. Many surface injuries of the eye are acutely painful and often disabling. In contrast, internal eye injury is commonly almost completely free from pain. Absence of pain does **not** necessarily exclude the presence of a serious eye injury.

Bleeding from or within the eyeball is certainly a sign of serious injury (Fig. 7-1).

Certain types of injury are particularly likely to cause serious damage. Most likely to be overlooked are the perforating injuries of *small, high-speed particles* such as are produced by explosives, by machining metal, or by hammering stone or metal. If the patient has been struck by *glass fragments* (as from a windshield or broken bottle) or if his spectacle glasses have been broken, the possibility of laceration of the eye by slivers of glass must be excluded. *Chemical burns* and *contusions* are two other common forms of injury, the occurrence of which can easily be established from the patient's history.

77

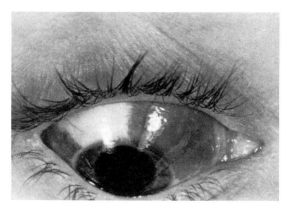

Fig. 7-1. Subconjunctival hemorrhages are more densely red than any other condition of the ocular surface. Initially the unaffected portion of conjunctiva may be normally white, but with time, diffusion of hemoglobin will cause reddish or yellowish discoloration of adjacent areas. (From Havener, William H.: Synopsis of ophthalmology, ed. 3, St. Louis, 1971, The C. V. Mosby Co.)

Since proper first-aid care of the injured eye is so very important, emergency management of the common types of eye injury will be presented in detail.

PENETRATING INJURY

Emergency care is always necessary for penetrating eye injuries (Fig. 7-2). Most important of all is the avoidance of further damage to the eye, which is extremely vulnerable to pressure. Unfortunately wiping away blood (Fig. 7-3), tears, or discharge from an injured eye seems to be an instinctive impulse. Unless prevented from doing so, the injured patient, his friends or relatives, and even some nurses will cause additional damage by wiping or pressing upon the eye.

The fundamental principle of first-aid care of an eye with a penetrating injury is to shield it against pressure. If available, a metal shield should be taped securely over the eye. (Fig. 5-3.) The edges of such a shield rest against the bony facial contours, and its center is outcurved so as to avoid any contact with the eye (Fig. 7-4). The patient and his attendants must be warned against pressure upon the eye.

As soon as possible, day or night, the patient should be taken to the nearest ophthalmologist. The patient may walk or may be transported sitting up in an automobile. However, unnecessary exertion of any type should be avoided. The patient should not be permitted to carry his own suitcase.

Definitive care includes massive antibiotic dosage, tetanus prophylaxis, removal of any retained intraocular foreign bodies, suturing of lacerations, and appropriate analgesics for relief of pain.

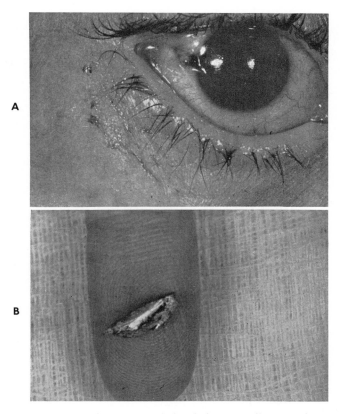

A

B

Fig. 7-2. A, A large penetrating wound of the limbus is easily recognized. This eye still contains the huge piece of metal shown in **B.** Pressure carelessly directed into the eye during examination could destroy it. Delay in recognition and in starting antibiotic therapy would probably result in serious infection. Proper care restored 20/20 vision. (From Havener, William H.: Synopsis of ophthalmology, ed. 3, St. Louis, 1971, The C. V. Mosby Co.)

CHEMICAL BURN

The delicate corneal and conjunctival surfaces can be severely and permanently damaged by contact with toxic chemicals (Fig. 7-5). Particularly dangerous are strong alkalis or acids, solvents, poisons, and similar caustic and irritating substances. Such substances are located not only in industrial plants and laboratories but also may be found in every home in the form of powerful cleaning solutions or powders. The alkali crystals used to clean toilet bowls contain particularly potent corrosive and toxic chemicals.

Do **not** call a doctor if such chemicals accidentally splash into an eye. By the time the patient reaches his office even the most skilled eye physician cannot help the eye as much as could any good first-aider at the time

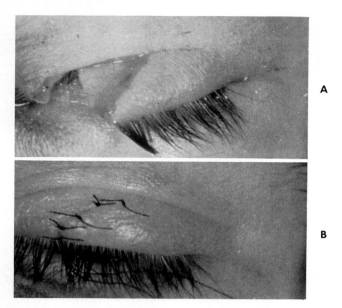

A

B

Fig. 7-3. A, Although lid lacerations bleed freely, pressure upon the lid should **not** be used to stop bleeding since the underlying eye might be damaged. **B,** Repair of lid lacerations requires exact approximation with delicate (No. 6-0) sutures.

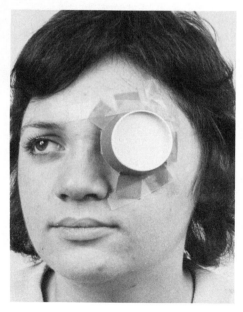

Fig. 7-4. An eye shield improvised from a paper cup.

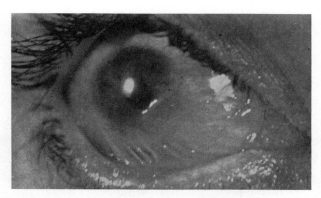

Fig. 7-5. Alkali burns are especially likely to cause permanent corneal scarring. Immediate and prolonged washing with ordinary water would have saved this man from a lifetime of blindness. (From Havener, William H.: Synopsis of ophthalmology, ed. 3, St. Louis, 1971, The C. V. Mosby Co.)

of the accident. **Immediate, prolonged washing with plain water** will prevent permanent scarring more effectively than will any other treatment. The eyelids should be separated so that the water may be poured gently upon the eyeball itself, thereby directly rinsing the toxic chemical from the corneal and conjunctival surfaces. Regardless of the type of chemical, emergency treatment is always the same. **Do not** search for specific antidotes such as baking soda or vinegar. Even seconds are precious if the cornea is to be saved from a strong chemical. Ordinarily, traces of irritant chemicals will persist despite ten minutes of irrigation; hence it is wise to continue washing for fifteen to twenty minutes. Be particularly careful to remove solid particles of chemicals such as lime. Seek medical care only **after** this thorough first-aid irrigation.

ULTRAVIOLET BURNS

Student nurses not uncommonly visit the eye clinic because of ultraviolet burn of the cornea suffered during exposure to a sunlamp. The corneal epithelium is quite susceptible to ultraviolet burn, and therefore the open eyes should never be exposed to a sunlamp for even a few minutes. Either the eyelids should be closed or protective goggles should be worn. Characteristically, several hours pass before a sunburn becomes painful. So also there is a delay of some hours before the pain of an ultraviolet corneal burn. Often the patient is awakened from sleep by the pain, whereas she was comfortable when she went to sleep right after reading under the sunlamp. Pain is severe and usually requires medical attention, but it rarely lasts more than a day. Cold compresses and aspirin or codeine will help the pain. Topical antibiotics should be used to prevent infection if the burn is severe.

Other sources of ultraviolet burns are germicidal lamps, electric flashes, and arc welding.

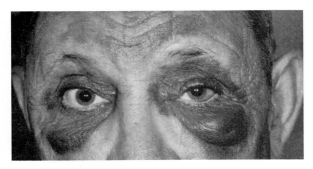

Fig. 7-6. If an injury has been severe enough to cause a black eye, it may also have damaged the underlying eyeball and therefore should receive medical attention.

CONTUSION

A severe blow to the eye, as by a fist, golf ball, BB shot, explosion, etc., will commonly cause extensive internal damage. Intraocular hemorrhage, rupture of the sclera, lens dislocation, macular edema and degeneration, retinal detachment, and other serious complications may develop immediately or many months after the accident. It is not possible to exclude internal injury without the use of the ophthalmoscope; therefore medical evaluation is important if an eye has been bruised sufficiently to cause a "black eye" (Fig. 7-6).

SUPERFICIAL ABRASION OR FOREIGN BODY

The commonest of all eye injuries are the small surface scratches or foreign bodies (cinder, bug, etc.) (Fig. 7-7). These injuries are usually correctly diagnosed by the patient himself, for they characteristically hurt and "feel like something got in the eye." The patient cannot differentiate between a scratch or foreign body, since both cause the same type of local pain.

It is important to recognize whether a foreign body is located upon the cornea or conjunctiva. Particles lying upon the conjunctiva are not of serious significance and may safely be cared for by the first-aider. They may easily be wiped out of the eye with a pointed spindle of clean cotton or facial tissue or work out spontaneously as the lid is blinked (Fig. 7-8). If available, an irrigating syringe may be used to wash out small particles. The natural resistance of the conjunctiva is high, and infections almost never develop. The patient with a superficial foreign body should be warned against rubbing his eye, for such pressure may cause a hard particle to abrade the cornea or become embedded within it.

In contrast, corneal injuries are much more dangerous, since resistance to infection is low, and even small scars may seriously impair vision if centrally located. Medical care is necessary because corneal foreign bodies cannot be removed without a local anesthetic and because topical anti-

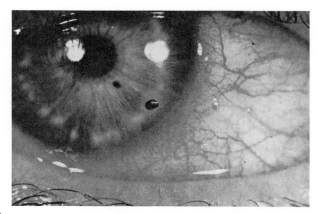

Fig. 7-7. A large foreign body is embedded in the peripheral cornea at about 4:30. Its removal requires topical anesthesia and sterile technique and therefore should be done by a physician. (From Havener, William H.: Synopsis of ophthalmology, ed. 3, St. Louis, 1971, The C. V. Mosby Co.)

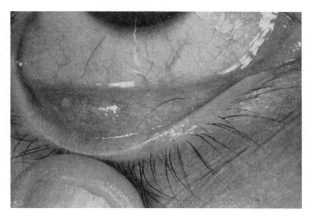

Fig. 7-8. Foreign bodies (such as this eyelash) in the lower conjunctival sac are easily seen when the lower lid is pulled downward. Such a conjunctival foreign body may be removed with a tissue or small cotton swab. Anesthesia and antibiotics are not required. (From Havener, William H.: Synopsis of ophthalmology, ed. 3, St. Louis, 1971, The C. V. Mosby Co.)

biotic treatment is indicated. Pain is much more severe with corneal foreign bodies than with conjunctival ones. Tiny foreign particles or abrasions are difficult to see and their recognition may require special equipment.

Everting the upper lid. One of the common sites where foreign bodies lodge is on the inner surface of the upper tarsal plate, where they are

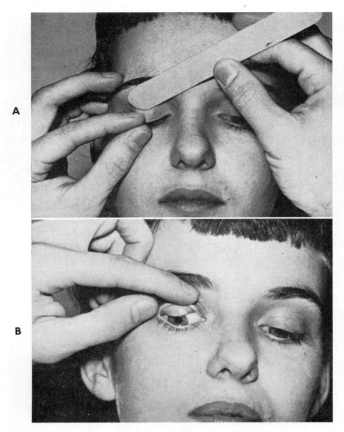

Fig. 7-9. A, The key step in everting the upper lid is downward pressure applied 1 cm. above the lid margin. **B,** The everted lid. (From Havener, William H.: Synopsis of ophthalmology, ed. 3, St. Louis, 1971, The C. V. Mosby Co.)

particularly irritating to the cornea. Everting the lids is the simplest approach to their removal. This procedure is easily done by the nurse.

Five simple steps will greatly facilitate eversion of the lids:

1. The patient must look down. This relaxes the levator muscle, which is attached to the upper border of the tarsal plate. When the patient looks up, the tarsal plate is retracted into the orbit, a position from which eversion is impossible.

2. The patient must not squeeze the lids shut. Such contraction of the orbicularis muscle effectively blocks eversion attempts. To ensure relaxation and avoid squeezing, reassure the patient, move slowly, and do not hurt him.

3. Hold the upper eyelashes. Grasping them is facilitated by lifting the upper lid, thereby causing the lashes to protrude straight forward. Do not pull on the lashes—this only causes the patient to squeeze his lids. Eversion is not accomplished by pulling the lashes upward or using them to roll

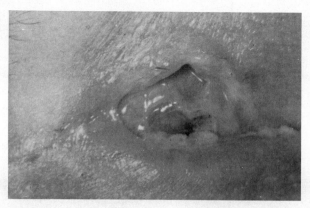

Fig. 7-10. Some types of injury are so destructive that eyesight can be saved only by prevention of the injury. This worker was splashed with molten metal while he was **not** wearing his required safety goggles.

the lid over a stick. In fact pulling gently down and forward simplifies the subsequent procedure.

4. Push down on the upper tarsal border with a small stick, such as an applicator or tongue blade (Fig. 7-9). The upper tarsal plate extends 12 mm. above the lid margin; therefore, pressure must be applied at least 1 cm. above the edge of the lid margin. You will find that this simple maneuver of pushing down the upper tarsal border is the key to easy lid eversion.

5. As soon as the lid is everted, appose the fingers holding the lashes to the brow, and the lid thus may be held securely in eversion during inspection of the conjunctival surface.

SAFETY PRECAUTIONS

Exposing an unprotected eye to occupational hazards can only be described as stupid. Most large companies enforce rigid safety programs that require the constant wearing of protective goggles in areas where metal is being machined, melted (Fig. 7-10), or welded, where flying particles of sand or cinders are anticipated, or where caustic solutions are being used. Similar goggles should be worn by workers in small companies or in home workshops.

Furthermore, all eyeglasses should be shatterproofed to prevent eye lacerations if the lenses are accidentally broken.

SUMMARY

Decreased vision, bleeding, or continuing pain after eye injury usually indicates that a serious injury exists. Proper first-aid care is often vitally important and may prevent blindness. Eyes with penetrating wounds must be protected from pressure. Eyes with chemical burns must be immediately irrigated with water. Eyes with surface foreign bodies should not be rubbed.

Protection of eyes with safety goggles may entirely avoid the injury and should be strongly advised for persons working in hazardous circumstances.

SUGGESTED READING

New Orleans Academy of Ophthalmology: Symposium on industrial and traumatic ophthalmology, St. Louis, 1964, The C. V. Mosby Co.

CHAPTER EIGHT Infections

The surface layers of the eye and eyelids are commonly infected by ordinary bacteria such as staphylococci. Infections of the interior of the eye and the orbit are much rarer but also much more serious. These infections will be described as they affect individual anatomic structures; however, it should be clearly understood that infection may readily spread from one structure to involve adjacent parts.

MINOR SUPERFICIAL LID INFECTIONS
(MARGINAL BLEPHARITIS, STY, AND CHALAZION)

Marginal blepharitis. Infection of the eyelid margins (Fig. 8-1) is extremely frequent. Its symptoms include crusting and irritation of the eyes. More severe cases cause redness and sometimes ulceration of the eyelid and may result in loss of eyelashes or unsightly thickening of the eyelids.

Sty (hordeolum). Bacterial invasion of the eyelash follicles and the accessory glands of the anterior lid margin results in the formation of small abscesses along the lid edge (Fig. 8-2). The most important practical fact about styes is that the patient should not squeeze them, lest the infection be spread into the thin lid tissues to cause a cellulitis.

Chalazion. A series of sebaceous glands (meibomian glands) lie deeply within the tarsal framework of the lids. Infection of these deep glands is termed a chalazion (Fig. 8-3). Acute chalazia are treated in the same way as are other superficial lid infections, but unfortunately they do not all clear with treatment. A chronic chalazion is an unsightly and slightly annoying hard lump within the lid. Incision and curettage (Fig. 8-4) under local anesthesia are necessary to cure a chronic chalazion.

Treatment. Treatment of the minor superficial lid infections (marginal blepharitis, sty, acute chalazion) requires thorough cleansing of the lid margins. This is best done by applying a hot moist compress for five minutes several times daily. When the moist heat has softened adherent crusts, gentle rubbing will mechanically remove this infected debris. After cleaning, a thin layer of antibiotic ointment should be applied to the lid margins. Treatment should continue until infection is eliminated (usually about a week). The same germs causing the lid infection are usually found

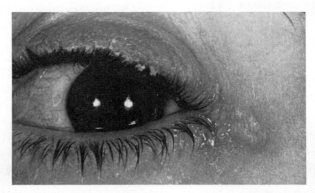

Fig. 8-1. An acute marginal blepharitis has caused this prominent crusting of the lid margins and lashes and the macerated area of the outer angle. Conjunctival redness and discharge are also present. Before antibiotic application all of these crusts should be scrubbed off mechanically. Hot soaks greatly facilitate removal of crusts. (From Havener, William H.: Synopsis of ophthalmology, ed. 3, St. Louis, 1971, The C. V. Mosby Co.)

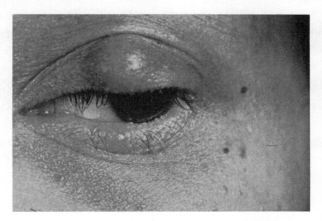

Fig. 8-2. Compare the appearance of the chalazion in the upper lid with the hordeolum in the lower lid. Note that the chalazion arises deep within the lid, whereas the hordeolum is situated on the anterior margin. Their locations directly opposite each other clearly indicate a common infectious origin. (From Havener, William H.: Synopsis of ophthalmology, ed. 3, St. Louis, 1971, The C. V. Mosby Co.)

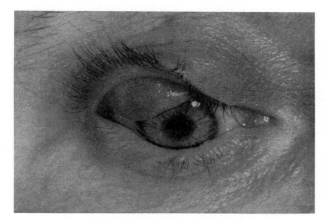

Fig. 8-3. The tarsal conjunctiva underlying a chalazion is red and inflamed. This is a useful confirmatory sign in diagnosis. Eversion of the upper lid is the best way to inspect the upper tarsal conjunctiva. (From Havener, William H.: Synopsis of ophthalmology, ed. 3, St. Louis, 1971, The C. V. Mosby Co.)

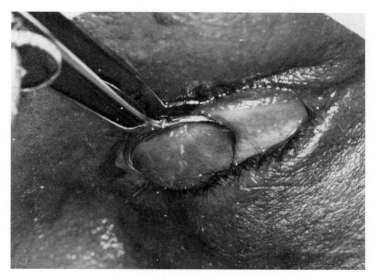

Fig. 8-4. A clamp everts the eyelid during surgery for chalazion. The incision will be made on the inner lid surface to avoid scarring. The viscous contents of the chalazion will be removed with a curette.

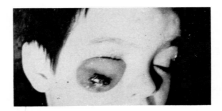

Fig. 8-5. Infection readily spreads through the thin skin of the lids. Unwise squeezing of a sty caused this severe cellulitis of the right lower lid.

elsewhere upon the body surface (ears, nose, scalp, and skin); hence re-infection may readily develop. The patient should be cautioned not to rub his eyes. Incidentally, all nurses should be aware that the germs acquired from their patients may be transmitted to the nurse's own eyes by careless rubbing. Do not rub or pick at your own eyes unless you have just washed your hands thoroughly. The delicate eye tissues are more susceptible to infection than is the tough skin of other parts of the body.

LID CELLULITIS

The subcutaneous tissue of the lids is very loose and permits easy spread of infection to involve the entire lid area. Unwise squeezing of a sty is the usual cause of such cellulitis (Fig. 8-5), although it may arise from a penetrating wound. Lid cellulitis is potentially a very dangerous condition, because loss of an eyelid is not only disfiguring but also compromises the protection of the cornea. Furthermore, the vascular drainage of the lids enters the cavernous sinus of the brain, to which infection may spread. Treatment requires vigorous use of systemic antibiotics.

DACRYOCYSTITIS

Although infection of the lacrimal sac must reach the lacrimal drainage system from the lid and conjunctival surfaces, dacryocystitis usually does not occur as a complication of surface infections alone. Almost invariably the nasolacrimal duct, which carries tears from the sac to the nose, must be blocked before dacryocystitis will develop (Fig. 8-6).

Congenital failure of the nasolacrimal duct to open into the nose is quite common. The first sign is tearing of the involved eye. Since tears are not formed until some weeks after birth, the eye does not water immediately. If dacryocystitis develops, the watery discharge becomes muco-purulent (Fig. 8-7). Fortunately the occluded nasolacrimal duct spontaneously opens within the first three months of life in most patients. If spontaneous opening fails, passage of a small lacrimal probe will usually open the obstruction. Antibiotic drops are used as necessary to control the infection.

Chronic dacryocystitis in adults is usually more difficult to treat, since the obstruction of the nasolacrimal duct is usually resistant to opening

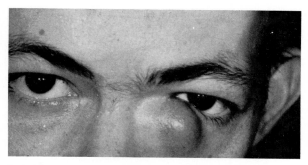

Fig. 8-6. Chronic infection of the lacrimal sac (dacryocystitis) causes a swelling of the lower inner corner of the eye socket.

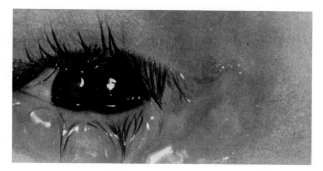

Fig. 8-7. This very large amount of mucopurulent discharge was expressed from an infected lacrimal sac by firm pressure directed into the lower inner corner of the orbit. One must not press on the side of the nose. The lacrimal sac is situated in the lacrimal fossa, which is posterior to the orbital rim. Confirmation of the diagnosis of suspected dacryocystitis is made through expression of purulent material from the sac. (From Havener, William H.: Synopsis of ophthalmology, ed. 3, St. Louis, 1971, The C. V. Mosby Co.)

by simple probing. Usually dacryocystorhinostomy is required. This is an operation that creates a new, large opening between the lacrimal sac and the nose.

CONJUNCTIVITIS

The exposed mucous membranes of the eyes are quite susceptible to infection by a great variety of microorganisms (Fig. 8-8). Acute conjunctivitis is commonly known as "pink eye." This common infection is very contagious among children. Fortunately general hygienic measures and topical antibiotic drops will eliminate most types of conjunctivitis without any residual scarring or abnormality of the eye.

A few organisms, such as the gonococcus (Fig. 8-9), may invade and destroy the intact cornea. Since the gonococcus is quite contagious, genital

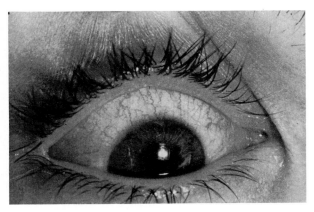

Fig. 8-8. The redness of acute bacterial conjunctivitis is just as marked in the cul de sac as near the limbus. Superficial vessels become dilated and conspicuous and therefore seem more numerous. Characteristic crusting of the lids is absent in this picture because the patient cleaned the lids before visiting the physician. Practically always the patient with bacterial conjunctivitis will report that the lids are "sticky" upon awakening. (From Havener, William H.: Synopsis of ophthalmology, ed. 3, St. Louis, 1971, The C. V. Mosby Co.)

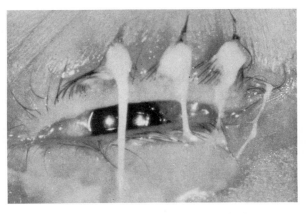

Fig. 8-9. Gonococcal infection of the conjunctiva causes serious damage to the eye itself and characteristically produces profuse mucopurulent secretion.

discharge from patients should never be permitted to touch the nurse's skin and certainly should not be wiped or splashed against the eye. Accidental splashing of such potentially infectious material into the eye should be treated immediately with saline irrigation and by prophylactic use of topical antibiotics. Prophylactic treatment of the eyes of newborn infants with silver nitrate or antibiotic drops is legally required throughout the United States and is an effective way of preventing gonococcal conjunctivitis.

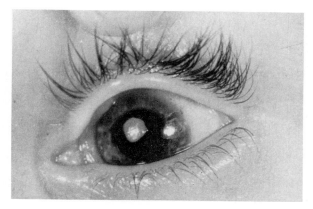

Fig. 8-10. Infectious ulcers of the cornea may rapidly cause permanent scarring and visual loss and require emergency evaluation and treatment.

Chronic redness of the conjunctiva may result from a great variety of conditions, including allergy, intraocular disease, and external irritants (e.g., smoke), as well as from infections. The differential diagnosis and treatment of a red eye should be left to the physician, since a number of these conditions are quite serious.

KERATITIS

Infections of the cornea should always be considered as serious, for they may cause blindness by impairing corneal transparency or may destroy the eye by corneal perforation. Most small infections of the corneal surface feel as if there was a foreign body in the eye. Some corneal infections may be extremely painful. Unfortunately absence of pain does not reliably exclude corneal infection, since some types of virus disease may destroy the nerves, thereby producing corneal anesthesia. Discharge and crusting of the lid margins is typically found in bacterial keratitis (and conjunctivitis) but is usually absent or minimal with viral keratitis. Virtually all types of infectious keratitis cause redness of the eye. Since corneal infection damages transparency (Fig. 8-10), the red eye with a corneal opacity should be considered a serious disorder.

When the presence of keratitis is suspected, prompt medical attention is necessary. Medical care can also be helpful in preventing corneal infection, if the doctor is consulted whenever a cornea is abraded sufficiently to cause persistent pain.

ORBITAL CELLULITIS

By extension from the adjacent sinuses, infection may enter the eye socket. Orbital infection may also occur at the time of a penetrating wound, by lymphatic drainage from a surface infection, or via the bloodstream. Inflammatory swelling of the orbital tissues causes the most characteristic fea-

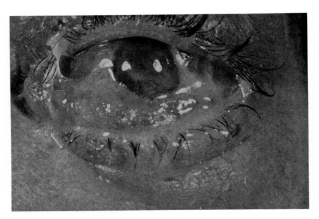

Fig. 8-11. Spontaneous rupture of the necrotic cornea represents the ultimate stage of destruction. Such loss of an eye can often be prevented through recognition of injury or infection and proper early care. (From Havener, William H.: Synopsis of ophthalmology, ed. 3, St. Louis, 1971, The C. V. Mosby Co.)

tures of orbital cellulitis, forward displacement of the eye, and severe swelling of the lids (Fig. 8-11). Damage to the extraocular muscles may cause limitation of eye movements and double vision. Often the optic nerve is damaged, causing loss of sight. Extension of infection backward into the brain may cause thrombosis of the large cerebral venous sinuses and death.

The progress of orbital cellulitis is rapid if untreated and may cause permanent ocular damage within a few days.

ENDOPHTHALMITIS

Microorganisms may enter the eye through a penetrating wound, via the bloodstream, or from surrounding orbital tissues. After a penetrating wound of the eye intensive antibiotic therapy will substantially decrease the risk of endophthalmitis. Once well established, intraocular infection invariably destroys sight.

Infection of the anterior part of the eye causes pain, redness, and visible purulent infiltration of the normally transparent cornea, anterior chamber, and lens. Infection of the posterior part of the eye may be relatively painless.

UVEITIS

A special kind of endophthalmitis results from infection of the uveal tract by organisms of slow growth or low virulence. The uveal tract is the vascular layer of the eye and includes iris, ciliary body, and choroid. Because of anatomic nearness, the iris and ciliary body are usually inflamed simultaneously, and the condition is called iridocyclitis. Similarly, choroidal inflammation almost invariably damages the retina; hence this is termed chorioretinitis. Organisms known to cause uveitis include tuberculosis, toxoplasmosis, histoplasmosis, and assorted viruses. Uveitis often occurs in association with sarcoidosis, severe arthritis, and collagen diseases.

Unfortunately the specific cause of most cases of uveitis cannot be diagnosed. This is because biopsy or culture examination of the interior of the eye is not possible without damaging the eye. Possible specific causes (e.g., syphilis, toxoplasmosis, etc.) of uveitis may be suggested by indirect studies such as roentgenography, blood examinations, and skin tests.

Corticosteroid treatment of uveitis is helpful because it often reduces the amount of intraocular scarring. Dilation of the pupil is routine in iritis in order to prevent adhesions between the iris and lens. If a specific etiology is suspected, definitive treatment may be given (e.g., pyrimethamine and sulfonamides for toxoplasmosis). Despite treatment, uveitis is a serious condition that may partially destroy sight.

OPTIC NEURITIS

Inflammation of the optic nerve may accompany meningitis or encephalitis or it may occur as an isolated infection. The etiology of a given case of isolated optic neuritis is always difficult to establish. Especially in northern climates, multiple sclerosis may be a cause of optic neuritis. Vascular disorders may also be a cause. The patient recognizes the presence of an abnormality because vision is blurred and the eye is painful when moved. Thorough medical, neurologic, and ophthalmologic examination is in order. Corticosteroid treatment is commonly used.

SCLERITIS AND EPISCLERITIS

Scleritis and episcleritis are usually benign, transient inflammations of the sclera and its surface, usually of unknown etiology. Rarely a patient with severe arthritis will have scleritis sufficiently severe to cause thinning of the sclera and local bulging and discoloration of the eye.

CHAPTER NINE # Strabismus

Crossing of the eyes is an easily recognizable sign of serious disease. Such crossing (called strabismus) may be caused by eye disease alone or may indicate disturbance of the central nervous system (Fig. 9-1). Because crossed eyes are quite common, affecting about 1% of the population, many laymen erroneously regard the condition as harmless and delay seeking medical advice. Actually prompt medical examination and care can often prevent later unpleasant or crippling defects.

Two types of strabismus exist, *paralytic* and *nonparalytic,* which are quite different in their characteristics and significance. *Paralytic* strabismus results from the inability of one (or more) of the extraocular muscles to move the eye. It may be caused by nerve damage (third, fourth, or sixth cranial nerve) or by involvement of the muscle itself (Fig. 9-2 and Table 1). Since tumor (Fig. 9-3), infection, or injury of the brain or orbit may be responsible for paralytic strabismus, this type of crossed eye is a warning signal that requires careful evaluation.

The characteristic symptom of paralytic strabismus is double vision (diplopia). Normally both eyes look at the same object and send similar messages to the brain, where the images are fused into a single picture. If a muscle paralysis causes the two eyes to cross, the brain receives the confusing sensation of seeing two separate pictures, which is called diplopia.

Some people experience transient diplopia when they are tired. This is not caused by muscle paralysis but results from temporary relaxation of the fusion mechanism of the brain. Since no muscle is paralyzed, the amount of separation of the double images does not change when the eyes are moved to different positions. Furthermore, these persons can make the double vision disappear promptly by looking more attentively. The double vision of alcoholic intoxication is another well-known example of diplopia resulting from a failure of the fusion mechanisms. Although this type of diplopia is not serious, it is mentioned here in order to differentiate it from the diplopia of a paralyzed muscle.

Recognition of a very crossed eye is quite easy by simple observation of the faulty position. If the eye is turned in toward the nose, the condition is called a convergent strabismus (or esotropia). If the eye is turned outward, it is called divergent strabismus (or exotropia). Hypertropia refers to an eye that is higher than it should be.

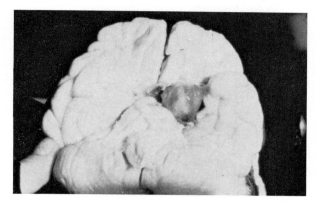

Fig. 9-1. Aneurysms at the base of the brain, such as the lesion that killed this patient, often cause paralysis of the extraocular muscles.

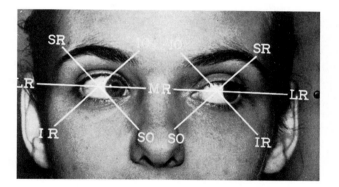

Fig. 9-2. Cardinal positions of gaze. Inability to move the eye into the positions specified indicates paralysis of the corresponding extraocular muscle. (From Havener, William H.: Synopsis of ophthalmology, ed. 3, St. Louis, 1971, The C. V. Mosby Co.)

Table 1. Six cardinal positions of gaze

Position to which eye will not turn	*Paretic muscle*
Straight nasal	Medial rectus (third nerve)
Up and nasal	Inferior oblique (third nerve)
Down and nasal	Superior oblique (fourth nerve)
Straight temporal	Lateral rectus (sixth nerve)
Up and temporal	Superior rectus (third nerve)
Down and temporal	Inferior rectus (third nerve)

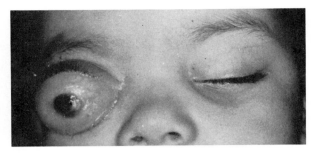

Fig. 9-3. An orbital tumor has caused enormous protrusion of this eye. Before the diagnosis was so evident, the condition seemed to be a case of strabismus. Early medical evaluation of all cases of strabismus will detect such disorders when they are most likely to respond to treatment.

If the crossing is very slight, a flashlight will greatly aid its recognition. The observer's eyes should be directly behind the flashlight, which is aimed at the patient. The patient is instructed to look directly at the light. Normally the bright reflection of the light will appear to be centered symmetrically within each pupil. If one eye is convergent, its light reflex will be displaced temporally (Fig. 9-4). Nasal displacement of the light reflex indicates divergent strabismus. Proper use of a flashlight in this manner will permit accurate recognition of even small amounts of strabismus (but not less than 5 degrees) and will identify straight eyes associated with facial configurations simulating strabismus.

Epicanthus is a fold of skin, very common in childhood, that runs from the upper lid to the nose, giving the eyes a sloped, oriental appearance. Convergent strabismus is often suspected in these children because this lid fold hides the inner corner of the eye, which often does look quite crossed. The flashlight inspection just described will identify the true straightness of such eyes. Epicanthus spontaneously disappears with growth and is without significance except for the unwarranted concern over straight eyes that appear as if crossed (Fig. 9-5).

As the name implies, *nonparalytic* strabismus is not caused by a paralyzed muscle. It is a defect of the position of the two eyes relative to each other caused by an inherited abnormality (Fig. 9-6) of the convergence or divergence mechanism within the brain. This type of strabismus is comparable to faulty alignment of the front wheels of an automobile. If a right front automobile wheel is imagined to turn in while the left is straight, it is evident that manipulating the steering wheel to straighten the right wheel will result in turning the left wheel in. The abnormal position of these wheels to each other cannot be changed by turning the steering wheel, since both are always simultaneously turned the same amount. As in this crooked automobile, in nonparalytic strabismus the amount of crossing does not change when the eyes move from one position to another.

Obviously the patient with nonparalytic strabismus cannot use the two eyes together as does the normal person. He may look straight (fix) with

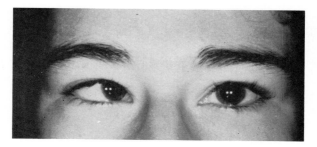

Fig. 9-4. Note the light reflections are centered in the left cornea and to the side of the right cornea. The positions of the corneal reflections of a light being observed by the patient help in the recognition of strabismus.

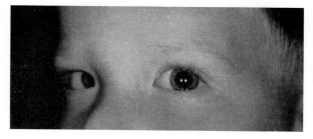

Fig. 9-5. Epicanthus simulates esotropia, especially when the head is turned so that the eye is hidden behind the lid fold and nose.

either the right or the left eye but not with both simultaneously. The eye that is straight at a given time is called the fixing eye; the other is the deviating eye. If the patient fixes first with one eye, then with the other, he has *alternating* strabismus. Fixation may alternate freely between the two eyes, or the patient may prefer to use one eye rather than the other. If this preference is so great that the patient always fixes with one eye and permits the other to deviate, he has *monocular* strabismus.

It is possible to predict what the brain is doing with the information sent by the two eyes if we know whether the strabismus is alternating or monocular. Information received from the fixing eye is always perceived clearly, just as if a normal person were looking with one eye, the other being covered. In alternating strabismus the information sent to the brain from the deviating eye is disregarded (suppressed). *Suppression* is the ability of the brain to discard conflicting information, as when the eyes send two different pictures. Suppression happens normally in everyday use of normal eyes and can be demonstrated by the following experiment. Close your left eye and look with the right eye at a doorknob or similar small object across the room. Hold one finger about a foot in front of the right eye so that the finger completely conceals the doorknob from view. Now

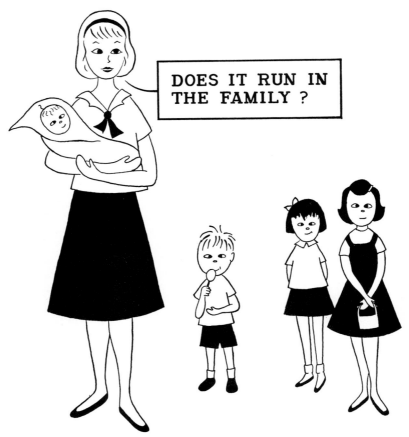

DOES IT RUN IN THE FAMILY ?

Fig. 9-6. Inheritance is the usual cause of nonparalytic strabismus. (From Havener, William H.: Synopsis of ophthalmology, ed. 3, St. Louis, 1971, The C. V. Mosby Co.)

open both eyes. The doorknob will be seen clearly, apparently right through a transparent spot in the middle of your finger! Since the brain has received conflicting pictures, a doorknob from the left and a finger from the right eye, it has automatically suppressed the part of the finger in front of the doorknob. In exactly this same way the brain suppresses conflicting information from the deviating eye of a patient with alternating nonparalytic strabismus. Suppression is a very efficient method of avoiding diplopia, which is rarely recognized by the patient with nonparalytic strabismus (in contrast to paralytic strabismus, the main symptom of which is double vision).

If a patient never uses a crossed eye, the constant suppression of this deviating eye may actually impair vision. This type of impairment is called *suppression amblyopia.* Suppression amblyopia may reduce the vision of the bad eye to as low as 20/200 (the big E). Occurring in approximately

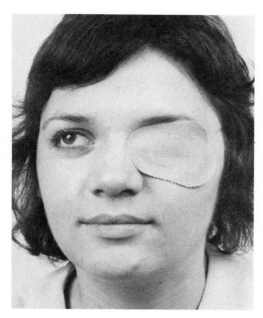

Fig. 9-7. Constant occlusion of the good eye in a child with suppression amblyopia will often restore vision to the bad eye. Ideally, supression should have been avoided through prompt referral of the squinting child. The sooner occlusion is begun the more rapid the restoration of lost vision. Occlusion is useless after the age of 6 years, a fact that underscores the importance of preschool vision testing in detection of suppression while it can still be treated. Proper management of occlusion is somewhat complicated and should be supervised by an ophthalmologist. Occlusion of an adult, as pictured here, is a waste of time.

1% of the population, suppression amblyopia is the most common cause of partial blindness in children. Usually by the age of 6 years a deviating eye has become suppressed to such a degree that it will not respond to a reasonable amount of treatment. Most tragic is that this permanent visual loss could have been prevented by prompt attention when the eyes were first noted to cross.

During early childhood, suppression amblyopia may be successfully treated with occlusion therapy. In principle this consists simply of constantly covering the good eye (Fig. 9-7) and thereby forcing the child to use the bad eye. The earlier occlusion is begun, the more rapid will be visual improvement. By the time the child reaches school age, occlusion is of little benefit. For this reason early recognition and care of strabismus and of suppression amblyopia are important. Mass screening of the vision of preschool children with an E block is one of the most valuable methods for the detection of suppression amblyopia (Fig. 9-8). This screening test can be easily performed by nurses or trained volunteers in nursery schools, Sunday schools, or other centers for preschool children.

Straightening the eyes of a patient with nonparalytic strabismus may

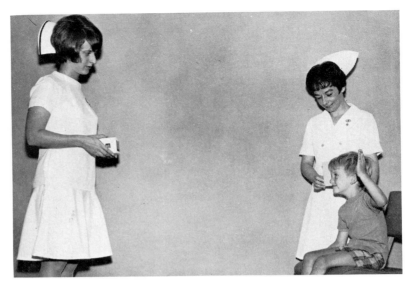

Fig. 9-8. Preschool vision screening with an E block.

be done by glasses, drops, orthoptics, or surgery, depending upon the case. Simply straightening the eyes does **not** correct already established suppression amblyopia.

The wearing of proper glasses will correct crossed eyes in patients with *accommodative* convergent strabismus. This condition causes about 15% of the cases of cross-eyed children. It occurs in farsighted children who accommodate and converge excessively. Accurate correction of this farsightedness eliminates the need for excessive accommodation. Ordinarily such patients must wear their glasses constantly, and the eyes tend to cross again as soon as the glasses are removed. Proper refraction of a cross-eyed child requires cycloplegic eye drops and therefore must be done by an ophthalmologist rather than by an optometrist. Furthermore, ophthalmologists, because of their medical training, are able to recognize and manage the serious ocular or general diseases that may cause strabismus as an early symptom.

Eye drops may also be used to correct the accommodative type of convergent strabismus. These drops are the long-acting miotics, such as echothiophate. Instilled once daily or perhaps every other day, echothiophate causes sustained contraction of the ciliary muscle, thereby correcting the farsightedness by means of chemically induced accommodation. Sometimes combined use of glasses and echothiophate will more effectively control strabismus than either method alone.

Orthoptics is training in the proper use of the two eyes together. This training may consist of muscle exercises designed to strengthen the ability of the eyes to move in a given direction. Even more important is fusion training. *Fusion* refers to the ability of the brain to combine information

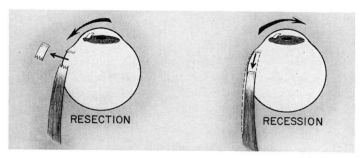

Fig. 9-9. In resection, part of the muscle tendon is removed. This procedure rotates the eye toward the operated muscle. In recession, the tendon is moved backward on the eye, permitting the eye to rotate away from the operated muscle. (From Havener, William H.: Synopsis of ophthalmology, ed. 3, St. Louis, 1971, The C. V. Mosby Co.)

from two eyes into a single mental picture containing information about the world such as distance, size, position, depth perception, etc. Fusion, really a rather remarkable achievement, is the most important factor maintaining straightness of the eyes. Orthoptic training can increase fusion ability and thereby contribute to the straightening of eyes.

Surgical correction of strabismus (Fig. 9-9) is simply a mechanical alteration of eye position by appropriate transfer of the muscle attachments. Any of the extraocular muscles may be cut from its insertion on the eye and reattached elsewhere upon the eye. A *recession* is surgical transfer of a muscle insertion backward from the original attachment on the eye. This weakens the action of the recessed muscle. For example, recession of a medial rectus muscle would permit the eye to turn more laterally and would tend to correct a convergent strabismus. *Resection* is the shortening of a muscle by removal of part of the tendon. This pulls the eye in the direction of the shortened muscle. To correct convergent strabismus, a lateral rectus muscle might be resected. Choice of the specific type and amount of muscle surgery is subject to a number of technical specifications and to the judgment of the ophthalmologist in a given case. In at least 75% of patients the eyes should be adequately straightened by a single operation. In general, surgery is advised only if the simpler methods of glasses, drops, and orthoptics do not satisfactorily correct the crossed eyes.

By whatever methods necessary, strabismus should be corrected before school age. Other children are sometimes cruel and readily accept the opportunity to comment upon an obvious deformity such as crossed eyes. Almost without exception a cross-eyed child will be quite sensitive about his handicap. Withdrawn, belligerent, or other antisocial behavior is common.

Consultation with an ophthalmologist should **not** be deferred until school age but is indicated as soon as the strabismus is recognized, even in the early months of life. The fact that serious disease of the eye or of the brain may cause strabismus is often overlooked. Strabismus is the first symptom in one third of all retinoblastomas (malignant intraocular tumor of childhood). Destructive inflammation, injury, or degeneration of one eye often results in its deviation, as may also brain tumor, injury, infection, or congenital anomaly. Thorough examination of the dilated eyes and their innervation is mandatory in the study of every cross-eyed child.

In *summary,* the objectives of treatment for strabismus are normal visual acuity, binocular vision, and good cosmetic appearance. These objectives may be achieved by early detection, occlusion therapy, orthoptic treatment, refraction, miotic therapy, and surgery.

CHAPTER TEN

Glaucoma

Glaucoma designates a group of diseases that cause the pressure inside an eye to increase above normal. This group includes chronic simple glaucoma, secondary glaucoma, and acute glaucoma. Glaucoma is important because it is common, because it causes blindness, and because proper early detection and treatment will prevent loss of eyesight.

Intraocular pressure is determined by the rate of aqueous humor production by the ciliary body and the resistance to outflow of aqueous humor from the eye. Intraocular pressure increases when the normal circulation of fluid within an eye is blocked. The aqueous fluid, formed by the ciliary processes, flows forward through the pupil, then filters out of the eye via a meshwork located in the circular space where the peripheral iris and cornea approach each other (Fig. 1-4). Most cases of glaucoma are caused by a block of this meshwork. The cause of the block is the feature that identifies the various types of glaucoma. Secondary glaucoma is caused by a clogging up of the meshwork by blood, fibrin, inflammatory cells and debris, pigment, etc. and is "secondary" to such diseases as injury or infection. Chronic simple glaucoma (the most common kind) is caused by a thickening of the meshwork itself, which occurs spontaneously as an eye with a hereditary predisposition to glaucoma becomes older. Acute glaucoma occurs only in the uncommon eyes in which the iris is displaced abnormally far anteriorly and is caused by the iris pressing against and covering the filtration meshwork. Whatever the cause, increased intraocular pressure gradually kills the optic nerve.

Glaucoma is the most common preventable cause of blindness. It is responsible for the disability of one of every ten blind persons in the United States. Surveys indicate that two of every hundred Americans over 40 years of age have glaucoma. (This means that if you are a member of a class of twenty-five nurses, one of the parents of this group is statistically expected to have glaucoma.) About one million cases of glaucoma exist in the United States today. Many of these cases are in early stages and still undiscovered by the patient.

How does a person discover that he has glaucoma? The first way is to realize gradually that he cannot see and to learn that no treatment can then restore his sight. The second way is to detect the disease early by a medical eye examination and to learn that proper treatment will maintain good vision.

Because it gradually destroys vision **without symptoms,** chronic simple glaucoma is never spontaneously discovered by the patient himself until he is partially blind. This disease is usually completely painless and does not cause redness or other alarming external appearances. The characteristic loss of side vision progresses slowly over a period of years and is unrecognized until the final stages of damage encroach upon central vision. For maximum benefit to the patient the presence of increased intraocular pressure must be discovered much earlier than this.

DIAGNOSIS

Fortunately intraocular pressure can be measured easily, painlessly, and safely by an instrument called the tonometer (Figs. 2-9 and 2-17). The basic principle of the tonometer (Fig. 10-1) is indentation of the cornea by slight pressure. Obviously, if intraocular pressure is high, the cornea will resist indentation more than if the pressure is low. The scale of the tonom-

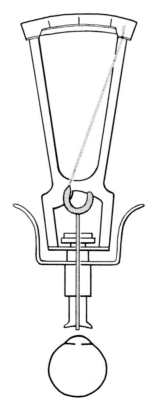

Fig. 10-1. The central plunger of a tonometer moves freely within the handle. The amount of corneal indentation caused by the weight of the plunger is determined by the pressure within the eye.

eter is calibrated to measure accurately the amount of indentation, from which the pressure is determined.

The technique of tonometry is very simple. The patient is tilted back in an adjustable chair and looks straight upward. A single drop of 0.5% Ophthaine is instilled into each eye and produces corneal anesthesia within a minute. The sterile tonometer is placed gently upon the center of the cornea for several seconds, during which the scale reading is determined. This simple test is the key to the prevention of blindness from glaucoma. Applanation tonometry is a more accurate method, in which the testing instrument is applied to the cornea during observation with the biomicroscope.

After tonometry the patient should be cautioned against rubbing his eyes for about fifteen minutes. During this period the cornea is still anesthetized and could be painlessly abraded. The patient may safely pat the *closed* eyelids with an absorbent tissue to remove tears. Unless cautioned, patients will almost invariably rub their eyes after tonometry because of the peculiar numb sensation of anesthesia. Minor but painful corneal abrasions not uncommonly occur if this warning is neglected.

All persons over the age of 40 years should have their intraocular pressure checked every five years, since the incidence of glaucoma is 2% in this age group. Because chronic simple glaucoma is very definitely hereditary, the over 40-year-old members of a family in which even one other case of glaucoma has occurred should have a tonometer check every two years. Tonometry is often an important part of the examination of patients with various eye diseases, with unexplained headaches, or with unsatisfactory vision despite repeated changes of glasses. Most ophthalmologists routinely check intraocular tension in all older patients and in any younger patient if there is any reason to suspect pressure abnormality (Fig. 10-2).

Several other methods are used to check intraocular pressure, but their limitations should be clearly understood. Finger tension refers to gentle alternating pressure upon an eye with two fingers. With this method a physician may detect a very hard or a very soft eye. The pressure in most

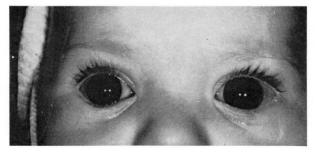

Fig. 10-2. Congenital glaucoma increases the size of the soft infant eye. A child with unusually large corneas should have a prompt and thorough eye examination. (From Havener, William H.: Synopsis of ophthalmology, ed. 3, St. Louis, 1971, The C. V. Mosby Co.)

cases of glaucoma is **not** high enough to detect by finger tension. Not even the most sensitive and skillful fingers are accurate enough for reliable screening of all eyes. Recently a very delicate electronic tonometer has been devised for use upon the unanesthetized cornea. This appears to be quite accurate and can be used successfully in many patients without anesthesia. Scleral tonometry is a method of estimating intraocular pressure by placing a spring-loaded plunger against the sclera. The sclera is covered by conjunctiva and fascia and varies considerably in thickness. Therefore, scleral tonometry is notoriously unreliable. In one study of patients with known high pressures, 80% were missed by scleral tonometry.

MEDICAL MANAGEMENT

If glaucoma could not be helped by treatment, early diagnosis would be of little value. Fortunately the great majority of early cases respond well to medical therapy. In contrast, advanced cases often fail to be controlled by either medical or surgical means. In most eyes simply the instillation of miotic drops several times daily will control pressure adequately. Miotics are medications that cause the pupil to become small and improve aqueous outflow, thereby reducing intraocular pressure. Commonly used miotics are pilocarpine, eserine, carbachol, and echothiophate. Various concentrations, frequency of dosage, or combinations of these drugs are used, depending upon the patient's response. Usually drops are instilled two to four times daily; however, just as no given dose of insulin can be predicted in advance for a diabetic patient, so also the miotic requirements of a glaucoma patient are subject to regulation by clinical trial.

Glaucoma is **not** cured by miotics, but pressure is controlled as long as therapy is maintained. The patient with glaucoma ordinarily requires miotics for the rest of his life. During vacations and hospitalizations, as well as during everyday life, miotic drops must not be neglected. The mistaken use of dilating drops may make glaucoma much worse; therefore the nurse must always be very careful to instill the correct kind of eye drops.

Another medical method of controlling intraocular pressure is to reduce the rate of aqueous formation. This can be done by carbonic anhydrase inhibitors (acetazolamide [Diamox], methazolamide [Neptazane]), which stop the action of an enzyme, necessary for the production of the aqueous. They are taken by mouth. Although these medications also increase the flow of urine, this action is entirely separate from their eye pressure–lowering effect. Other diuretics, such as meralluride (Mercuhydrin) or chlorothiazide (Diuril), do not reduce intraocular pressure.

Whether or not a case of glaucoma is being adequately controlled is determined by regular checks (usually every three months, although this varies with the ease or difficulty of control of the given case) of visual acuity, intraocular pressure, visual field, and ophthalmoscopic appearance of the optic nerve. The management of glaucoma is moderately complicated and should be supervised by a physician specializing in eye care.

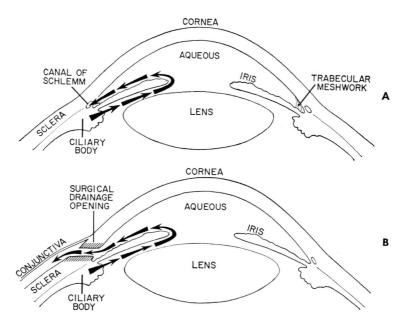

Fig. 10-3. A, Originating from the ciliary processes, the aqueous flows through the pupil into the anterior chamber and normally leaves the eye via the canal of Schlemm. **B,** In glaucoma the normal aqueous outflow is blocked. The purpose of glaucoma surgery is to create a new channel through which aqueous can leave the eye. (From Havener, William H.: Synopsis of ophthalmology, ed. 3, St. Louis, 1971, The C. V. Mosby Co.)

SURGICAL MANAGEMENT

Surgery is ordinarily used only if medical treatment fails to control intraocular pressure. Several procedures are available. The most common group are called filtering operations (iridencleisis, trephine, and sclerectomy). These create an opening between the anterior chamber and the space beneath the conjunctiva, thereby bypassing the blocked trabecular meshwork (Fig. 10-3). The aqueous fluid released from the eye by such surgery does not flow to the outside like tears but is absorbed into the subconjunctival tissues. If the iris itself is responsible for the block of aqueous flow, a piece may be excised (iridectomy). Rarely, surgery is intended partially to destroy the ability of the eye to secrete aqueous. This operation (cyclodiathermy) destroys part of the ciliary body. The postoperative care after glaucoma surgery is comparable to that for other types of intraocular surgery.

MISCONCEPTIONS

Frequently unnecessary restrictions are self-imposed by the concerned patient or advised by an overly cautious physician. The fear of possible blindness and the necessity for endless use of drops are sufficient nuisance without adding others. The following statements are intended to debunk a number of common misconceptions.

Use of the eyes is not harmful. A partially sighted patient may fatigue more rapidly than normally, but he cannot damage the eyes by reading or by any other seeing activity. One cannot "save eyesight" by rationing its use. As a matter of fact, it has been demonstrated that aqueous outflow is actually slightly improved during reading.

Drinking fluids under normal circumstances will **not** increase intraocular pressure. There is a diagnostic test for glaucoma, in which the patient fasts for twelve hours and then drinks a quart of water within five minutes without eating any food. Although it is true that this may briefly raise the pressure of a glaucomatous eye, these exact circumstances would never ordinarily occur. Drinking smaller amounts of water less rapidly, eating at the same time or within a few hours before, drinking beverages containing sugar or other chemicals in solution—any of these alterations from the diagnostic test situation will completely eliminate any significant pressure elevation. There is no logical reason for a patient with glaucoma to limit his fluid intake.

Restriction of coffee depends upon the individual patient. Only one of seven patients will have an elevation of intraocular pressure caused by by caffeine. This may easily be detected by tonometry before and after drinking several cups of coffee. Most patients may drink coffee without changing their intraocular pressure. Smoking and drinking alcoholic beverages do not significantly change eye pressure.

General physical exercise is not harmful to a glaucomatous eye. Bright lights or darkness do not affect an eye under miotic treatment, since the pupil always remains small. With the single exception of the atropine-like drugs, medications taken for other diseases will not interfere with the treatment of glaucoma.

Nurses commonly believe there is a relationship between vascular hypertension and ocular hypertension (glaucoma). No such relationship exists.

ACUTE GLAUCOMA

Acute glaucoma, a relatively rare condition, is one of the most dramatic and rapidly destructive diseases of the eye. It characteristically produces severe pain, at first localized in the eye but later radiating to any part of the head. Nausea and vomiting are common and sometimes mislead the patient and nurse into believing that the primary complaint is abdominal. Corneal edema causes vision to become blurred. The many tiny droplets of fluid in the edematous cornea disperse light into its spectral components and result in the rainbow-colored halos seen around lights. During an attack of acute glaucoma, the eye appears very inflamed.

Acute glaucoma can occur only in a structurally predisposed eye. In such an eye, aging causes a progressive narrowing of the peripheral angle of the anterior chamber. Ultimately the iris approaches so closely to the trabecular structures that slight dilation of the pupil caused by darkness, excitement, or a dilating drop results in apposition of the iris to the filtration spaces, with complete block of the aqueous outflow mechanism. Aqueous secretion continues, and intraocular pressure rises rapidly. Death of the nerve fiber results when the intraocular pressure reaches such heights that the central retinal artery can no longer maintain circulation. Untreated, a severe attack of acute glaucoma may cause permanent blindness within a few days.

SUMMARY

Glaucoma (increased pressure within the eye) is the most common preventable cause of blindness. The most frequent kind of glaucoma is inherited and affects older persons. Since it causes no symptoms, early detection is possible only by routine measurement of eye pressure with a tonometer. Use of eye drops can prevent this kind of blindness in most persons—if started early.

SUGGESTED READING

Kolker, Allan E., and Hetherington, John, Jr.: Becker and Shaffer's diagnosis and therapy of the glaucomas, ed. 3, St. Louis, 1970, The C. V. Mosby Co.

CHAPTER ELEVEN # Cataract

The term "cataract" is frightening to the average person and often seems to be used as a synonym for blindness. When asked about eye disease in their family, many patients will report some distant relative with "cataract." On closer questioning the patient admits he does not know what was wrong but has called the problem "cataract" because sight was lost. Medical personnel should be aware that "cataract" does have this alarming implication to many people.

Actually, cataract is preferable to most other damaging diseases because vision lost from cataract can be restored by surgical removal of the cataract. In contrast, blindness caused by glaucoma or senile macular degeneration is irreversible. Furthermore, cataract extraction is almost always a successful operation.

ETIOLOGY

Cataract (Fig. 11-1) is a loss of transparency of the normal lens within the eye. It is not a growth upon the outside of the eye, as is believed by many lay persons. Most cataracts are caused by the slow degenerative changes of age and are called senile cataracts. The tendency to develop senile cataracts is inherited. Although most senile cataracts do not require surgery until the patient is over 50 years of age, they may occasionally develop much earlier.

The next most common cause of cataract is injury to the eye. Either a penetrating wound or a contusion may sufficiently damage the lens to destroy its transparency. Some poisons may cause cataract. Such poisons include naphthalene (a constituent of mothballs) and dinitrophenol (a chemical used in the manufacture of explosives). Cataracts present at birth are called congenital. Most congenital cataracts are hereditary, but they may be caused by virus infections such as German measles, if contracted by the mother during the first three months of pregnancy. Endocrine cataracts result from a deficiency of parathyroid hormone, which may result if the parathyroid glands are inadvertently removed during thyroidectomy. Complicated cataracts follow severe intraocular infections or are associated with some types of eye disease, such as retinitis pigmentosa. Roentgenograms or electric shocks may cause cataract.

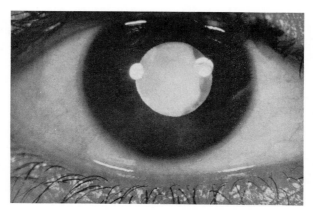

Fig. 11-1. A dense cataract is visible as a white discoloration just behind the pupil.

SYMPTOMS

The symptoms of cataract are various types of loss of sight. Gradual blurring of vision is the most common complaint. Most types of cataract cause scattering of light, resulting in an unpleasant glare when the patient is in bright light. This is somewhat comparable to the glare of the morning sun upon a frosty windshield. Irregularities within the lens may cause distortions of sight or sometimes double vision. One type of senile cataract causes progressive nearsightedness. Changes in the glasses worn for distance are uncommon in older persons and usually result from cataract formation. Cataract do not cause floating spots, loss of part of the visual field, rainbow halos about lights, or pain.

Visual loss caused by cataract is gradual. The rate of cataract development is impossible to predict, although some types grow faster, others slower. Senile cataract characteristically affects both eyes, but often one cataract is considerably worse than the other. Not infrequently gradual loss of vision in one eye is not recognized by the patient until he accidentally covers the better eye—discovery of visual loss in this way may be misinterpreted as a sudden loss of sight.

Other conditions besides cataract may cause gradual loss of vision with increasing age. The worst of these is glaucoma, visual loss from which is irreversible. Serious general diseases such as diabetes, high blood pressure, and brain tumor may also gradually damage eyesight. Because the elderly patient with failing vision cannot tell whether he has cataract or a much more serious disease, loss of vision in the older person requires a medical eye examination. All too often the onset of blindness is wrongly accepted as a natural change of old age.

MANAGEMENT

In many patients with early cataract a change of glasses will restore useful vision. Later, however, the cataract becomes more dense and new glasses are only a waste of money. Except in the very rare cases of cataract caused by hypoparathyroidism or galactosemia, medical treatment is of absolutely no value in retarding the progress of cataract. Many types of drops, vitamins, and other nostrums have been recommended, but none is of any use at all. Patients often fear to read or otherwise use their eyes lest they be damaged. There is no basis for such fears—use of the eyes will neither accelerate nor hinder cataract formation.

The proper time for cataract surgery is determined by the patient's eyesight, occupation, general health, personal wishes, and convenience. An almost true generalization is that the cataract should be operated on when the patient is sufficiently dissatisfied with the vision of his better eye. Usually a patient with unilateral cataract is happier without surgery. A cataract is not like a cancer, which should be removed immediately simply because it exists. Until vision is impaired, cataract surgery will not benefit the patient. However, a patient does not need to suffer complete blindness before he can be helped by surgery.

If sight is very poor in both eyes, removal of both cataracts at the same hospitalization (but one week apart) is desirable. If the better eye still sees usefully, the average patient is happier to postpone surgery on the second eye until the first operated eye has completely recovered and is fitted with glasses.

With the multiple-suture intracapsular technique of cataract extraction (described later in the chapter), severe restrictions upon the patient's postoperative activity are unnecessary. Sandbag immobilization of the head and bedpans are no longer required after cataract surgery. The average patient is able to be up and to care for himself on the same day surgery is performed. The duration of hospitalization is less than a week. Reading and light activity are permitted immediately upon return home. Heavy work

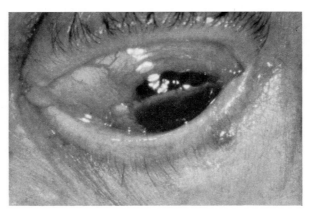

Fig. 11-2. Three weeks after cataract surgery this patient rubbed his eyes, causing the incision to burst open. Because the newly operated eye is very delicate, it must be protected carefully against any possible injury for at least a month.

should not be undertaken until four to six weeks after surgery. The operated eye is atropinized (a drop of 1% atropine each day) for one to two
weeks. Home cleaning of the eye is most easily done with hot compresses
(see Chapter 5). A metal shield must be taped securely over the eye each
night for a month to avoid accidental damage to the eye by rubbing it during sleep (Fig. 11-2). The patient should be careful not to bump his eye
accidentally. Wearing glasses during the day will help to protect the eye.

Office visits will be necessary at about one week after discharge from
the hospital and one and three months after surgery. More frequent visits
will be advised if any problems occur. The patient should call the office at
any time if he feels the eye is not healing properly. Some irritation is expected until the stitches (which may be catgut) spontaneously dissolve after
about three or four weeks.

GLASSES

After cataract surgery the eye will never see clearly without glasses.
Three months of healing are necessary before prescription of permanent
glasses. Helpful temporary glasses may be prescribed as early as one to four
weeks after surgery, depending upon the rate of healing and the amount of
vision in the other eye. Because the curvature of the cornea continually
changes during the first few months after surgery, the expensive permanent glasses are usually not prescribed until three months postoperatively.
Some patients will want to wear contact lenses; these may be fitted at three
months.

Cataract glasses restore sight and are greatly appreciated. The better
quality glasses are far superior to cheaper ones and are more free of
problems. Some problems are inherent in strong glasses (Fig. 11-3) and cannot be completely avoided. The weight of thick lenses is quite uncomfortable to some people. Skilled preparation of the glasses can greatly reduce
this weight. Plastic lenses are much lighter than glass ones. Cataract glasses
magnify, so that everything seen through such a glass appears about one-
fourth larger than normal. This magnification gives the illusion that everything is one-fourth closer than it actually is. For example, a cup sitting
on the table appears closer than it is, so the person wearing cataract glasses
may pour his coffee on the table in front of the cup. After about a month
most people adapt to this magnification and no longer are troubled by
distance judgment (provided that both eyes have been operated—with only
one eye accurate distance judgment is always difficult).

Accurate adjustment and positioning of cataract glasses is essential. Even
slight changes in the position of the glass can cause very annoying distortions of vision. Inexpensive glasses may cause abnormal curvatures, so that
the edges of a door, for example, seem to curve outward at top and bottom.

Cataract glasses will **not** focus both eyes together if the cataract has been
removed from only one eye. Such a patient may be fitted with glasses so
as to focus either the operated or the unoperated eye (depending on which
sees better), but he cannot be fitted to use both eyes together. Only when

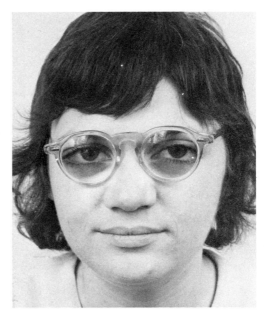

Fig. 11-3. Following cataract surgery, strong glasses are necessary to compensate for the loss of the focusing power of the lens of the eye.

fitted with a contact lens can an operated eye work together with its un-operated mate.

If a dense cataract develops in one eye only, its removal and subsequent fitting of a contact lens may restore binocular vision. A regular cataract eyeglass cannot be used because its magnification causes intolerable double vision. Contact lenses completely eliminate the cataract eyeglass problems of magnification limited side vision, distortion, uncomfortable weight, and cosmetic faults of thick lenses. Most younger persons prefer contact lenses after cataract extraction. Older persons usually do not adapt well to the problems of contact lenses.

Contact lenses require three to six training sessions to learn their use. Reasonable dexterity is necessary to handle these small lenses (not practical for an old person with trembling hands). More care and time are necessary in the maintenance of contact lenses than in simply putting on a pair of spectacles. Contact lenses cost about twice as much as a pair of spectacle eyeglasses.

COMPLICATIONS

Can other problems follow cataract surgery? Certainly. Whether oper-ated or not, an older eye is more likely to fail than a young, healthy eye. The most common serious diseases are glaucoma and retinal detachment. A careful medical examination of the eye is important one year after surgery and every several years thereafter. Early detection of some of these serious problems permits much more effective care; also, a change of glasses may sometimes improve vision.

If vision fails after cataract surgery, the patient should seek prompt medical attention. For example, the sudden appearance of very many floating spots or a progressive dark shadow beginning at the side and advancing toward the center of vision are symptoms characteristic of retinal detachment. Most ophthalmologists would prefer to have their patients call rather than ignore any unusual eye symptoms after cataract surgery.

The chances are nineteen out of twenty that a patient with an otherwise healthy eye will have no further troubles after a successful cataract operation. After complete healing and fitting with glasses he may be normally active with no restrictions. Physical exertion, including heavy work, will not harm the eye. Use of the eyes for reading, sewing, or any other activity cannot cause damage. Naturally fatigue will follow prolonged use of the eyes, whether operated or not, but this is not harmful.

Dark glasses may be used by the aphakic patient for comfort, just as by anyone else. Do not attach clip-on sunglasses to cataract glasses, since the center of the lenses will be scratched. Do not lay the glasses down so that the glass part touches a hard surface, or scratches will result.

Often older persons are advised by well-meaning but mistaken friends that they must forever restrict their activity after cataract surgery. This is a serious error; normal physical and social activity is necessary for good health and morale. Unnecessary restriction of activity leads to physical and mental deterioration. The patient should be *fully active* after complete healing of a cataract operation.

SURGERY

A brief description of the technique of cataract extraction may be of general interest. The operation is usually done under local anesthesia. Sensory block and immobilization of the extraocular muscles are obtained by injection into the orbit behind the eye. The lids are prevented from closing by injection of the seventh nerve fibers as they enter on the lateral side. A lid speculum is used to provide good exposure of the eye.

The conjunctiva is dissected away from the upper limbus throughout the entire upper half of the eye. The incision into the eye is made just at the junction of cornea and sclera and extends through the entire upper 180 degrees of circumference. This large incision is necessary because of the size of a cataract. A triangular knife, called a keratome, may be used to start the incision, which is then enlarged with scissors. Most nurses are surprised to see the sutures placed into position across the incision before the cataract is extracted. This is done because the cataract helps to hold back the fluid intraocular contents and therefore is not extracted until after all is in readiness for immediate tying of the sutures. Currently available sutures are unbelievably fine. Our 10-0 suture is only 22 μ thick—three times the diameter of a red blood cell.

When the lens is removed from an eye, the vitreous tends to come forward and block aqueous flow through the pupil. Such a pupil block may be prevented by creating an additional opening through the iris. Either a peripheral or a sector iridectomy may be performed. A peripheral iridectomy is a small opening (perhaps 1 mm. diameter) in the outer rim of the upper iris. A sector iridectomy is the removal of a segment of the upper iris, extending completely from the periphery to the pupil. Either type of iridectomy is done just before delivery of the lens.

Lens extraction is accomplished by a combination of push and pull. The pull may be exerted by means of a delicate forceps or by a small vacuum cup (erisophake). The push is applied through the lower cornea with a muscle hook or similar small blunt instrument. A popular method of lens extraction is called "tumbling" because the bottom edge of the lens is rotated (tumbled) up and comes out of the eye first. The reason for this rotation is that it permits a few zonular fibers at the bottom to be broken first, then a few more along the sides, progressively, until finally the top remnants are broken. If an attempt were made to rupture all the zonular fibers simultaneously, their combined strength would be too great, and the lens capsule would tear instead.

In another method of lens extraction, a small probe is caused to adhere to the wet surface of the cataract by freezing to it. This is called cryoextraction (Fig. 11-4).

Intracapsular extraction refers to removal of the lens within its intact capsule and is the method of choice because it leaves a perfectly clean and open pupil. Extracapsular extraction happens when the capsule is accidentally broken during delivery. This is undesirable because more or less of the pupil may be blocked by remnants of the lens cortex or capsule.

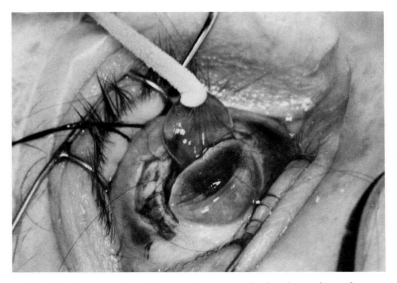

Fig. 11-4. A cryoprobe adheres to the cataract by freezing to its surface.

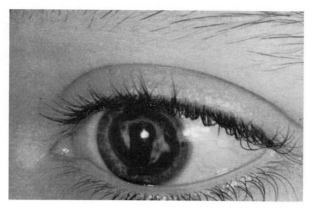

Fig. 11-5. A secondary cataract, remaining after a "needling" operation. Needling is a technique of cutting apart the cataract with a tiny knife.

The frequency of extracapsular extraction may be reduced by irrigating the eye with alpha-chymotrypsin, an enzyme that dissolves the zonular fibers without causing significant damage elsewhere within the eye. Such zonulolysis is particularly useful in surgery for traumatic cataracts in persons between 20 and 40 years of age.

In persons younger than 20 years and particularly in children, the vitreous is adherent to the lens and prevents uncomplicated intracapsular extraction. Cataracts in very young persons are usually partially removed by "needling" (Fig. 11-5), which is a cutting of the capsule with a very tiny knife. The substance of the cataract may be partially aspirated through a small hollow needle. In the newest variant of the cataract surgical technique, the substance of the lens is broken up by ultrasonic vibrations before it is aspirated.

PROGNOSIS

The prognosis for uncomplicated senile cataracts is good, since about 95% of such patients will regain satisfactory vision postoperatively. Of course, if some other condition such as senile macular degeneration or diabetic retinopathy has destroyed the central retina, cataract extraction will not restore useful vision. The serious unexpected complications most frequently encountered during or after routine cataract surgery are infection, hemorrhage, wound rupture, epithelial downgrowth, retinal detachment, and glaucoma. Postoperative intraocular infection is usually disastrous; hence meticulous sterile technique is necessary during all intraocular surgery. Although hemorrhage and wound rupture may occur spontaneously, they are usually caused by injury and may be prevented by avoiding falls and by faithful use of the metal eye shield. Downgrowth of surface epithelium through the incision is catastrophic because it characteristically spreads uncontrollably throughout the eye. Such downgrowths usually follow faulty wound closure. Retinal detachment or glaucoma may develop despite perfect technique because of other degenerative ocular changes accompanying the cataract. Needless to say, inexpert surgical technique can and does destroy eyes. Cataract extraction is a precision operation requiring faultless technique.

SUMMARY

Cataract, the opacification of the lens of the eye, is usually caused by age, injury, toxic influences, or inheritance. Only medical examination can differentiate cataract from more serious blinding diseases with similar symptoms. Extraction of an uncomplicated cataract should restore good vision in about 95% of patients.

SUGGESTED READING

Havener, William H., and Gloeckner, Sallie:
Atlas of cataract surgery, St. Louis, 1972,
The C. V. Mosby Co.

CHAPTER TWELVE # Retinal detachment

When the retina (the part of the eye that sees) falls away from its normal position in the back of the eye, it is said to be "detached." Most detachments result from holes in the retina. The fluid contents of the eye leak through these retinal holes and displace the retina from its normal position. A retinal detachment is somewhat similar to a flat tire. Just as the air leaks out through a puncture in the inner tube of the tire, so the interior fluid of the eye leaks slowly through the retinal hole to cause a retinal detachment.

ETIOLOGY

The most common cause of holes in the retina is a slowly developing fault within the eye resulting from aging changes. A delicate transparent framework called the vitreous humor occupies the inside of the back part of the eye. In an older eye the vitreous framework shrinks. Sometimes this shrinking framework is attached to a part of the retina and pulls on it sufficiently to tear a hole. Almost always such retinal holes are the spontaneous result of the internal changes of the vitreous and are **not** caused by accidents. Very commonly, in attempting to explain their eye problem, patients wrongly attribute the detachment to a recent accident.

Severe injuries to the eye may, of course, result in retinal holes and subsequent detachment; penetrating wounds and direct contusions of the eye are examples of such injuries. Because months or years may pass before the appearance of a detachment, regular medical eye examinations are desirable after a severe injury.

Some types of nearsighted eyes are predisposed to retinal detachment. Even young children may suffer from this kind of detachment. Not uncommonly the symptoms of detachment are misinterpreted as being some type of contact lens or spectacle problem. Actually the symptoms of refractive error are entirely different from those of a retinal detachment.

Infrequently retinal detachments are caused by inflammations of the interior of the eye. After such inflammations the vitreous framework may shrink and tear holes in the retina.

121

SYMPTOMS

What are the symptoms of a retinal detachment? Many (not all) patients know when the retinal hole developed. The tearing of a hole in the retina commonly ruptures small blood vessels, permitting a small amount of internal bleeding into the eye. Blood suspended within the vitreous framework casts small shadows upon the retina. These shadows drift about as the eye is moved. Hence the patient with a retinal tear may perceive a large number of floating spots, which appear to be loosely suspended in front of the affected eye. These spots usually appear quite rapidly—within a few hours. (To prevent unnecessary alarm we must state here that almost everyone can see a few floating filaments when looking at a light background—these are normal.) The sudden appearance of very many floating spots is a danger signal for which an ophthalmologist should be promptly consulted. Almost always the floating spots that precede a detachment will decrease for several days or weeks, thereby falsely reassuring the patient that he is getting better.

Stimulation of the retina by vitreous pull may cause a sensation of flashes of light, especially prominent when the eye is moved. These flashes resemble a distant lightning flash, seen to one side. The flashes usually disappear spontaneously within several days or weeks, just as do the floating spots.

The retina cannot perceive pain, therefore retinal tears and detachments do not hurt.

Since the peripheral edge of the retina is thinnest, retinal holes and detachments usually start peripherally and only gradually extend. The area of the retina that is detached is separated from the part of the eye that nourishes it (choroid). Lacking nourishment, the detached part of the retina becomes blind. The patient recognizes the beginning detachment as a shadow, which usually starts somewhere to the side and gradually increases in size. Often this shadow is misinterpreted as a block of vision caused by dirt upon the eyeglasses, a drooping eyelid, or perhaps a swollen nose. Vision of the eye may remain good straight ahead so long as the center of the retina is uninvolved. When the center of the retina is damaged by a detachment, eyesight becomes distorted, wavy, and indistinct. Unless the retinal holes (often more than one) are sealed, the retina will progressively detach, and in most cases total blindness of the eye ultimately results. Days, weeks, or months may pass before the retina entirely detaches. Unfortunately retinal detachments do not spontaneously cure themselves, as a patient "gets over" a cold with time.

SURGERY

Surgery is necessary to seal most holes in the retina. The operation is usually done with a general anesthetic. Just as a flat tire is fixed by sealing the hole in the inner tube, so a retinal detachment is repaired by sealing the retinal hole. The hole is sealed by causing a scar to form in the outer layers of the eye, which become adherent to the hole, thereby closing it. The scar may be formed by heat, electrical current, or cold. The scar is

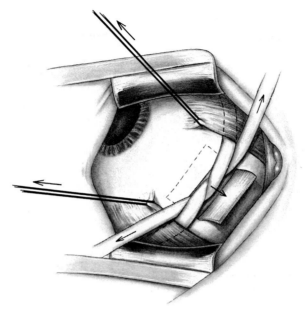

Fig. 12-1. In retinal detachment surgery the volume of the eye is decreased by removal of the subretinal fluid and by encircling the equator of the eye with a belt of foreign material, such as donor fascia lata. This technique mechanically aids in reapposing the retina to its normal position against the choroid. (From Havener, William H., and Gloeckner, Sallie: Atlas of diagnostic techniques and treatment of retinal detachment, St. Louis, 1967, The C. V. Mosby Co.)

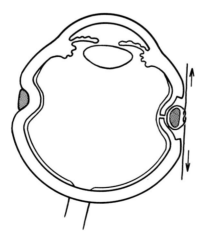

Fig. 12-2. Cross section of eye, to illustrate the decreased vitreous volume following encircling procedure for retinal detachment. (From Havener, William H., and Gloeckner, Sallie: Atlas of diagnostic techniques and treatment of retinal detachment, St. Louis, 1967, The C. V. Mosby Co.)

held firmly against the retinal hole by local pressure, which may be achieved by a variety of surgical techniques, depending upon the individual circumstances. In one such technique a reinforcing band of fascia or plastic may be circled about the equator of the eye to enhance the local pressure (Figs. 12-1 and 12-2).

If retinal holes are detected very early, before a detachment has developed, they may be treated with a flash of light. The light must be very intense and is produced by instruments such as the laser or photocoagulator. These instruments are simply giant flashlights, which can focus a very bright light precisely at any pinpoint spot within the eye. Such a light will produce enough heat to induce scar formation about the hole, thereby sealing it. Light coagulation does not damage other parts of the eye and does not require surgical incisions. Unfortunately most detachments lift the retinal holes too far away from the back of the eye to permit successful "spot welding" with the photocoagulator.

PROGNOSIS

All retinal detachments are serious problems that may result in blindness despite the best surgical efforts. Naturally some eyes are much more diseased than others, hence the prognosis will be worse for some eyes than for others. In general, about two out of three retinal detachments will be corrected by a single operation. About one patient out of three will require repeated surgery because of the development of new holes, failure of original holes to heal properly, or unusual complications such as hemorrhage. Perhaps one eye out of ten fails to remain reattached despite repeated surgery. In such failures the eye usually remains cosmetically normal in appearance, although it is blind.

Restoration of sight depends mainly upon the extent and duration of detachment prior to surgery. If the center of the retina was not damaged by the detachment, successful surgery will maintain perfectly normal vision. Permanent distortion of straight-ahead vision usually follows detachment of the central retina. Obviously, better vision results if the detachment is is detected and treated early. Almost normal side vision and partial central vision often can be restored even after detachment has existed for many months. However, a detached retina slowly dies unless replaced, and after several years of uncorrected detachment blindness is irreversible.

About three months will pass before maximum vision is achieved after surgery. Often a change in eyeglasses is necessary at this time. Uncommonly, complications such as hemorrhage will delay recovery.

GENERAL INFORMATION

Admission to the hospital is usually arranged as soon as possible. On admission the patient will have a complete physical examination, and laboratory tests of blood and urine will be required before anesthesia. While waiting for surgery, the patient may be advised to limit his activity. These instructions will vary considerably, depending upon the individual eye problem. Some patients should hold their head in certain positions before surgery. Because comparable positioning is required of everyone for several days after surgery, these principles will now be discussed.

The patient's head is usually positioned so that the retinal hole is in the lowest part of the eye. Gravity causes the hole to fall downward. Hence, if the head is positioned so the hole is at the top of the eye, the detachment will tend to worsen. Conversely, if the hole is down, the detachment usually will not become worse, or if surgery has already been performed, the hole will not fall out of position before healing occurs. For example, if the hole is in the upper right side of either eye, the patient should lie down in bed with his head turned to the right. While his head is in this position, he should move his body and extremities freely in order to maintain his strength. Such movement cannot harm the properly positioned retina, either before or after surgery. When traveling to and from the hospital, the proper head position should be maintained by lying down in the back seat of the automobile.

Surgery is performed under a general anesthetic, therefore the patient may not eat or drink after midnight on the night before surgery, nor on the day of surgery. If he eats breakfast on the day of surgery, the operation must be postponed. Appropriate sedatives are given before surgery. The patient is awake until after entering the operating room, but then he will seem suddenly to fall asleep and will remember nothing until awakening in the recovery room. The relatives should be aware that the patient will normally spend four to six hours in surgery and the recovery room, otherwise they will worry unnecessarily about his long absence. Postoperative nausea or vomiting is not unusual and may be made worse by eating or drinking too much at first.

To prevent the retina from falling out of position before it can heal, both eyes may be covered for several days after surgery. During this time the patient must usually stay in bed. His head is positioned to place the retinal hole down, as previously explained. Exercising arms and legs in bed is encouraged. Visits by relatives or use of a bedside radio will help to pass the time. The nursing personnel are adequate to care for the patient during this time, and special nurses are unnecessary.

Usually by the second postoperative day the eye has healed sufficiently to permit the patient to be up carefully with his good eye uncovered. He may be up to meals and bathroom and may sit in a chair. When first arising from bed, the patient will usually be surprisingly weak and unsteady and must be helped to prevent falling. Sitting up in bed for five minutes, followed by dangling his legs from the bed for another five minutes will help to accustom the patient to being up and will decrease the possibility of fainting. Strength will be regained rapidly, and most patients will be ready to go home by the third day.

Instructions and eye drops are given to the patient upon discharge. He should travel lying in the back seat of the automobile, with his head properly positioned on a pillow.

The patient may completely care for himself at home. He may be up for meals and bathroom and may dress, shave, brush his teeth, comb his hair, and perform any other activity required for personal care. Accidental falls and bumps must be avoided during the first several weeks, so during this time he should stay in the house and do nothing except care for himself.

Rapid eye movements, as in reading, may be harmful and should be avoided for several weeks. Looking straight ahead, as in talking with friends or watching television, is not harmful and will help to pass the time.

The operated eye and lids are expected to be somewhat uncomfortable, swollen, and discolored for a week or two. The eye will water and crusts will adhere to the eyelashes. Gentle application of a warm compress to the closed eyelids will aid in cleaning the eye and will be comforting. For this purpose a clean washcloth may be moistened in ordinary hot tap water, squeezed free of excess water, and laid upon the eyelids. Hot compresses should be applied at least four or five times a day for ten to fifteen minutes at a time.

Most patients should instill a drop of atropine into the eye once daily for several weeks. This dilates the pupil and reduces inflammation.

An eye pad on the operated eye neither aids nor retards healing but is usually comforting for several days. The retina is in the back of the eye and heals equally well whether the eye is covered or open. The wearing of dark glasses is entirely optional.

The eye should be examined by the ophthalmologist ten to fourteen days after discharge from the hospital. If all is well at that time, the patient may begin to do light activity about the house, visit friends, attend church, etc. At three weeks light work is allowed (for example, secretarial or administrative work). Six weeks after surgery heavy work and athletic activity are permitted, within reason. The operated eye should be refracted at three months and fitted with a new lens if necessary.

Eye checks by the ophthalmologist will be advised at increasing intervals after surgery. Ultimately examination every year or two will be adequate. If at any time a new retinal hole is found on routine examination, it should be prophylactically sealed to prevent another detachment. Other changes such as glaucoma or cataract are more common in eyes that have suffered a detachment and may be detected on routine examination by the ophthalmologist.

The patient should be taught to recognize the symptoms of retinal holes and detachment. These have been previously described as the sudden onset of many new floating spots, many flashes of light, and appearance of a progressive shadow starting from the side. If any of these symptoms should appear in either eye of a patient who has had a retinal detachment, he should be considered to have developed a new retinal hole until proved otherwise by careful medical examination through a widely dilated pupil. The ophthalmologist should be notified immediately of the new symptoms and reminded of the preceding history of retinal detachment. No doubt some of these calls will be false alarms, but the opportunity for early care of retinal detachment is too important to be lost by delay.

SUGGESTED READING

Havener, William H., and Gloeckner, Sallie: Atlas of diagnostic techniques and treatment of retinal detachment, St. Louis, 1967, The C. V. Mosby Co.

CHAPTER THIRTEEN

Uncommon eye conditions

There are a considerable number of unusual eye conditions (Fig. 13-1), most of which are of little interest except to the ophthalmologist. Representative examples of these rare conditions will be mentioned in this chapter.

KERATOCONUS

Keratoconus is a degenerative thinning of the central cornea, occurring usually during adolescence. The cornea develops a conical contour that causes severe optical distortion. In late stages the central cornea may lose its transparency. The disease is usually bilateral.

Ordinary spectacles do not adequately correct the high astigmatism of keratoconus. By substituting a smooth front surface for the irregular cone contact lenses effectively restore vision in most early cases. If corneal scarring develops, corneal transplantation is necessary.

In conditions such as keratoconus or for other localized corneal scars caused by injury or infection, vision can be restored by transplanting a fresh clear donor cornea as a substitute for the opaque and scarred cornea. Many persons falsely believe that the whole eye is transplanted—actually only a 6 mm. disk from the center of the cornea is transplanted. The donor cornea is obtained by the eye bank with permission of the relatives of a recently deceased patient. To contribute the gift of sight to another person is an inspiring way of permitting a part of yourself to live on usefully even after your death.

SENILE MACULAR DEGENERATION

The central portion of the retina is subject to selective deterioration with age in some families. This causes gradual loss of clear central vision, with resulting inability to read, to drive, or to do other activities requiring good acuity. Fortunately the peripheral retina is never affected by this disorder, and therefore the patient always retains side vision and the ability to care for himself. Both eyes are usually affected, although not necessarily equally. No treatment will halt the progress of this degenerative change, however spontaneous partial improvement in vision may sometimes occur.

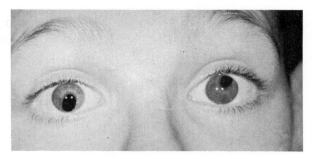

Fig. 13-1. Coloboma of the iris is a defect, usually located inferiorly. It is usually an inherited congenital fault but may result from maternal infection such as rubella, as in this patient.

RETINITIS PIGMENTOSA

Degeneration and clumping of the retinal pigment, which can be seen with an ophthalmoscope, occur in some families. The earliest symptom is night-blindness. Whereas the normal person adapts to the dark and is able to see well enough to get about in semi-darkness, these patients cannot do so. Later their peripheral field of vision is lost, even in daylight. Ultimately in severe cases total blindness may ensue.

CANCER (Fig. 13-2)

Intraocular neoplasms may originate in the retina or the uveal tract or metastasize to the eye from elsewhere in the body.

Retinoblastoma is a highly malignant childhood cancer arising from the retina of one or both eyes. Almost invariably the first eye involved is so seriously damaged by the time of discovery (Fig. 13-3) that it must be removed. Careful, repeated examinations of the second eye are essential to detect possible tumor within it at an early stage. Retinoblastoma may be hereditary; therefore siblings of affected children should also be examined thoroughly. Should the affected patient survive to have children, about half of these offspring will have retinoblastoma and therefore must be examined repeatedly from earliest infancy to school age.

X-ray therapy, chemotherapy, and photocoagulation may save the second eye if a small tumor is found early. Photocoagulation is a new technique whereby an extremely bright light may be focused precisely through the transparent part of the eye upon the retinoblastoma. This light is so intense that it burns up the tumor just as a piece of paper may be burned by sunlight focused by a magnifying glass.

Melanoma (Fig. 13-4) is pigmented tumor arising from the iris, ciliary body, or choroid. Older persons are more likely to be affected. Enucleation is usually necessary, although sometimes a small iris melanoma may be removed by iridectomy.

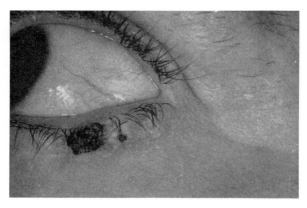

Fig. 13-2. Basal cell carcinoma of the skin is a persistent, crusting lesion that may bleed slightly when the crust is removed. Early recognition permits surgical removal with minimal cosmetic disfigurement.

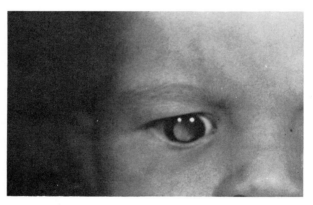

Fig. 13-3. One fourth of the cases of retinoblastoma are first seen for the complaint of strabismus. This patient also shows the yellowish pupil reflex caused by growth of tumor within the eye. Thorough examination of the eyes themselves is necessary in all strabismus. (From Havener, William H.: Synopsis of ophthalmology, ed. 3, St. Louis, 1971, The C. V. Mosby Co.)

After enucleation the cosmetic appearance of the patient is restored with an artificial eye. Such a prosthesis is a thin shell, which fits between the lids. Upon its surface is painted an iris matching that of the normal eye. The artificial eye may be removed simply by separating the lids and gently pulling upon it with a suction cup. Minor surface infection and discharge is common in the patient with an artificial eye. Topical instillation of an antibiotic drop, cleaning with warm compresses, and general hygienic care will eliminate most such infectious problems. Neither leaving the eye in the socket for long periods of time nor leaving it out (as might happen during a serious illness) is harmful. Ordinarily the patient will care for his own artificial eye, and this will not be a nursing responsibility.

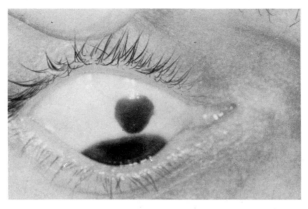

Fig. 13-4. A malignant melanoma of the eye may extend to the surface and appear as a dark plaque upon the eye.

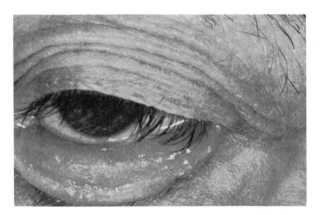

Fig. 13-5. Ectropion, or turning out of the lid, is most commonly caused by senile relaxation of the eyelid framework.

OPTIC ATROPHY

Partial or complete death of the optic nerve is usually caused by central nervous system disease, although it may also result from eye diseases such as glaucoma or arterial occlusion. Once dead, the optic nerve can never regenerate; therefore it is important that this cause of reduced vision be detected early in order that treatable lesions may be corrected before irreversible damage is done.

ECTROPION AND ENTROPION

Faulty position of the lower eyelid occurs most often because of age or injury. Sagging of the lid away from the eye is called ectropion (Fig. 13-5). The

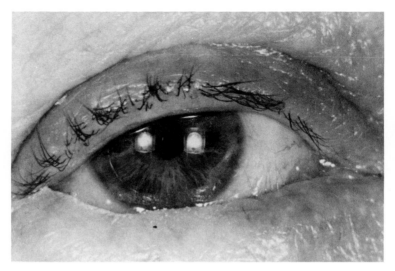

Fig. 13-6. Entropion, inward turning of the eyelid, is the result of relaxation of the framework of the eyelid, combined with excessive contraction of the orbicularis muscle.

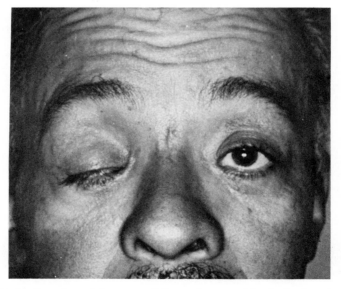

Fig. 13-7. Ptosis (drooping of the upper lid) may be caused by faulty function of either muscle or innervation.

main disturbance caused by ectropion is overflow of tears down the patient's face. This is because the tear punctum is in faulty position, thereby preventing normal drainage. The exposed conjunctiva of the lower lid may also become irritated. Entropion (Fig. 13-6) refers to an inrolling of the lower lid. This causes the lashes to rub on the cornea, which is very irritating. Plastic surgery is required to correct these faults of lid position.

PTOSIS

Drooping of the upper lid (ptosis) may result from congenital or acquired weakness of the levator muscle (Fig. 13-7). Paralysis of the third cranial nerve, which innervates the levator, may be due to a variety of intracranial diseases. Partial ptosis can be caused by malfunctions of the sympathetic portion of the autonomic nervous system—this is called Horner's syndrome and is accompanied by a small pupil on the affected side. In contrast, a paralyzed third nerve causes the pupil to enlarge.

Surgical shortening of the levator muscle will elevate the lid and is often beneficial to patients suffering from ptosis.

SUMMARY

In addition to the many common eye diseases, there exist a considerable variety of rare problems. Some of these have been described. Since these conditions may cause many queer symptoms, patients with unusual ocular complaints should not be considered as having functional disorders before they are thoroughly evaluated by an ophthalmologist.

CHAPTER FOURTEEN # Prevention of blindness

It is not through chance that the United States has the lowest incidence of blindness in all the major nations. Only two per 1,000 inhabitants of the United States are blind, as contrasted to forty per 1,000 Arabs living in the Middle East (Fig. 14-1). The main reason for this difference is the careful application of medical knowledge. *Blindness is preventable!* This chapter will outline the magnitude of the problem of blindness, refer to rehabilitation, describe representative examples of preventable blindness, and make specific suggestions for further reducing the incidence of blindness.

STATISTICS

More than 300,000 men, women, and children in the United States are now legally blind. Each year 30,000 new persons become blind. The enormous sum of $150 million is spent annually to care for these blind persons. How much money and productivity is lost through their inability to work can only be guessed. The personal tragedy of blindness can be fully realized only through acquaintance with an unfortunate person whose life has been cruelly altered by loss of sight. Appalling though these statistics are, they are dwarfed by the number of people who are handicapped by loss of vision in one eye. About five per 100 Americans see less than 20/200 (the big E on the eye chart) with one eye, and this vision cannot be improved with glasses.

Rehabilitation methods are often remarkably successful in restoring a blind person to a considerable degree of self-sufficiency. Guide dogs, white canes, Braille writing, and suitable occupational training are familiar approaches to this rehabilitation. National, state, and private agencies for this purpose seem uniformly enthusiastic and helpful and should be contacted for further specific information.* In general, a newly blinded person should *immediately* be brought to the attention of such agencies in order to avoid development of psychologic attitudes that will interfere seriously with his

---

From Havener, William H.: Synopsis of ophthalmology, ed. 3, St. Louis, 1971, The C. V. Mosby Co.

*See Appendix.

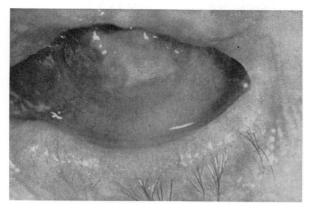

Fig. 14-1. Trachoma is a chronic, destructive disease of the cornea and conjunctiva and tends to cause serious corneal scarring. This disease is rampant in the **Middle East** because of poor medical care and unsanitary conditions. (From Havener, William H.: Synopsis of ophthalmology, ed. 3, St. Louis, 1971, The C. V. Mosby Co.)

rehabilitation. Remarkable as these rehabilitation achievements may be, they are a poor second-best approach as compared to prevention of the original cause of blindness.

MEDICAL KNOWLEDGE

It is estimated that nearly one half of the present blindness could have been prevented by ideal *application of presently existing medical knowledge*. Pills lying idle on the druggist's shelf cure no disease. A person with a sick eye not seen by a physician is no better off than a similar person in darkest Africa beyond the reach of the miracles of twentieth-century medicine. The goal of elimination of preventable blindness will not be reached until every patient with persistent eye symptoms realizes he should consult a competent physician. The following are examples of the prevention of blindness through medical care.

Silver nitrate drops are now, by law, instilled in the eyes of every newborn infant (Fig. 8-9). This destroys the germs of gonorrhea, which once blinded hundreds of helpless babies. Vaccination (Fig. 14-2) has all but wiped out smallpox—a disease that through its destructive scarring was once the leading cause of blindness. The blood tests required during pregnancy detect and lead to the treatment of syphilis, thereby eliminating another cause of childhood (and also adult) blindness. Deliberate exposure of little girls to German measles will give them permanent immunity, thereby ensuring they cannot catch it during their later pregnancies, when measles can destroy the eyes of an unborn child. An effective vaccine is now available.

Premature babies become blind when given too much oxygen. Five thousand American babies lost their sight permanently before research

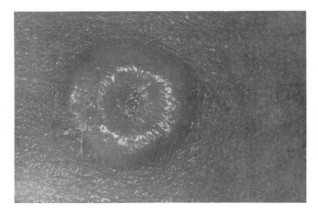

Fig. 14-2. The familiar appearance of a vaccination is not usually thought of as a preventive of blindness, yet the corneal scarring of smallpox was a leading cause of blindness. Care must be exercised to avoid ocular inoculation of vaccinia through scratching. (From Havener, William H.: Synopsis of ophthalmology, ed. 3, St. Louis, 1971, The C. V. Mosby Co.)

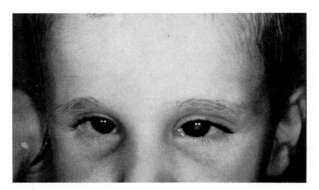

Fig. 14-3. Retinopathy of prematurity is recognized by the bilateral appearance of a dense white membrane behind the lens in premature children who have received excessive oxygen. Since retinoblastoma and inflammation may cause a similar appearance, an expert opinion should be obtained. (From Havener, William H.: Synopsis of ophthalmology, ed. 3, St. Louis, 1971, The C. V. Mosby Co.)

discovered the cause of this disease, called retrolental fibroplasia (Fig. 14-3).

Diabetes, high blood pressure, brain tumors and other diseases of the nervous system, poisoning, and a host of other diseases that affect the whole body may cause blindness. Sometimes eye damage is the first sign permitting the physician to recognize the presence of these diseases.

Infection of the cornea of the eye may easily occur after even a small injury (Fig. 14-4). Any cinder or other foreign particle embedded in the

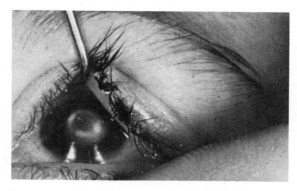

Fig. 14-4. This destructive corneal ulcer followed infection of the epithelial defect remaining after removal of a small corneal foreign body. Prophylactic antibiotics every
several hours would probably have prevented this misfortune. (From Havener, William
H.: Synopsis of ophthalmology, ed. 3, St. Louis, 1971, The C. V. Mosby Co.)

clear cornea should be cared for by a physician, who will know how to
prevent such infections with antibiotics. Severe pain is the warning signal
to the patient of injury to the cornea and should not be ignored, since a
blinding scar may follow.

The outlawing of fireworks, BB guns, and arrows greatly decreases the
number of children's eyes needlessly put out. Safety goggles in industry
and shatterproof automobile glass likewise protect adult eyes.

Glaucoma (increased pressure inside the eye) causes 12% of all blindness in the United States. It is aptly termed the "thief in the night" because
it steals away eyesight unknown to the victim until he is almost blind.
Two people in every 100 over 40 years of age now have glaucoma and do
not know it. The only way to detect glaucoma before it has done permanent damage is to measure the eye pressure with a *tonometer*—a method
routinely used by all ophthalmologists.

Blindness of disuse damages the crossed eye of a cross-eyed child so
often that 1% of our population is handicapped with a poor eye from this
cause. Parents could prevent this simply by taking their child for medical
treatment as soon as they recognize that his eyes are not straight.

Consulting a physician for eye symptoms will permit early care of potentially serious conditions. Redness of an eye occurs in many serious eye
diseases that may lead to blindness without proper medical care. Similarly,
decrease of vision is an ominous sign that may precede blindness. It is unfortunate that many laymen think that "a change of glasses" is all that their
eyes ever need. The symptoms of refractive error closely simulate the early
symptoms of blinding eye disease, those of serious general bodily illness, or
even those of mental illness. Every patient with persistent eye complaints
deserves a medical eye examination. A study of case histories of preventable

blindness all too often discloses the pattern of early symptoms disregarded by the patient, unrecognized by the nonmedical optometrist, and occasionally misinterpreted by a hurried physician.

MEDICAL RESEARCH

Medical research has already pointed the way to the prevention of many forms of blindness. A few of these examples have been cited in preceding paragraphs. If proper support is given to presently existing programs of research, continuing progress in our fight against blindness will surely be seen in the coming years.

EDUCATION

Safety precautions and first-aid knowledge are practical manifestations of the teaching approach to the prevention of serious accidents of all types, including those to the eyes. Teaching of the warning symptoms of eye disease, proper eye care, and first aid for eye injury should be as widespread as possible.

Seven eye danger signals. The seven eye danger signals for which a physician should be consulted are the following:

1. Persistent *redness* of the eye—The physician and nurse should consciously evaluate a red eye for the presence of these features, which suggest that major disease is present. Since diseases with these findings may cause blindness, accurate diagnosis and prompt, specific therapy are mandatory. The following are findings in a red eye suggesting major disease:
   a. Vision loss
   b. Pain
   c. Opacities of the clear parts of the eye
   d. Pupil irregularities of size and shape
   e. Distribution of redness encircling the cornea
   f. Pressure abnormality—hard or soft
   g. History of previous serious eye disease
   h. Response to therapy—failure to respond to adequate treatment within three or four days
2. Continuing discomfort or pain about the eye, especially after injury
3. Disturbances of vision
   a. Trouble seeing *near* or *distance*
   b. *Fogginess* of vision or *rainbow-colored* halos around lights
   c. Loss of *side vision*
   d. Persistent *double vision* (seeing two things when there is really only one there)
   e. Sudden development of many *floating spots* before the eyes
4. Crossing of the eyes, especially in children
5. Growths on the eye or eyelids or opacities visible in the normally transparent parts of the eye
6. Continuing discharge, crusting, or tearing of the eyes
7. Pupil irregularities (unequal size in the two eyes or distorted shape)

Eye examinations. How often should eyes be checked? No specific answer can be given to cover all patients, but the following general outline summarizes presently recommended optimal times for medical eye examination.

1. Whenever one of the seven eye danger signals appears, at any age
2. At birth (to detect malformations, injuries, and infections)
3. Between 4 and 5 years of age (to detect "lazy eyes," which occur in 1% of children and must be treated before school age)
4. Every five years after the age of 40 years (because by far the highest incidence of blindness is in older age groups)
5. As often as your own medical physician recommends (For example, after certain eye operations or serious inflammations much more frequent examinations are necessary. Annual checks of eye pressure are necessary after the age of 40 years if cases of glaucoma occur in your family.)

FIRST AID IN EYE INJURY

Knowledge of these simple principles will prevent blindness. *Wrong first aid causes blindness.*

1. Chemical eye burns (acids, caustics, poisons, etc.)—*Wash immediately with plain water* and continue washing for at least fifteen minutes. Pour the water right into the open eye. Do not go to a doctor or any-

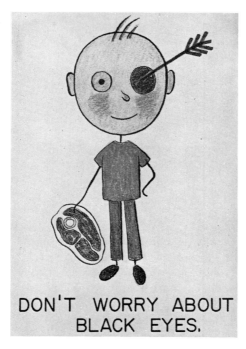

DON'T WORRY ABOUT BLACK EYES.

Fig. 14-5. A common misconception. (From Havener, William H.: Synopsis of ophthalmology, ed. 3, St. Louis, 1971, The C. V. Mosby Co.)

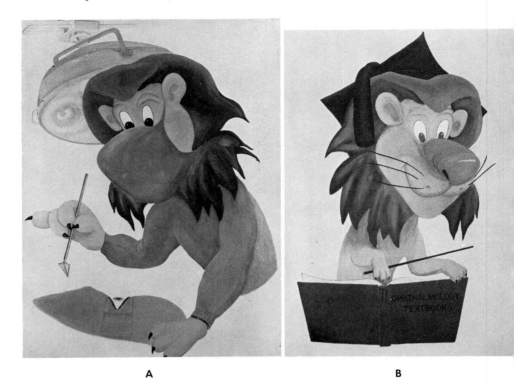

A B

Fig. 14-6. A, Application of presently existing medical knowledge can prevent blindness.
B, Teaching of the importance and methods of proper eye care will prevent blindness.
(From Havener, William H.: Synopsis of ophthalmology, ed. 3, St. Louis, 1973, The C. V.
Mosby Co.)

where else until the eye has been washed thoroughly for *at least fif-*
teen minutes.

2. Wounds penetrating into the eyeball—*Do not touch* these eyes in any
   way! Seek medical care as an immediate emergency. If possible, cover
   the eye with an out-curved metal shield, which will protect against
   any accidental pressure on the eye.
3. Bleeding from the eye or eyelids—*Let it bleed!* The eyeball itself may
   be damaged if pressure is applied to stop bleeding.
4. Foreign body or scratch on the clear cornea—*Do not rub* your eye or
   pick at it. This must be treated with sterile instruments and protected
   against infection by antibiotics. See your physician promptly.
5. Foreign particle on the conjunctiva (white of the eye)—If the particle
   is easily seen, it may be carefully picked out with something clean.
   Do not use a dirty handkerchief. Do not touch the clear cornea!
   If removal is successful and the person is perfectly comfortable and
   sees well, no further treatment is necessary.

6. "Black eye"—See your physician to be certain the eyeball itself has not been damaged (Fig. 14-5).

SUMMARY

Although the United States has the lowest incidence of blindness among major nations, there are now over 300,000 legally blind men, women, and children in the United States, and 30,000 new cases of blindness occur each year. Application of *presently existing medical knowledge* (Fig. 14-6, *A*) could prevent much of this blindness, and our best efforts must be directed toward this goal. *Medical research* must be aggressively directed toward developing as yet undiscovered means of preventing blindness. *Teachers* (Fig. 14-6, *B*) at all levels should tell how, with proper medical care, BLIND-NESS IS PREVENTABLE!

CHAPTER FIFTEEN **Common misconceptions**

The nurse will often encounter erroneous beliefs concerning health and disease. Although many such "old wives' tales" are harmless, some may lead to mismanagement and neglect of serious conditions. Identification of some of the common misconceptions may be helpful as well as interesting.

"The child will outgrow crossed eyes" (Fig. 15-1). This is one of the worst of the old wives' tales, since it is partially true and therefore is widely believed. One form of crossed eyes, resulting from childhood farsightedness, will disappear as the maturing eye becomes less farsighted. This is also the type of crossed eyes that is most effectively corrected by the early prescription of glasses. Unfortunately, if one eye crosses and is not used for a prolonged time during childhood, it will lose vision (suppression amblyopia). Prompt early treatment will restore good vision to such a suppressed eye, but delay till 6 years of age usually dooms the patient to having only one good eye for the rest of his life.

Most crossed eyes will not spontaneously disappear but will require correction by surgery or glasses.

"The child is too young to take to the eye doctor" (Fig. 15-2). This misconception is based upon two false premises—first, that the eye of an uncooperative child cannot be adequately examined and, second, that children are too young to have serious disorders. Actually, since the eye is mostly transparent and therefore can easily be seen, thorough examination can be performed even in very young children. Even measurement for glasses can be done accurately without any need for the child to read a chart or to choose between several lenses.

Serious inflammations, injuries, congenital deformities, and also eye cancers occur in even the youngest children. Approximately one third of children with retinoblastoma (a highly malignant eye cancer) are brought to the doctor because of the complaint of crossed eyes.

"Cataract is a film growing over the surface of the eye." Most people are unaware that cataract is a loss of transparency of a normal part of the eye (lens) and consider the disease to be some type of newly formed membrane. Often the term "cataract" is used as a synonym for any type of blindness.

"Cataracts can be dissolved" (Fig. 15-3). The widespread belief that eye

142

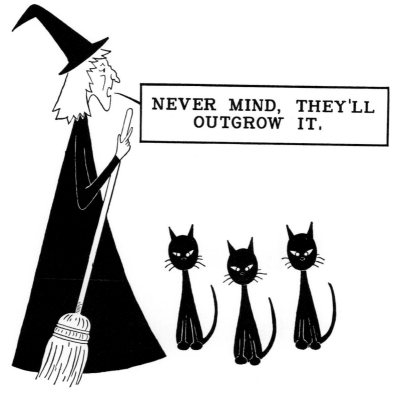

Fig. 15-1. The worst of the old wives' tales advises delay in care of crossed eyes in the mistaken belief that this condition will spontaneously clear.

drops will dissolve cataracts or at least retard their progress originates from the declining but still common medical practice of prescribing eye drops for cataract patients. Most physicians who still prescribe such drops freely acknowledge this as being a placebo, intended to comfort the patient and reassure him that he is "taking care of his eyes." No drops are known that will retard the development of cataracts.

"*A cataract must ripen before surgery.*" With older methods a cataract could not be removed successfully until it was sufficiently far advanced that its interior was partially liquefied. Since the technique of intracapsular extraction has been perfected, the lens may be removed from any patient over 20 years of age at any time. The time for surgery is when the lens is opaque enough to interfere with necessary vision, and it is no longer necessary for an eye to become almost completely blind before the cataract can be removed.

"*The surgeon takes out the eye to operate on it*" (Fig. 15-4). Surprisingly often patients do not believe delicate eye surgery can be performed without removing the eye and placing it on the operating stand. Recently a young

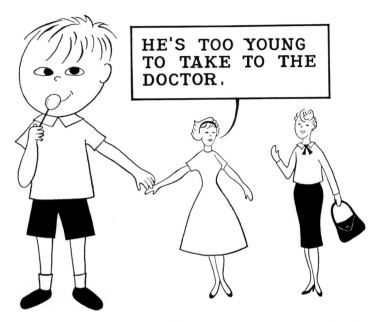

Fig. 15-2. The time to take a cross-eyed child for medical eye examination is as soon as the crossed eyes are first recognized. Even the youngest child can be adequately examined—and is particularly likely to benefit from early care!

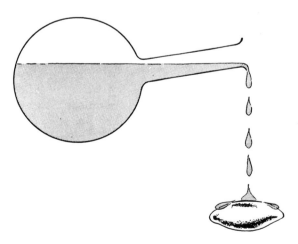

CATARACTS CAN BE DISSOLVED.

Fig. 15-3. Although some doctors do dispense "drops for cataract," these are placebos, intended only to treat the emotional needs of a nervous patient.

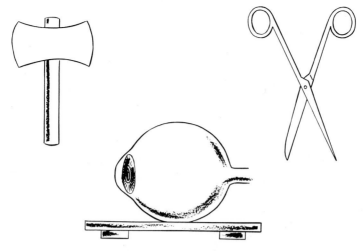

TAKE OUT EYE TO OPERATE

Fig. 15-4. It is surprising how many people believe an eye is removed during surgery and later replaced. This would certainly make eye surgery more convenient, but unfortunately it is impossible.

nursing student asked, "How do you put back the eye when you've finished operating on it?" Naturally the delicate vessels and nerves would be irreparably damaged by removal of the eye, and its replacement is impossible.

"The eye can be transplanted." Only the central part of the cornea can be transplanted. The back part of the eye is much too delicate to tolerate transplant surgery.

"Don't worry about black eyes" (Fig. 14-5). Fortunately eyes are sturdily constructed and often withstand injury without permanent damage. Nevertheless, any blow sufficiently forceful to cause bleeding within the lids may also damage the interior of the eye and warrants medical examination, especially if vision is blurred.

"Redness is a common and insignificant eye change that can safely be disregarded" (Fig. 15-5). Although many minor disorders cause redness, so also do most of the serious diseases of the anterior portion of the eye. Redness probably indicates serious disease if present simultaneously with one or more of the following findings: decreased vision, pain, opacity of the clear parts of the eye, or pupil irregularities.

"Serious eye disease is rare" (Fig. 15-6). Statistics on blindness refute the fallacy that serious eye disease is rare. One in five hundred Americans dies blind in both eyes. One in twenty-five becomes legally blind in one eye during his lifetime. A much greater number of persons suffer partial visual loss or, through prompt seeking of expert medical care, are successfully saved from blindness. In almost every class of medical students there usually will be found several young men who have already lost the sight of one eye. In the sophomore class of fifty, taught during the week this chapter

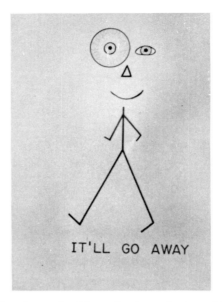

Fig. 15-5. An inflamed, red eye should not be ignored, since this may be one of the signs of serious eye disease.

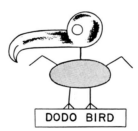

SERIOUS EYE DISEASE IS RARE.

Fig. 15-6. Everyone thinks, "It can't happen to me"; however, 30,000 persons will become blind next year in the United States. Many more will lose the sight of one eye.

was written, one student had an artificial eye and another had an eye useless because of suppression amblyopia.

"Eye symptoms merely require a change of glasses" (Fig. 15-7). The great majority of patients expect (or hope) to find that their recently acquired eye trouble, whatever it may be, can easily be corrected by prescription of proper glasses. Actually the only symptoms likely to be corrected by glasses are discomfort directly related to use of the eyes and decreased visual acuity. Furthermore, these two symptoms may also be caused by serious eye disease.

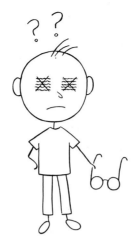

EYE SYMPTOMS JUST
NEED NEW GLASSES.

Fig. 15-7. The symptoms of disease and of refractive error may be similar. Thorough medical eye examination is the only way to be sure of the condition of your eyes.

"Wrong glasses damage eyes" (Fig. 15-8). Fortunately eyes cannot be damaged by wearing faulty glasses or by not wearing necessary glasses. Discomfort or blurred vision may result, but no structural damage or disease will develop. The probable origin of this misconception is the frequency with which nonmedical refractionists overlook the early stages of a serious eye problem and simply prescribe a new pair of glasses. Subsequent to the wearing of these glasses the patient loses eyesight because of the progress of the original disease. Obviously this eye damage is not caused by wearing glasses but by the delay in seeking capable medical attention.

"Wearing glasses makes the wearer dependent upon them." Glasses should not be prescribed or worn unless a real need exists for their use. Frequently the natural course of this condition is slowly progressive (e.g., presbyopia or myopia). Naturally if the condition is progressive, the patient will need glasses more after he has worn them for a year (or, for that matter, if he did not wear them for a year!). Furthermore, having experienced the clear vision obtainable with glasses, most patients with substantial refractive errors are not satisfied with the blurred vision they had previously tolerated.

If unnecessary glasses are prescribed, they will not harm the eye, but eventually they will be discarded because their nuisance value outweighs their benefits. Ophthalmologists know that most of the minor refractive errors present in almost every eye do not require correction. Patients are commonly encountered who have been sold a pair of "window glasses," which are designed to correct an insignificant refractive error. Such prescriptions are a waste of money.

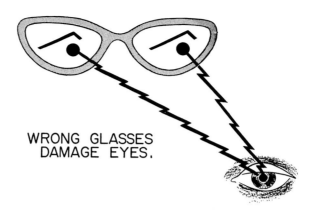

WRONG GLASSES
DAMAGE EYES.

Fig. 15-8. This is one of the most common misconceptions. Although faulty glasses may induce discomfort and fatigue, they cause no damage to the eyes.

"Exercises will correct refractive errors." Errors of refraction are determined by the length and curvatures of the eye. These are genetically controlled characteristics, just as is a person's height. Refractive error and height are characteristics that cannot be altered by exercises. Charlatans abound in all health fields, preying upon the gullible, and among their claims is "discard glasses through exercises."

"Misuse of eyes in childhood results in a need for glasses in old age." Presbyopia forces everyone to wear reading glasses in old age—unless they are myopic, in which case they need glasses for distance. This would be more accurately phrased, "Not dying before 45 years of age results in a need for glasses"!

"Ignore blurred vision" (Fig. 15-9). Not only is blurred vision an unnecessary handicap (if it can be corrected with glasses), but it may be an effective warning signal (if caused by serious disease). The function of the eyes is to see, and malfunction of such an important sense cannot safely be disregarded.

"Reading in the dark is harmful to eyes" (Fig. 15-10). Clarity and efficiency of vision is certainly reduced by inadequate lighting, and fatigue may result from prolonged, poorly lighted work. However, no structural damage to the eye results from such use. Children do not "ruin their eyes" by reading in dim light after bedtime.

"Television hurts eyes" (Fig. 15-11). The light rays emerging from a television tube do not contain any harmful radiations different from the radiant energy of ordinary sunlight. Certainly the intensity of light from a television set is only a tiny fraction of the brightness of sunlight—which we do not fear as being harmful to eyes. Excessive watching of television whodunits may stunt intellectual development but will not damage eyesight.

"Reading on your stomach hurts eyes." Reading on your stomach does

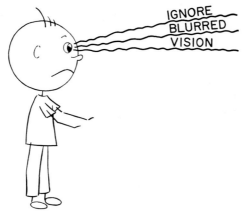

Fig. 15-9. Blurred vision is a warning signal of eye disorder. Although often caused by refractive error, blurring may be an early sign of serious disease.

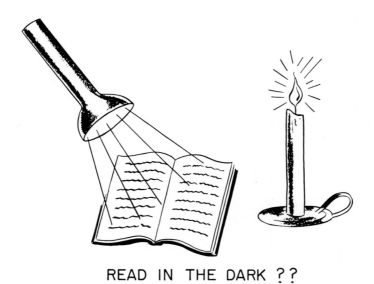

READ IN THE DARK ??

Fig. 15-10. Contrary to popular belief, reading in the dark is not harmful to the eyes.

not hurt your eyes, neither does reading with the book "too close" or "too far away," or on a train, or in bed, or before breakfast, etc.

"If one eye has been lost, use of the remaining eye will strain or damage it." Many serious eye diseases are often bilateral (e.g., glaucoma, senile macular degeneration, and retinal detachment); hence loss of one eye may be followed by deterioration of the second. This sequence of events may be misinterpreted as resulting from use of the eyes. Approximately one person in every twenty-five has only one useful eye. These individuals should exer-

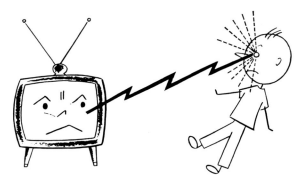

TV HURTS EYES.

Fig. 15-11. Although constant watching of television may be of doubtful benefit to intellectual development (especially some programs!), this will not damage eyesight.

cise every care to avoid injury to their remaining eye, but they may use it freely for visual purposes.

"Sight-saving classes help eyes." This is simply a more cheerful way of saying "classes for half-blind children." These classes use books with large print and rely more heavily upon nonvisual teaching methods. These specialized teaching methods certainly help the education of a handicapped child but neither help nor harm his eyes.

"A person with failing sight should save his eyes." One of the most tragic mistakes possible results when a person faced with slowly progressive and inevitable blindness because of an incurable disease "saves" his eyes. This misconception needlessly wastes the months or years of reading, sewing, or other visual pleasures that should be enjoyed while sight permits. Loss of these pleasures will come all too soon from the slowly progressive darkness and will not be postponed one moment by not using the eyes. Such patients should be encouraged to use their eyes as much as they are able, without fear of accelerated damage.

"Try my good eye drops." Some people trade prescriptions for eye drops just as they exchange home remedies for headache or athlete's foot. This practice naïvely presupposes that all eye ailments are identical. When the exchanged drop happens to be atropine, the recipient learns the hard way (through loss of accommodation for a week or more) that this practice is unwise.

"Vitamins are good for your eyes" (Fig. 15-12). Since the discovery that vitamin deficiencies can cause night blindness (vitamin A), corneal damage (vitamin A), optic neuritis (vitamin B), and many other disorders, the promotion and sale of vitamins has become a national scandal. No evidence exists that more than the required amount of vitamins will enhance eye health. In fact, excessive vitamin A may cause increased intracranial pressure and papilledema. Since flour, milk, and other foods have been enriched

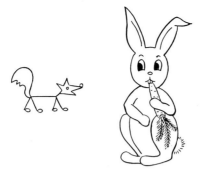

VITAMINS ARE GOOD FOR YOUR EYES.

Fig. 15-12. Vitamins are like water in an automobile radiator. Enough is vitally necessary; an excessive amount is wasted and may do more harm than good. Vitamin A intoxication, for example, damages the optic nerve. Vitamin supplements do not help any eye disorder, except the rare specific deficiences.

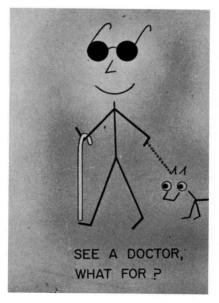

Fig. 15-13. It is amazing how long some people will put off seeking medical care.

and fortified with additional vitamins, it is almost impossible to find a vitamin-deficient patient in the United States.

"There's no use in seeing an eye doctor" (Fig. 15-13). The National Society for the Prevention of Blindness estimates that fully half of the blindness in the United States is needless and is preventable by early use of existing medical knowledge.

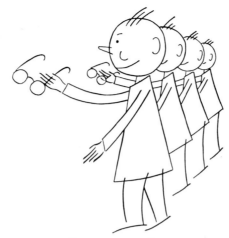

ALL EYE "DOCTORS" ARE THE SAME.

Fig. 15-14. Great variation exists in the skill and training of eye "doctors."

"All eye doctors are the same" (Fig. 15-14). Considerable variations exist in the ability and skills of different persons, to say nothing of the differences in educational backgrounds. The best way (although not perfect) to select an eye specialist is to find a man certified by the American Board of Ophthalmology. The background attested to by such certification is more likely to prevent blindness than any other type of training program in the United States today. It must be emphasized here that the optometrist is not a physician and is not medically trained or qualified.

SUMMARY

Although some of these misconceptions are quite amusing and really harmless, others result in serious errors in eye care. Many well-educated persons accept a surprising number of these fallacies as truth. Educational programs for nurses should include sufficient information about eye health and disease to permit the nurse to advise her friends, relatives, and patients intelligently concerning eye care.

The patient with ear, nose, and throat disorders

The nurse's role in otolaryngology is an important and diverse one; one reason is that the field itself is the broadest of the surgical specialties, encompassing virtually all diseases of the head and neck with the exception of the brain and eye. Medical or nonsurgical treatment is also an important part of otolaryngology since patients are seen daily with headache, vertigo, tinnitus, cough, sore throat, loss of hearing, sinusitis, earache, and a host of other complaints related to the head and neck area. On the surgical side of the specialty there are operations involving major resection and reconstructions such as laryngectomy, radical neck dissection, glossectomy, parotidectomy, mandibulectomy, and maxillectomy; operations utilizing special endoscopic instrument for study of the larynx, trachea, and bronchoesophageal areas; operations on the middle and inner ears requiring extremely delicate instruments and 10 to 16 times magnification; and facial plastic surgery such as otoplasty, rhinoplasty, and facelift. Most major head and neck tumor surgery is now performed by an otolaryngologist.

To be effective in this setting, nurses, both student and graduate, require basic understanding of the structure and function of the organ systems involved. They need knowledge of the disease processes affecting these systems, and information about treatment. Nurse practitioners in the hospital, both those working on an otolaryngology service and those on other services, nurses serving in extended care and other community facilities, nurses working as office assistants, nurses in the operating room—all should be acquainted with the fundamentals of otolaryngology.

CHAPTER SIXTEEN   # Oral cavity and pharynx; salivary glands

Examination of the ears, nose, and throat is basically a study of epithelium. Using brilliant illumination, the physician is able to inspect directly or indirectly most parts of the upper respiratory passages. A few parts, such as the nasal accessory sinuses and the middle ear, cannot be visualized. Nevertheless, the examiner is usually able to infer their condition by the appearance of adjacent mucous membranes.

The basic set of instruments needed for examination is rather simple (Figs. 16-1 and 16-2). Instruments are cleaned and sterilized after use but are not sterile when used on the next patient. Some special instruments, not used regularly, will be illustrated later.

ORAL CAVITY

The oral cavity is lined with squamous mucosa. This type of mucous membrane is several layers thick and therefore relatively resistant to trauma. It is admirably suited to the oral cavity where there is more opportunity for trauma, for example, from eating and chewing, than there is in most other parts of the body lined by mucous membrane. It connects above with the nasopharynx and below with the hypopharynx, which leads into the lower respiratory and food passages. The ducts of the major and minor salivary glands empty into the oral cavity; they provide saliva for assistance in mastication and provide enzymes as part of the digestive process. The disorders affecting the oral cavity include congenital malformations, trauma, inflammation and infection, neoplasms, and of course all of the disorders that affect the teeth.

The nurse must have knowledge of the normal appearance of the oral cavity since she frequently is required to look into the mouth and make observations during both health and disease. She should know such things as the normal color of the oral mucous membranes, the location of the tonsils, the appearance of the tongue and teeth, and the sites where the major salivary glands drain into the oral cavity. Only then will she be able to appreciate the common abnormal conditions such as acute tonsillitis, bleeding from the nose which may appear in the mouth, or bleeding after tonsillectomy, ulcerative tumors, etc. Fortunately the oral cavity is relatively easy for the nurse to examine using only a bright light and a tongue blade.

155

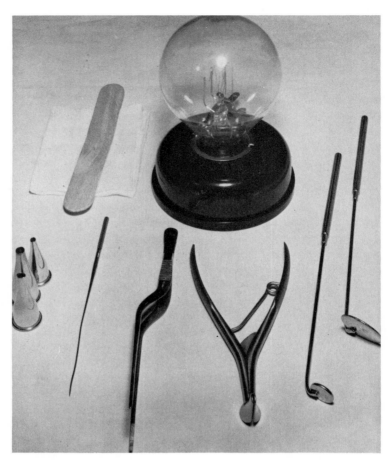

Fig. 16-1. Instruments used in ear, nose, and throat examination: three aural specula, tongue depressor and gauze, cotton applicator, bayonet forceps, nasal speculum, No. 0 mirror, No. 5 mirror, and 150-watt clear bulb.

The tongue

Normal appearance. The tongue is covered on its dorsal surface with several different papillae: filiform, fungiform, and circumvallate. Normal variations and pathologic changes in these papillae may vary or alter the surface appearance of the tongue. If the filiform papillae became keratinized, the tongue has a white coating. If they are stained by tobacco or chromogenic organisms, the tongue looks brown or black.

The undersurface of the tongue is smooth and is attached anteriorly to the floor of the mouth by the frenum. On each side of the frenum and just behind the lower central incisor teeth are the two openings of the ducts of the submandibular salivary glands (Wharton's ducts). Posteriorly the tongue

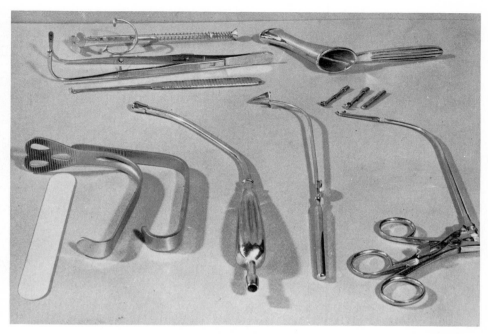

Fig. 16-2. Some special instruments. **Top:** Soft palate retractor, cotton holder for anesthesia of larynx, tonsillar pillar retractor, and direct nasopharyngoscope. **Bottom:** Wooden and two metal tongue depressors, tonsil and adenoid sucker, epiglottis retractor, and laryngeal biopsy forceps.

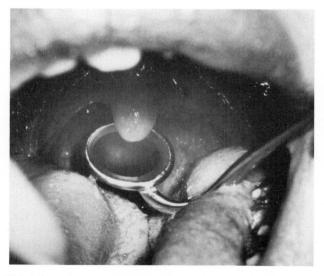

Fig. 16-3. Mirror in place behind uvula for examination of nasopharynx.

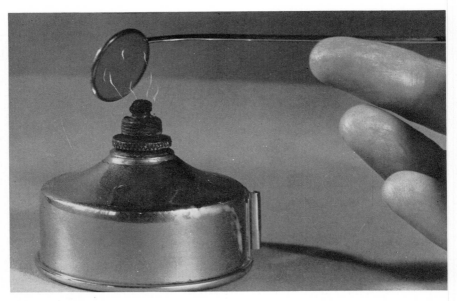

Fig. 16-4. Warming the mirror. (From DeWeese, David D., and Saunders, William H.: Textbook of otolaryngology, ed. 4, St. Louis, 1973, The C. V. Mosby Co.

is joined to the soft palate, the epiglottis, and the pharynx by folds of mucous membrane and by muscle.

The normal color of the dorsum of the tongue varies from day to day and from person to person, depending upon what has been eaten and also upon the degree of keratinization of the filiform papillae. Not much emphasis should be placed on the color of the tongue as an indication of general health. A dry tongue may indicate a general condition of dehydration, or it may mean only that the patient is a mouth breather because of nasal obstruction.

Lesions of the tongue

Black hairy tongue. Sometimes the papillae are greatly elongated and infected with fungi. Usually such a tongue is dark, and we say the patient has *lingua nigrans,* or *black hairy tongue* (Fig. 16-6). If patients with hairy tongue smoke, they should stop. If they are using antibiotic lozenges or taking antibiotics systemically, they also should stop because antibiotics, by reducing the bacterial flora, permit an overgrowth of fungi and favor development of hairy tongue. Clearing the patient of his hairy tongue is not always easy. The elongated hairlike papillae may have to be shaved or scraped off. Brushing of the tongue at the time of cleaning the teeth may help to remove an undesirable coating. Frequently the condition recurs.

Median rhomboid glossitis. In median rhomboid glossitis (Fig. 16-7)

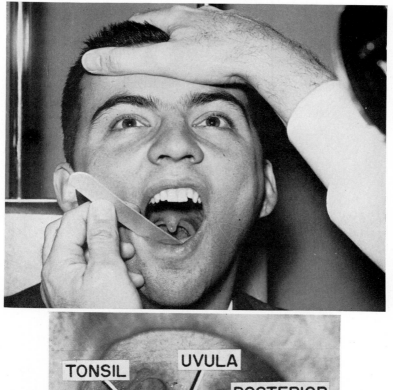

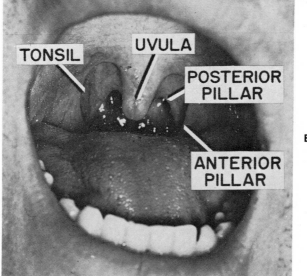

TONSIL UVULA POSTERIOR PILLAR ANTERIOR PILLAR

Fig. 16-5. A, Depressing the tongue. The tongue blade is held in the left hand, which leaves the right hand free for positioning of the head and the use of other instruments. The hand is braced on the patient's check as the tongue is depressed and scooped forward. **B,** Landmarks of the pharynx. (**A** from Saunders, William H.: Ears, nose, and throat. In Prior, John A., and Silberstein, Jack S.: Physical diagnosis, ed. 4, St. Louis, 1973, The C. V. Mosby Co.)

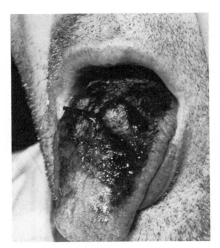

Fig. 16-6. So-called "black hairy tongue," or lingua nigrans; these are elongated filiform papillae.

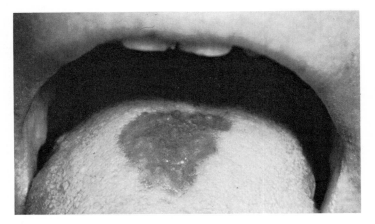

Fig. 16-7. Median rhomboid glossitis.

there is a lozenge-shaped area on the back of the tongue that fails to develop papillae. The surrounding tongue looks normal, but the one area is slick and red because blood vessels in the submucosa shine through the thin epithelium. There are no symptoms.

Geographic tongue. In geographic tongue (Fig. 16-8), a rather common condition, some of the filiform papillae desquamate, and the remaining papillae stand out in contrast with the desquamated or denuded areas to produce a pattern. Eventually other parts of the tongue desquamate while previously denuded areas heal. Because the pattern changes, geographic tongue is also called migratory glossitis. There are no symptoms, and it does not predispose to infection or malignancy.

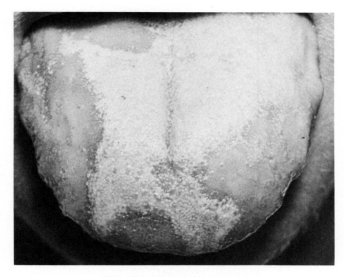

Fig. 16-8. Geographic tongue.

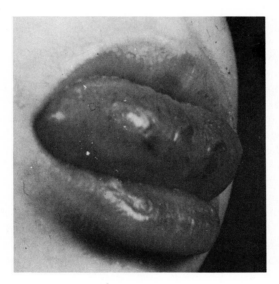

Fig. 16-9. Lingual abscess.

Lingual abscess. Lingual abscess (Fig. 16-9) is a very painful and potentially dangerous condition. It may result from trauma or a foreign body or spread from an adjacent infection. If the tongue swells enough, tracheotomy may be necessary to provide an airway. The nurse should observe the patient carefully for signs of increasing respiratory obstruction such as noisy respiration, cyanosis, or increasing apprehension. Treatment of lingual abscess is by incision and drainage and administration of appropriate antibiotics.

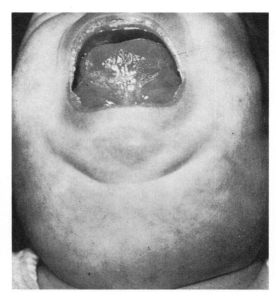

Fig. 16-10. Cystic hygroma, or cavernous lymphangioma. Note how the tongue is pushed up from the floor of the mouth.

Mouthwashes might be of some assistance, but irrigations with hot saline would help more. If an incision has been made to drain the abscess, it should be kept open. Irrigations help to do this, and once a day a hemostat may have to be inserted into the incision. It is rather difficult to get a drainage tube to stay in place in an organ as mobile as the tongue.

Cavernous lymphangioma. Cavernous lymphangioma (Fig. 16-10) is an abnormal condition caused by massive overgrowth of the normal lymphatic system so that the glands and lymph vessels become masses of dilated lymphatics forming a tumor. In the tongue these dilated and proliferating lymphatics cause great enlargement (macroglossia). The condition in the tongue is sometimes part of a similar lymphangioma of the cervical region called *hygroma colli.* Treatment is by excision of part of the tongue.

Tumor. A tumor at the base of the tongue may obstruct lymphatics or cause hemorrhage into the tongue and impair the airway (Fig. 16-11). A more common cause of macroglossia is a hematoma (Fig. 16-12) from trauma, such as might follow an automobile accident or a fight. Again tracheotomy may be necessary.

Paralysis. Paralysis of the tongue (Fig. 16-13) is caused by interference with its motor nerve supply, the hypoglossal or twelfth cranial nerve. This nerve runs through a foramina at the base of the skull and crosses the upper neck to eventually supply the musculature of the tongue, one nerve on each side. Paralysis may result from invasion of the nerve by neoplasm, infections such as poliomyelitis, or trauma. A cerebral vascular accident also may cause paralysis of the hypoglossal nerve.

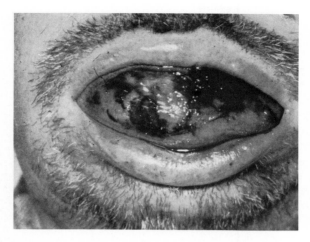

Fig. 16-11. Swelling of the tongue secondary to lymphatic obstruction by a tumor at the base of the tongue; also some bleeding into the tongue.

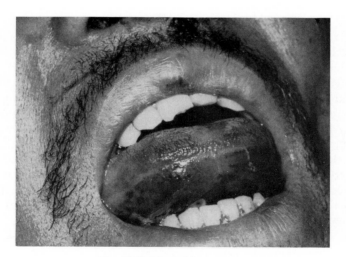

Fig. 16-12. Lingual hematoma.

When the normal tongue is protruded it ordinarily remains in the midline, but in hypoglossal paralysis the strong side pushes the paralyzed side away, and the tongue deviates toward the weak side. Unilateral paralysis produces, surprisingly, almost no symptoms. The patient can eat and speak normally. Bilateral paralysis, on the other hand, is extremely debilitating, and the patient has great trouble with speech or swallowing. Fortunately this is a rare condition.

Tongue tie. Tongue tie is less common than generally thought. If the patient can protrude his tongue even a little beyond the teeth, he will have no

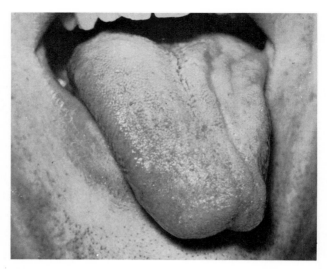

Fig. 16-13. Hypoglossal paralysis. One side of the tongue shows atrophy, and the tongue deviates toward the weak side.

speech difficulty. Clipping of the frenum, which binds the tongue to the floor of the mouth, is easy but rarely needed.

Laceration. Lacerations of the tongue are common. They should be sutured carefully or the edges will heal irregularly. Although almost any type of suture material can be used in the tongue, knots must be tied carefully because they frequently untie in this moist, mobile organ.

Care of the mouth during the healing period is important but should not be too vigorous, since the sutures must not be dislodged. Saline mouth irrigation is as good as anything. Commercial preparations recommended as bacteriostatic do not serve this purpose and can be considered only as local cleansing agents no more effective than saline. Preparations such as hydrogen peroxide, usually provided as a diluted mixture of one part peroxide to two parts water, are effective, particularly when anaerobic organisms are predominant. In certain instances the uses of so-called water pics or other pressure sprays may be of considerable value for improving oral hygiene of the gums. Application of cream or petrolatum to the lips will prevent cracking and chapping; this is particularly important in some patients who are mouth breathers or who must temporarily breathe through their mouths because of nasal fractures.

The palate

The palate has two parts—soft and hard. The soft palate is a muscular structure covered above (nasal surface) and below (oral surface) with mucous membrane. Its muscles are strong and serve to close off the nasal cavity during phonation of certain sounds (for example, "k," "kick") and during swallowing. When the patient has palatal paralysis as a result of cerebral vascular accident or tumor, or when the palate has a surgical or other defect, liquids may come out the nose when he drinks, and he has a "nasal voice." The nurse may instruct the patient that, by closing his nose with his fingers, drinking becomes easier. The palate also assists in the formation of intelligible speech. The palate, along with the lips and the tongue, forms part of the "molds of speech."

The hard palate is part of the maxillary bone and is covered above and below by mucous membrane. Its upper surface forms the floor of the nasal chamber, and its lower surface forms the anterior part of the roof of the mouth. It is the part of the mouth covered by an upper denture.

Lesions of the palate

Torus palatinus. Torus palatinus is an exostosis, or overgrowth of bone, in the midline of the hard palate (Fig. 16-14). A relatively common condition, most tori are not nearly as large as the one illustrated in Fig. 16-14. Ordinarily it causes no difficulty, but some times if the patient requires an upper denture, the torus must be removed. Similar exostoses associated with the mandible are called torus mandibulare. Usually there are two or three on each side of the mandible near the midline.

Nicotine stomatitis. Nicotine stomatitis, the result of excessive smoking, produces changes in both the hard and the soft palates (Fig. 16-15). At first there is a blanching of the hard palate but a hyperemia of the soft palate. Later, orifices of the mucous glands in the hard palate become red and surrounded by a raised border. Finally, there may be actual ulceration, and the palate looks parboiled and fissured.

Bifid uvula (Fig. 16-16). Bifid uvula occurs commonly. Its significance is that the patient may also have a submucous cleft of the soft palate. This means that, although the mucous membrane of the palate is intact, the muscular tissues of the two halves of the palate are not joined firmly in the midline, and so by palpating the soft palate in the midline one can feel a weakness or a cleft. In these patients a poor voice may result after adenoidectomy, since with an insufficiency of muscular tissue the palate is weak and cannot close forcibly against the posterior pharyngeal wall as it normally does. If the child has a large pad of adenoid, the soft palate does not have to stretch far in closing the nasopharynx, and usually there are no symptoms; but with the adenoid removed, the postnasal space is much larger, and the weak palate fails to close off the nasopharynx.

Some surgeons will not remove the adenoid in a patient with bifid uvula for fear of producing a poor voice. In any case, if the operation is to be done, the parents should be told of the difficulty that may develop postoperatively.

Acute edema of the uvula (Quincke's disease) (Fig. 16-17). In acute edema, the uvula may become greatly swollen in a short time as the result of unusual sensitivity to a drug or other allergen. Both uvula and soft palate look pale and swollen, and sometimes there is an associated hoarseness—an ominous symptom indicating laryngeal edema as well.

Treatment with epinephrine by injection is the treatment of choice.

Also useful are intravenous corticosteroids and antihistaminics. If there is also laryngeal edema, the physician must be prepared to pass an endotracheal tube or perform a tracheotomy to maintain the airway.

Squamous papilloma. Squamous papilloma (Fig. 16-18) of the soft palate and uvula is common. These wartlike growths hang from the free edge of

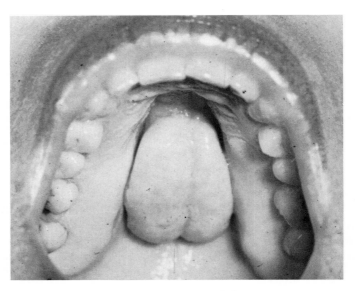

Fig. 16-14. Large torus palatinus.

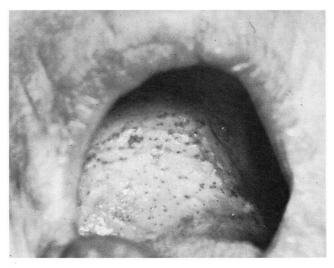

Fig. 16-15. Nicotine stomatitis. In some heavy smokers the hard palate develops a cooked appearance, and the orifices of the mucous glands stand out prominently.

the soft palate or uvula but cause no symptoms and never become malignant. They may be removed if the patient wishes, but it is unnecessary.

Pyorrhea. Pyorrhea, or periodontoclasia (Fig. 16-19), is a common disease and one that is largely preventable, since ordinarily it starts as a simple gingivitis. In late stages pyorrhea causes loosening and loss of teeth. Any

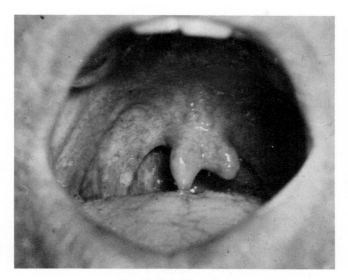

Fig. 16-16. Bifid uvula.

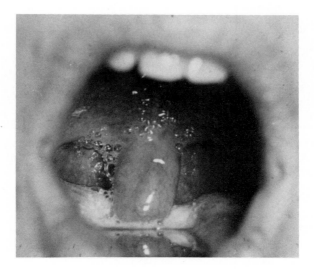

Fig. 16-17. Edematous uvula in patient with acute drug sensitivity.

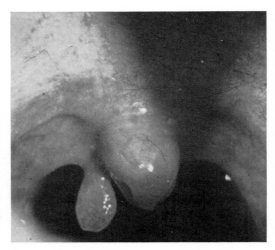

Fig. 16-18. Typical squamous papilloma. (From DeWeese, David D., and Saunders, William H.: Textbook of otolaryngology, ed. 4, St. Louis, 1973, The C. V. Mosby Co.)

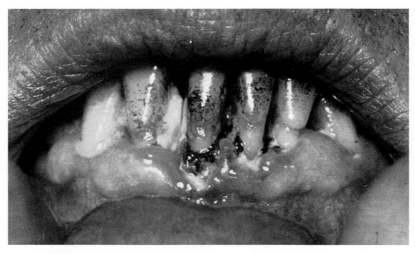

Fig. 16-19. Advanced pyorrhea. (From DeWeese, David D., and Saunders, William H.: Textbook of otolaryngology, ed. 4, St. Louis, 1973, The C. V. Mosby Co.)

patient with bleeding or swollen gums should be urged to see his dentist for treatment.

Hyperplasia. Hyperplasia of the gingiva is sometimes caused by drug toxicity. For example, diphenylhydantoin (Dilantin), which is an antiepileptic drug, sometimes causes massive hyperplasia or overgrowth of the gums. Pregnant women sometimes have bleeding from the gums, and there

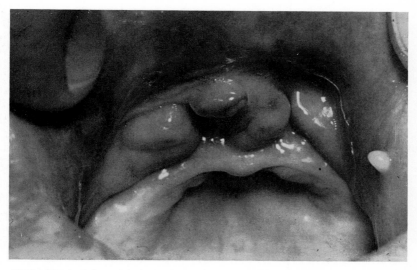

Fig. 16-20. Gingival hyperplasia resulting from an ill-fitting denture. (From DeWeese, David D., and Saunders, William H.: Textbook of otolaryngology, ed. 4, St. Louis, 1973, The C. V. Mosby Co.)

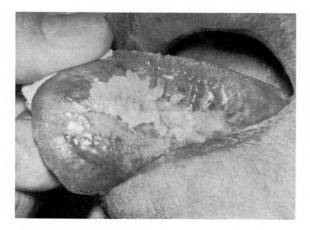

Fig. 16-21. Leukoplakia on the undersurface of the tongue.

may be localized gingival swellings, called *pregnancy epulis.* The condition recedes spontaneously after pregnancy. *Giant cell epulis,* which also causes bleeding from a tumor of the gingiva, is usually associated with a focus of osteomyelitis near a tooth root. Treatment is by excision of the epulis and correction of the underlying infection of the tooth or bone.

Recession of the gums with age. Normally as age advances there is a recession of the gums so that more and more of the tooth is exposed. The old expression "getting long in the tooth" refers to advancing age.

Ill-fitting dentures may produce masses of hyperplastic mucosa (Fig. 16-20) in the sulcus under the lip where the flange of the plate is loose and rubs and grinds. The same condition occurs in the mucosa of the palate covered by the upper plate. There is improvement after the denture is removed. The final treatment, of course, is for the patient to see his dentist for relining of his present denture or the making of a new denture.

Leukoplakia

Leukoplakia ("white plaque") may occur anywhere in the oral cavity, but it is most common on the tongue (Fig. 16-21), the gingiva, and the lower lip. It is considered a premalignant lesion. The cause is usually an irritant: the sun's rays on the lower lip (more exposed than the upper lip), smoking, a jagged tooth, or an ill-fitting denture. Everything possible should be done to remove such sources of irritation. When feasible, the leukoplakia is excised or destroyed with fulguration. Sometimes, however, leukoplakia is too widespread for local excision, and the most one can do is to observe the involved area periodically to make sure that carcinomatous changes do not occur.

Squamous cell carcinoma

Squamous cell carcinoma of the oral cavity is fairly common. Most physicians believe that smoking is a significant factor in the production of oral cancer, just as it is in laryngeal and lung cancer. Poor oral hygiene can result in gingivitis, dental caries, broken teeth, pyorrhea, and glossitis. These conditions, when improperly treated or ignored, are a source of chronic irritation—one of the precursors of carcinoma. Most physicians also feel that preexisting syphilis is one of the causes of oral cancer, especially cancer of the tongue. Therefore the nurse needs to *observe* the oral hygiene of her patients and to *teach* good oral hygiene. Patients with broken teeth, ill-fitting dentures, and gingivitis should be referred for dental care.

Oral cancer is usually found to involve the tongue (Fig. 16-22), the floor of the mouth (Fig. 16-23), the tonsillar pillars, or the lower lip (Fig. 16-24). Most forms of oral cancer are serious because they tend to spread rapidly and metastasize to regional lymph nodes in either side of the neck and also to the lung. If the lesions are found early, of course, the prognosis is much better than when they have become large. Because there is not always ulceration of the mucous membrane, palpation with the gloved finger is important in examining the patient for carcinoma. A mass that cannot be seen may sometimes be readily felt with the finger. Ordinarily, however, the patient with oral carcinoma presents all too familiar a picture. There is a large painful ulcer that bleeds easily, and its margins are indurated. Lymphadenopathy representing metastases is frequently present when the patient is first seen.

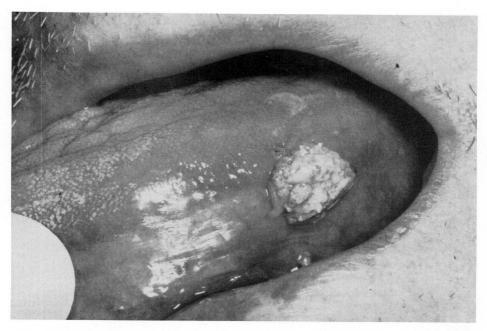

Fig. 16-22. Localized, exophytic squamous cell carcinoma. Some lesions looking like this will represent hyperkeratosis or other nonmalignant conditions. (From Saunders, William H.: Ears, nose, and throat. In Prior, John A., and Silberstein, Jack S.: Physical diagnosis, ed. 4, St. Louis, 1973, The C. V. Mosby Co.)

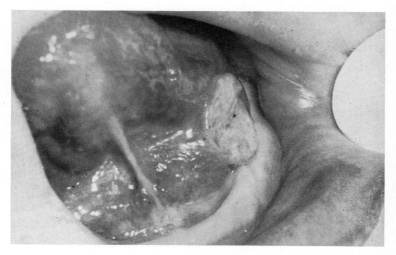

Fig. 16-23. Squamous cell carcinoma. This condition is treated by local excision, although often a radical neck dissection is done in conjunction with excision of the primary tumor.

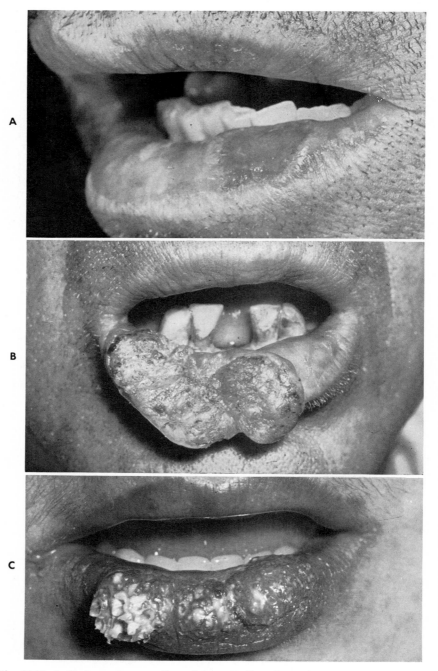

Fig. 16-24. A, Early squamous cell carcinoma. **B,** Far-advanced squamous cell carcinoma. Bilateral cervical metastases were present. **C,** Superficial squamous cell carcinoma and leukoplakia of the lower lip. (From DeWeese, David D., and Saunders, William H.: Textbook of otolaryngology, ed. 4, St. Louis, 1973, The C. V. Mosby Co.)

Most important of all is for the physician to recognize cancer when it occurs and to obtain promptly a specimen for examination. Removal of tissue (biopsy) in the oral cavity is easy and not likely to cause excessive bleeding. It is done as an office procedure using local anesthesia. Sutures are usually not required since the amount of tissue removed is small. The patient is not apt to have postoperative pain but he may require aspirin or other mild analgesics and should be told to eat soft food for a day or two if his regular diet causes pain.

Treatment is by surgical excision or by irradiation therapy. If surgical excision is used, the operation may be relatively minor, as in excising a small carcinoma from the lip or a small carcinoma from the anterior aspect of the tongue or floor of the mouth. Local excision with primary closure is effective treatment for small lesions but when the tumor has become large, a much more extensive and serious operative procedure is required. A large carcinoma of the lip, for example, may involve excision of almost all of the lower lip and then reconstruction, using a pedicle flap from the upper lip or other adjacent tissue. A large malignant lesion of the tongue often involves resection of more than half of the tongue and sometimes even all of the tongue (total glossectomy). Such an operation is usually combined with radical neck dissection of one or both sides since there is a likelihood of metastasis having occurred to the lymph glands in the neck.

Reconstructive techniques are of great importance in these cases, since the patient needs as much postoperative function as possible and as early as possible. Therefore preoperative planning often includes a careful laying out and diagramming of a suitable pedicle flap—for example, a forehead flap (Fig. 24-15, *D*), which can be used to close the operative defect in the oral cavity. The nurse should assess the patient's oral hygiene and institute care to ensure that the patient has a clean mouth, including his tongue and teeth. The nurse should also see that the patient's hair is shampooed and that he is clean-shaven just before surgery.

The nurse's postoperative responsibility is most important. Not only is this patient likely to have considerable pain, requiring the use of analgesics such as codeine and meperidine (Demerol), but also his airway is apt to be in danger. Frequently a tracheotomy is in place and this may be the patient's only airway for several days postoperatively. Therefore the nurse must make certain that the tracheotomy tubes are tied securely and that the inner cannula of the tracheotomy is kept free (see Chapter 26). She also can use mouth care very effectively in this instance. The patient often has many sutures in his oral cavity which require cleaning as they collect blood and mucus; this can be accomplished by gentle irrigation with saline or weak hydrogen peroxide solution or by the use of cotton applicators soaked with such medications. Since the lips are apt to chap and crack, they can be kept lubricated with petrolatum or cream. Bleeding from the resection site should be noted by the nurse and reported immediately. Fever in the postoperative period associated with tenderness and swelling in the neck indicates that a fistula is forming.

PHARYNX
Diseases and inflammations

From the standpoint of physical examination the pharynx should be thought of as being divided into three parts: epipharynx (nasopharynx), oropharynx, and hyopharynx. Proper examination of the oropharynx (Fig. 16-15) requires a bright light and a tongue blade; of the nasopharynx, a bright light and a mirror to look above the palate (Fig. 16-4); of the hypopharynx, a bright light and a large mirror. This concept of the need for three different instruments is important because often the mistake is made of examining only the oropharynx—a bare one-third of the total mucosal surface of the pharynx (Fig. 16-26).

The nasopharynx communicates with the nasal cavity through the posterior choanae, while the hypopharynx leads downward from the oropharynx toward the trachea and esophagus (Fig. 16-25).

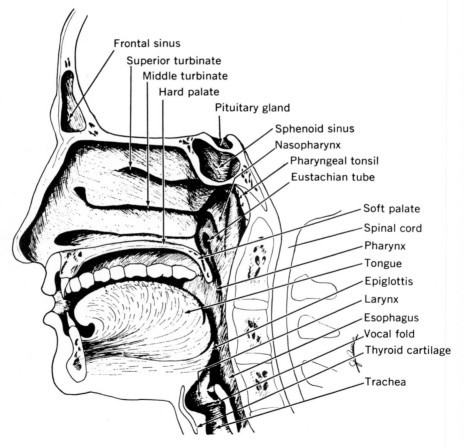

Frontal sinus
Superior turbinate
Middle turbinate
Hard palate
Pituitary gland
Sphenoid sinus
Nasopharynx
Pharyngeal tonsil
Eustachian tube
Soft palate
Spinal cord
Pharynx
Tongue
Epiglottis
Larynx
Esophagus
Vocal fold
Thyroid cartilage
Trachea

Fig. 16-25. Section of the head. Note the area of the pharynx, the relationship of other structures, and openings into the nasal canal. (From Gragg, S. H., and Rees, O. M.: Scientific principles in nursing, ed. 7, St. Louis, 1974, The C. V. Mosby Co.)

Waldeyer's ring is a collection of lymphoid tissue in the pharynx consisting of the adenoid or pharyngeal tonsil, the palatine or faucial tonsils, the lingual tonsils, and the lateral pharyngeal bands. Palatine or faucial tonsils are those collections of lymphoid tissue most persons refer to when speaking of their "tonsils." Infection in any of this lymphoid tissue is common. All parts of Waldeyer's ring are more prominent in children than in adults; in adults the adenoid frequently regresses almost completely.

Viral or bacterial infection. Acute infections of the pharynx are caused by viruses or bacteria. During the common cold, a viral infection, there is a feeling of burning and scratchiness in the nasopharynx. Infectious mononucleosis, probably a viral disease, is another cause of nasopharyngitis, and usually it causes severe mucous membrane ulceration, exudate, and systemic manifestations. Viral infections in children are especially common and account for more than 90% of all infections of the pharynx. Therefore one should not treat most cases of pharyngitis in children with antibiotics since these drugs are not effective against viruses.

Bacterial infections of the pharynx, especially those caused by the streptococcus, are also common; severe sore throat and chills and a temperature to 102° F. or higher are present. The patient may be unable to swallow because of pain. Treatment for streptococcal infection of the throat is with penicillin (the drug of choice) or other antibiotics. Treatment may prevent the occasional development of rheumatic heart disease or glomerular nephritis. Complications such as septicemia or infection of one of the potential spaces about the pharynx are seen occasionally, although they are much less common now than in the days before antibiotic drugs. Parapharyngeal abscess is one of these space infections and peritonsillar abscess or quinsy is another, more common one (see p. 177).

Acute tonsillitis (see also Chapter 17). Treatment of acute tonsillitis with antibiotics is usually successful. Throat irrigations with hot saline solution are also helpful. Tonsillectomy is indicated when a patient has recurrent tonsillitis. In children, adenoidectomy is usually done at the time of tonsillectomy, but in adults the adenoid has often atrophied and only tonsillectomy is required.

Lingual tonsillitis. Lingual tonsillitis, although not as common as infections of the palatine tonsils or of the adenoid, should not be overlooked. To see the lingual tonsils one must use a large laryngeal mirror; remember that one can see only a third of the pharynx with a tongue blade. Many patients with nasopharyngitis or lingual tonsillitis go without correct diagnosis because of the physician's failure to employ mirrors for examination. Acute lingual tonsillitis causes essentially the same symptoms as does acute palatine or faucial tonsillitis. The patient has a severe sore throat, difficulty in swallowing, fever, and malaise. Treatment is with penicillin, because the most likely organism is the streptococcus. If there seems to be any doubt, cultures should be made and antibiotic sensitivity tests done to determine the exact organism and the exact choice of antibiotic. Chronic lingual tonsillitis in adults causes persistent mild sore throat and low-grade fever. Treatment of recurrent acute or chronic lingual tonsillitis is lingual tonsillectomy under general anesthesia.

Chronic tonsillitis. Chronic tonsillitis is a term that is frequently misused. Often it is employed to describe any type of sore throat in a patient who still has his tonsils. Actually the diagnosis is hard to make for several reasons: patients thought to have chronic tonsillitis may have recurrent episodes of acute tonsillitis; the mere appearance of large tonsils does not mean that they are infected; and white, cheesy plugs of debris seen in many tonsils are not necessarily abnormal (this debris forms in tonsillar crypts by desquamation of the squamous mucosa lining the crypt).

Pharyngitis. Pharyngitis not associated with acute tonsillitis is also common. Patients should be told that after tonsillectomy they may again develop sore throats, since the mucous membranes and the remaining lymphoid tissue of the pharynx can also become infected. Treatment of pharyngitis is with antibiotics, if necessary, and saline irrigations. Gargling is less useful than irrigations, since in gargling, liquids do not reach the posterior parts of the pharynx. Many patients who complain of sore throat do not have an infection at all. Some are mouth breathers (especially at night), and the drying of their pharyngeal mucosa produces discomfort. Their throats feel scratchy and irritated in the morning but improve later in the day. In general, any patient with sore throat lasting only a few hours should not be considered to have an infection, since infections do not clear this quickly.

Humidification is of considerable help to some patients with chronic throat conditions. A forced-air humidifier that connects to the hot-air heating system is best. Small room or table-top humidifiers are of little value because they do not evaporate enough water.

Smoking. Smoking is another cause of sore throat that is unrelated to infection. Persons who smoke excessively often complain about irritation of the throat, which is usually worse in the morning, and postnasal discharge.

Fungal infection. Fungal infection of the oral cavity is sometimes seen during or after antibiotic therapy. Normally there is a certain balance between the flora of bacteria and fungi in the mouth, and when the bacterial elements are unduly depressed by antibiotics, fungi may overgrow and cause stomatitis and pharyngitis. Serious fungal infections, such as those caused by blastomycosis or actinomycosis, can result in osteomyelitis of the jaw, which leaves sinus tracts draining through the skin or mucous membranes. Fortunately these serious diseases are rare.

Tuberculosis. Tuberculosis of the pharynx and larynx is now uncommon because of modern methods of managing pulmonary tuberculosis. Formerly this disease was one of the "laryngeal triad"—syphilis, tuberculosis, and cancer. Whenever it does occur, it is always associated with far-advanced tuberculosis of the chest. The treatment, which is medical, is directed toward the pulmonary lesion.

Peritonsillar abscess. Peritonsillar abscess, or quinsy, is an exceptionally painful condition occurring as a complication after acute tonsillitis. Pus forms in the potential space behind the capsule of the tonsil. The voice becomes muffled because of the great swelling and interference with function of the palate. The patient is unable to eat, saliva drools from his mouth, and he has difficulty opening his mouth (trismus). Sometimes spontaneous rupture of the abscess occurs and quantities of pus drain through the anterior tonsillar pillar. Rather than waiting for spontaneous drainage, however, an incision should be made to evacuate the abscess. This incision is made with or without local anesthesia through the mucous membrane of the anterior tonsillar pillar. When the abscess is reached, pus pours out, with immediate relief of pain. Subsequently it may be necessary to reopen the incision every day for a few days to ensure continued drainage.

Retropharyngeal abscess. Retropharyngeal abscess is seen in children under 2 years of age. After a throat infection pus forms in the posterior midline of the pharynx. The child's cry is muffled, he has great trouble swallowing, and his airway is in danger. Drainage is usually done without anesthesia. The head is extended over the end of a table, and strong suction is used to aspirate the pus, which gushes from the incision. If care is not taken to aspirate pus instantly, it goes down the trachea and may asphyxiate the patient. The usual organism is the streptococcus and therefore penicillin is ordinarily the treatment of choice. Of course, cultures should be made and antibiotic sensitivity tests done to determine the specific antibiotic of choice.

Ludwig's angina. Ludwig's angina is an uncommon infection of the potential spaces that lie between muscles in the floor of the mouth. Usually there is little or no free pus. The tongue is pushed upward, and the neck feels woody. If the infection spreads, it may travel down the neck all the way to the clavicle, endangering the airway and making tracheotomy necessary. Treatment is with antibiotics and drainage through a generous external incision.

Infectious mononucleosis (glandular fever). Infectious mononucleosis is believed to be caused by a virus. Common clinical findings are cervical lymphadenopathy, pharyngitis and nasopharyngitis, splenomegaly, and fever. In other words, this is a systemic disease with local manifestations in the pharynx. There are mild and severe cases, and in the latter the patient may become so ill with fatigue, throat pain, and fever, as to require hospitalization. The aftermath of the acute stage of the disease may persist for weeks, and the patient only slowly returns to normal. The disease is most common in patients in their late teens and early 20s.

Diagnosis is established by the differential white blood count, which shows a preponderance of lymphocytes and atypical forms, plus a positive heterophil antibody test or Monospot test. The latter test is now used most commonly. Treatment is symptomatic and supportive because no antibiotic or other medication will cure the patient.

Thrush. *Candida albicans* is a fungus that may infect the throat. Discrete white patches of exudate form over the pharynx, the tonsillar pillars, and the base of the tongue. This infection was formerly seen chiefly in children and malnourished adults, but since the advent of antibiotics, it occurs in persons of all age groups because of the depression of normal bacterial flora of the oral cavity that allows overgrowth of *Candida.*

Treatment comprises local cleansing and the use of nystatin (Mycostatin), a fungicidal drug. Gentian violet (1% aqueous solution) painted on the pharyngeal lesions may also be beneficial. Gentian violet leaves a stain, but it comes off after a few days. The nurse must be careful, however, to protect the patient's clothes as well as her own, since the stain on clothing is hard to remove.

Vincent's angina. Vincent's angina, a disorder of the mucous membrane of the pharynx, is caused by a spirochete and fusiform bacillus acting in symbiosis. The gums are even more commonly infected than the throat, and then the disorder is referred to as "trench mouth." There is a fetid odor and a bad taste. Examination shows deep circumscribed ulcers of the tonsil with dirty gray bleeding bases. The ulcer crater does not involve the tonsillar pillars, and Vincent's angina rarely occurs in the pharynx after tonsillectomy. Ulceration and infection of the gums often accompany pharyngeal infection.

Treatment is by application of hydrogen peroxide, half strength, to the infected area. This may be done by holding cotton applicators on the ulcer or by using mouthwashes and gargles. One level teaspoonful of sodium perborate and one-half glass of warm water is also worthwhile. These oxygen-releasing preparations are of value because the spirochete of Vincent's angina is anaerobic and does not thrive well in the presence of high oxygen concentration.

Thyroglossal duct cyst. In the embryo the thyroid gland is situated at the foramen cecum near the base of the tongue. In development it descends along the course of the thyroglossal duct to reach its adult position in the neck just under the larynx. Sometimes remnants of the embryonic thyroglossal duct persist and form a cyst in the anterior midline of the neck (Figs. 16-26 and 22-1). Persistence of the thyroglossal duct may connect the cyst with the foramen cecum at the base of the tongue, but usually no tract can be demonstrated. Treatment is excision of the cyst, including removal of the body of the hyoid bone, since in embryonic life the hyoid forms around the thyroglossal duct and creates the possibility that some of the duct may persist if the body of the hyoid is left behind.

Lingual thyroid. Lingual thyroid is a rare condition in which thyroid tissue remains at the foramen cecum. There is a swelling on the posterior part of the tongue that may interfere with swallowing or with the voice. This is, of course, a congenital condition, but symptoms may not appear till later in life. If the lingual thyroid is to be removed, one should first make certain that there is additional thyroid tissue in the neck in its usual location. This determination may be made by use of scanning techniques after

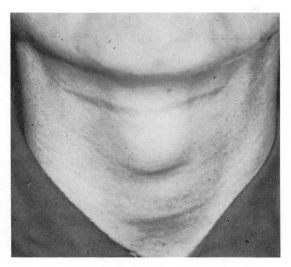

Fig. 16-26. Thyroglossal cyst. Marks on neck indicate from above downward hyoid bone, top of thyroid cartilage, and cricoid cartilage. The cyst is situated characteristically at the thyrohyoid interval.

administration of radioactive iodine. Such scanning will indicate thyroid tissue wherever it may be located. This precaution is necessary because removal of the lingual thyroid could account for all of the thyroid tissue that the patient has.

Throat irrigations

The nurse should know how to instruct the patient in throat irrigations (Fig. 16-27). Physiologic saline, as hot as the patient can tolerate (about 110° to 115° F.), is used to produce hyperemia of the mucous membranes—a treatment both soothing and of some therapeutic value. *Irrigations are much more effective than gargling* because in gargling, liquids do not reach the posterior parts of the oropharynx. To irrigate the throat, place an irrigation can filled with hot saline solution (two teaspoonfuls salt to one quart water) two feet above the patient's head and attach a glass medicine dropper as a tip on the end of the rubber hose leading from the can. This system directs a stream of hot saline solution at the posterior pharyngeal wall. The patient leans over a washbasin or holds a large pan to collect the water running in and out of his mouth. The procedure may be performed with the patient lying on his side, the solution running out the lower side of the mouth, or he may stand and let the water run from his mouth into a sink or basin. The patient should be instructed to hold his breath while the solution is running into the oral cavity and to stop the flow or signal the nurse to stop the flow when desiring to take a breath or rest. The patient's clothes should be protected, and he should be provided with a towel. Irrigations should be carried out several times a day.

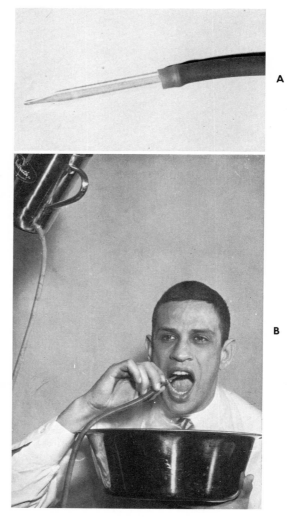

Fig. 16-27. Throat irrigation. (**B** from DeWeese, David D., and Saunders, William H.: Textbook of otolaryngology, ed. 4, St. Louis, 1973, The C. V. Mosby Co.)

SALIVARY GLANDS

There are six major salivary glands as well as many lesser salivary glands scattered throughout the oral cavity and pharynx. The major glands are the parotids, the ducts of which open *opposite the upper second molar teeth* (Fig. 16-28); the submandibular glands, with ducts opening opposite the frenum of the tongue just behind the lower central incisor teeth (Fig. 16-29); and the sublingual glands, the several ducts of which open into the floor of the mouth.

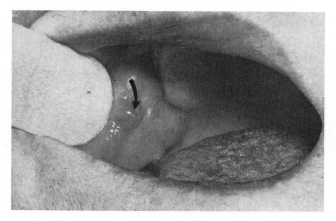

Fig. 16-28. Parotid orifice is indicated by arrow. Here it is swollen because of infection in the parotid gland.

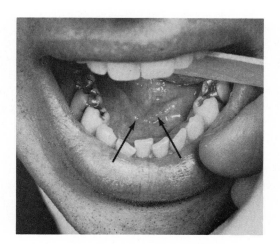

Fig. 16-29. Orifices of submaxillary ducts.

Methods of examination

Methods of examination of the major salivary glands include palpation, examination of the secretion from the duct, probing of the ducts, and x-ray examination with a technique called sialography. Lacrimal dilators are useful in probing the parotid and submandibular ducts—a No. 0 or 00 dilator is the one commonly used—but the sublingual ducts are too small for probing. Sialography is done by injecting radiopaque dye into the duct and exposing x-ray films. The dye outlines the duct and acini of the gland.

Inflammation

Inflammation of the salivary glands may be suppurative or nonsuppurative. Mumps (epidemic parotitis) is probably the most common nonsuppurative disease affecting the salivary glands. It usually affects the parotid gland, but sometimes it may affect the submandibular gland. Mumps is a viral disease and can cause complications such as oophoritis, orchitis, pancreatitis, meningitis, encephalitis, and unilateral deafness. Mumps viremia is known to occur in the absence of parotitis, and such a bloodstream infection may also cause these complications. There is no effective treatment for mumps.

Recurrent obstruction of the parotid duct by mucous plugs, by partial stricture caused by the patient biting the cheek, or from a tooth rubbing on the orifice of the parotid duct is common. In this case the parotid gland swells much as it does in mumps, but when pressure is made over the gland, ropy secretions come from the duct. The secretion in mumps is clear.

Suppurative infections of the parotid or submandibular gland are not uncommon. Any of the common bacteria that enter the duct in retrograde fashion may be the cause. Suppurative parotitis is a serious disease and one that may require external incision and drainage. Antibiotics are indicated. One type of suppurative parotitis is called *"surgical parotitis"* because it is seen in patients during postoperative periods. Overall dehydration is probably the most important single etiologic factor. Dry mouth, poor oral hygiene, and decreased salivation are important contributing causes of postoperative parotitis. The infective organisms is usually *Staphylococcus pyogenes* var. *aureus*. Although this condition is most likely to occur after abdominal surgery, it also occurs in patients who have had head and neck surgery.

The reason postulated for the greater incidence in patients who have had abdominal surgery is that after surgery these patients are usually allowed nothing by mouth until there is evidence of intestinal activity Nurses should be aware of the need for accurately recording the fluid intake of the patient and for reporting inadequate intake to the physician.

To prevent surgical parotitis it is recommended that the following steps be taken:
1. Frequent rinsing of the mouth, even during the initial "nothing by mouth" postoperative period
2. Frequent use of antiseptic mouthwash and cleansing of teeth with a *toothbrush* postoperatively
3. Accurate recording of the patient's intake and output

The nurse should observe the condition of the patient's oral mucosa and report changes. A tongue blade and flashlight are necessary for thorough inspection of the mouth. Various agents such as 1% hydrogen peroxide and alkaline mouthwashes are useful. After thorough cleansing and rinsing of the mouth the mucosa can be coated with a solution of mineral oil or glycerin diluted with water and lemon juice. Probably the single most important factor is the *frequency* of care rather than the agents used in improving oral hygiene.

Calculi

Calculus or stone formation is fairly common in the submandibular duct (Fig. 16-30) but less common in the parotid. If stones are recurrent or far back in the duct, it is necessary to excise the entire submandibular gland and duct.

The causes of salivary calculi are unknown. There is a history of pain and swelling under the ramus of the mandible during or just before eating. This is caused, of course, by the stimulation of salivary secretions from the taste and odor of food. Because the calculus obstructs the duct, the secretions cannot pass and they distend the duct and gland. Usually the swelling subsides after an hour or two, but it may remain longer. Depending somewhat on how tightly the stone obstructs the duct, swelling may or may not occur at each meal. The diagnosis can be made by palpation in the floor of the mouth, by probing the duct, and by roentgenography. Most, but not all, stones show on roentgenograms, since some do not contain enough calcium. A stone in the submandibular duct is usually not difficult to remove as an office procedure. Local anesthesia is sufficient. The duct can be opened either at the site of the stone or else split from its orifice back to the stone and the stone lifted from the duct (Fig. 16-31). It is not necessary to suture the duct, since the fistula that forms drains saliva into the floor of the mouth right where it should be.

Neoplasms

Most neoplasms of the salivary glands are benign mixed salivary gland tumors (Fig. 16-32), and most affect the parotid gland. Benign neoplasms enlarge slowly and painlessly and often are present many years before the patient seeks medical treatment. These benign tumors can be removed surgically, but great care must be taken during removal to preserve all branches of the facial nerve, which divides and branches within the parotid gland. This nerve, which first travels through the middle ear, leaves the temporal bone at the stylomastoid foramen just under the ear. At the time of surgery a nerve stimulator may be used to identify the fine branches of the nerve. One mistake which is sometimes made in parotid surgery is to make too small an incision so that one cannot actually identify the main trunk of the nerve and all of its branches (Fig. 16-33, *A* and *B*). Postoperative facial paralysis, which results if the nerve is injured, is a serious complication since it is deforming. The nurse can be of help in the immediate postoperative period by noting whether the patient's face moves on the operated side. If it does move initially, and then fails to move several hours subsequently, at least we know that the nerve has not been cut and that the paralysis will be temporary. Tests for facial function include having the patient wrinkle his forehead, purse his lips, smile to show his teeth, wrinkle his nose, and squeeze his eyes shut tightly. Weakness or total

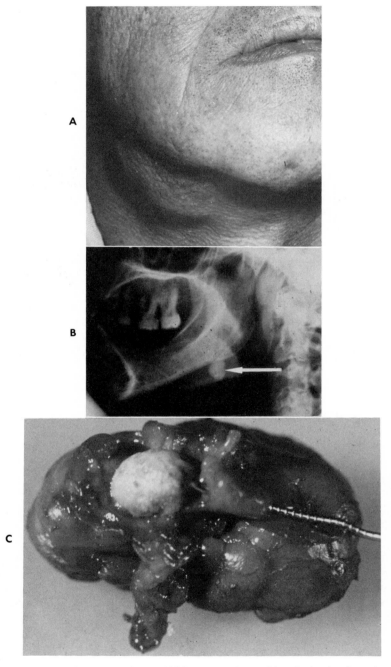

Fig. 16-30. A, Swelling below the mandible in a patient with calculus in the submaxillary salivary gland. **B,** Note the roentgenographic appearance of a dense round stone near the angle of the mandible. **C,** Gland excised, showing calculus. Probe enters the submaxillary duct.

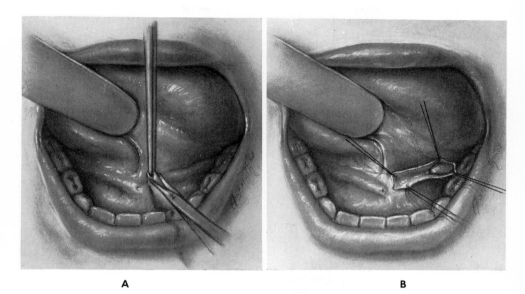

Fig. 16-31. A, Cutting off the submaxillary duct papilla. **B,** Submaxillary duct stone exposed before removal. (From DeWeese, David D.: Portland Clinical Bulletin 7:1, 1953.)

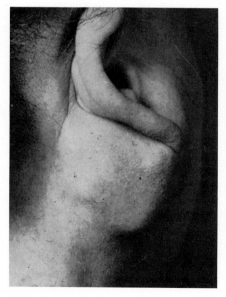

Fig. 16-32. Large mixed tumor of the parotid gland.

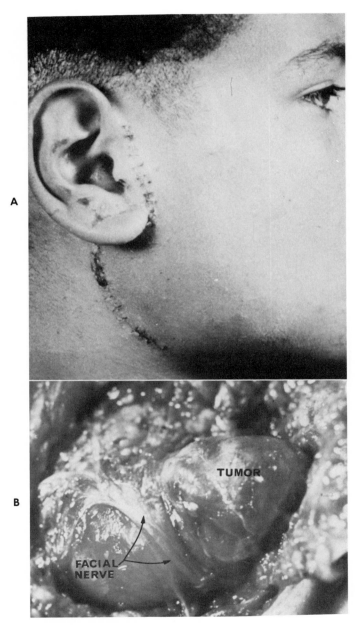

Fig. 16-33. A, Typical parotidectomy incision healing. No smaller incision will be adequate to expose the entire gland and facial nerve. **B,** Trunk of the facial nerve greatly stretched by a tumor of the parotid gland.

loss of function will interfere with one or all of these normal facial movements since the facial nerve innervates all of the muscles of facial expression.

Malignant tumors are less common (Fig. 16-33). The chief manifestations are pain, rapid increase in size of the tumor, and facial paralysis. Any swelling of the parotid gland associated with facial paralysis indicates a malignant neoplasm. The treatment of malignant tumors is surgical excision or irradiation therapy, but the prognosis is not good in either case. Often the facial nerve is sacrificed in order to completely excise the tumor. If the nerve is resected, sometimes grafting is done utilizing the greater auricular nerve (a sensory nerve) in the upper neck. This nerve is placed between the cut ends of the facial nerve, and regeneration occurs over a period of several months.

SUGGESTED READINGS

Becker, W., and others: Atlas of otorhinolaryngology and bronchoesophagology, Philadelphia, 1969, W. B. Saunders Co.

DeWeese, David D.: Diagnosis and treatment of submaxillary duct stones, Portland Clinical Bulletin 7:1, 1953.

DeWeese, David D., and Saunders, William H.: Textbook of otolaryngology, St. Louis, 1973, The C. V. Mosby Co.

Frazell, Edgar L., Strong, Elliot W., and Newcombe, Barbara: Tumors of the parotid, American Journal of Nursing **66:** 2702-2708, Dec., 1966.

Harmon, W. G.: Nursing care in surgery of the head and neck, Nursing Clinics of North America 2:475-481, Sept., 1967.

Keough, Gertrude, and Niebel, Harold N.: Oral cancer detection—a nursing responsibility, American Journal of Nursing **73:** 684-686, April, 1973.

Kesel, Robert G., and Sreenby, Leo M.: Toothbrushing, American Journal of Nursing 57:186-188, Feb., 1957.

Martin, Hayes: Radical neck dissection, Ciba Clinical Symposia 13:115-120, Oct., Nov., Dec., 1961.

Martin, Hayes: Surgical removal of parotid tumor, Ciba Clinical Symposia 13:121-131, Oct., Nov., Dec., 1961.

Newcombe, Barbara: Care of the patient with head and neck cancer, Nursing Clinics of North America 2:599-607, Dec., 1967.

Passos, Joyce Y., and Brand, Lucy M.: Effects of agents used for oral hygiene, Nursing Research 15:196-202, Summer, 1966.

Pizer, Marvin E., and Kay, Sanford: Mouth cancer—concepts of treatment, RN 35:12-16, Oct., 1972.

Saunders, William H.: Nicotine stomatitis of the palate, Annals of Otology 67:618, 1958.

Tassman, Gustave C., Zayon, Gilbert M., and Zafran, Jack N.: When patients cannot brush their teeth, American Journal of Nursing 63:76, Feb., 1963.

CHAPTER SEVENTEEN

Tonsils and adenoids

There are three distinct masses of lymphoid tissue in the pharynx called tonsil: (1) the pharyngeal tonsil or adenoid, (2) the palatine, or faucial, tonsil (the one commonly referred to as the "tonsil"), and (3) the lingual tonsil. In addition there are scattered buds of lymphoid tissue on the posterior pharyngeal wall and the so-called lateral pharyngeal bands behind the posterior pillars. Taken all together, this pharyngeal lymphoid tissue is called Waldeyer's ring. Its purpose is not definitely known, but removal of any or all of it does not affect the patient adversely.

INDICATIONS FOR TONSILLECTOMY AND ADENOIDECTOMY

Fewer tonsillectomies and adenoidectomies are done today than were done during the 1930's, when many were performed. The advent of the sulfonamide drugs in the 1930's and penicillin and other antibiotics in the mid-1940's has done a great deal to eliminate the need for tonsillectomy and adenoidectomy. One must not conclude, however, that either tonsillectomy or tonsillectomy and adenoidectomy is not distinctly worthwhile and that many patients do not need the procedure. Admittedly, however, it is sometimes difficult to tell just when the operation will be worthwhile. Certainly not all patients with histories of sore throats are cleared of their symptoms after tonsillectomy and adenoidectomy. The earlier belief that infected tonsils and adenoids caused many systemic ills is largely unfounded. At one time it was thought that there was a direct relationship between infected tonsils and rheumatic fever—a theory that also is doubted.

Tonsillectomy is indicated chiefly if there have been repeated attacks of acute tonsillitis or if peritonsillar abscess (quinsy) has occurred. The faucial, or palatine, tonsils probably never cause obstruction of the pharynx, although hypertrophy of the adenoid commonly causes obstruction of the nasopharyngeal airway. Recurrent attacks of acute otitis media or of serous otitis media are indications for tonsillectomy and adenoidectomy in a child. Persistent enlargement of cervical lymph glands, common in many children, usually indicates disease of the tonsils and adenoids, although this finding in itself may not be enough to warrant tonsillectomy and adenoidectomy (Figs. 17-1 and 17-2).

Often a child is brought to the physician with the request for tonsillectomy and adenoidectomy because the parents insist the child has sore throats. On close questioning the physician learns that the sore throats are present only briefly and, therefore, they probably are not bacterial. The child may breathe through his mouth at night and have a sore throat for a short time after he awakens, but the sore throat clears later in the day. Such a patient, unless obstructed by the adenoid that causes his mouth breathing, is likely to continue to have sore throats even though he has a tonsillectomy. The same is true of the adult. Other children are seen because their parents complain that they have various systemic illnesses or that they fail to gain weight, and it is thought that the tonsils and adenoids

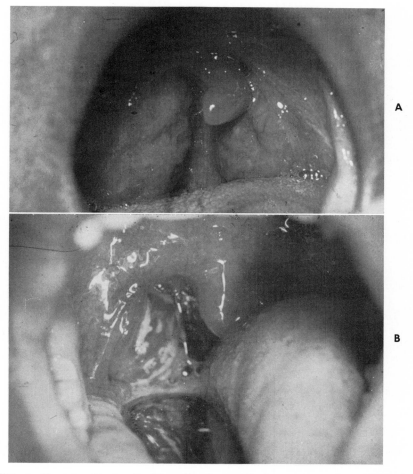

Fig. 17-1. A, Hypertrophic tonsils. Normally the tonsils do not protrude much beyond the margin of the tonsillar pillars. **B,** Acute follicular tonsillitis. Compare with Fig. 16-5, *B,* p. 159. (From Saunders, William H.: Ears, nose, and throat. In Prior, John A., and Silberstein, Jack S.: Physical diagnosis, ed. 4, St. Louis, 1973, The C. V. Mosby Co.)

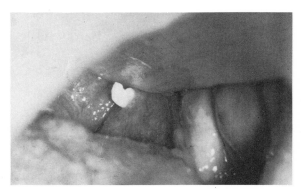

Fig. 17-2. One side of the oropharynx. The white plug of epithelial debris extrudes from a tonsillar crypt. This is not infection but a peeling off of the lining of the crypt. Patients with deep crypts may find small cheesy plugs in their mouths that annoy them.

are the cause. This may occasionally be the case, but usually it is not. Since there is always a risk in the operation, the careful otolaryngologist will not operate on patients who are unlikely to be improved.

The operation is never done when there is an acute infection or when there is an epidemic of any disease. Blood dyscrasias such as aplastic anemia, hemophilia, or leukemia also contraindicate tonsillectomy and adenoidectomy.

Preoperative care. The child undergoing tonsillectomy should be prepared psychologically for the operation. To help prepare the parent as well as the child for surgery, some health care facilities have "lemonade parties" a week or so prior to admission to provide information and to tour the areas that will be seen by the child. Information sheets or booklets are often given the parents to help them prepare the child for this experience. In making explanations, it is best to use terms such as "fix" or "remove" rather than "cut" since the child, especially, has fantasies and fears. Also, reassurance should be given that no other part of his body is to be removed and that no one is to blame for the condition. He should be informed as follows:

1. Why the procedure is being done
2. What the hospital routine is, as well as the functions of the doctors and nurses
3. That he will be put to sleep briefly, so he will not feel the operation
4. That for a short time afterward he will have a sore throat
5. That the doctors and nurses know how to make his throat feel better
6. That his mother (or father) will be with him immediately before and after the operation
7. What his postoperative course is expected to be

Special concerns of the child, depending upon his age and other factors, play an important part in his reaction to this experience. Play with a doctor's kit allows the child to express his concern. It is important that the nurse understand these reactions and how she can assist the child and his parents in adjusting to hospitalization with the least amount of trauma for all concerned. For further reading on how best to care for specific age groups, see references listed at the end of the chapter.

ACUTE TONSILLITIS

Acute tonsillitis is caused most frequently by the streptococcus organism, although many other bacterial organisms, some viruses, and even some fungi may be responsible. Sometimes acute tonsillitis is an isolated infection with no other part of the pharynx seemingly involved. At other times there is an associated generalized pharyngitis and nasopharyngitis. Symptoms of acute tonsillitis include mild to severe throat pain, difficulty in swallowing, fever, and lymphadenopathy in the submandibular area. Headache and muscle and joint pain may also be present, especially at the onset. Examination of the throat shows an acutely inflamed, red mucous membrane, often studded with white or yellow follicles. Often one tonsil is more involved than the other. Exudate is confined to the lymphoid tissue of the throat and ordinarily does not involve the tonsillar pillars or soft palate. If these latter parts are involved by membranous exudates, the examiner should suspect diphtheria. In any case, the use of a bright light and tongue blade should give the examiner a good view of the tonsillar area and therefore the correct diagnosis. One should remember, however, that, in addition to involvement of the palatine tonsils in the oropharynx (mesopharynx), there also may be involvement of the pharyngeal tonsils (adenoid) in the nasopharynx, or of the lingual tonsil in the hypopharynx, and that *mirror examination* will be required to show the latter areas. Conversely, a patient with a sore throat may have normal-appearing palatine or faucial tonsils but have a nasopharyngitis or lingual tonsillitis that cannot be seen if the examiner uses only a tongue blade.

Treatment consists of antibiotics (usually penicillin), throat irrigations, and analgesics such as codeine, 32 mg. every three hours. To provide this dosage of codeine, one may prescribe Empirin Compound with codeine phosphate No. 3, or Ascodeen-30. Children may also have codeine but in lesser dosages. Acetaminophen (Tylenol) liquid may be useful for children to provide an analgesic in an acceptable form. In severe cases the patient may have to be hospitalized in order to maintain proper fluid balance by intravenous therapy. It is very important that the antibiotic drugs be continued long enough, because if they are stopped too soon, recurrence is common. In general, antibiotics should be given for forty-eight hours after all symptoms and signs have cleared.

If the patient has repeated attacks of acute tonsillitis or if tonsillitis is complicated by peritonsillar abscess (quinsy), tonsillectomy is indicated. Tonsillectomy is never done during acute tonsillitis, and preferably a month or more should pass after all symptoms of acute infection have subsided before an operation is done.

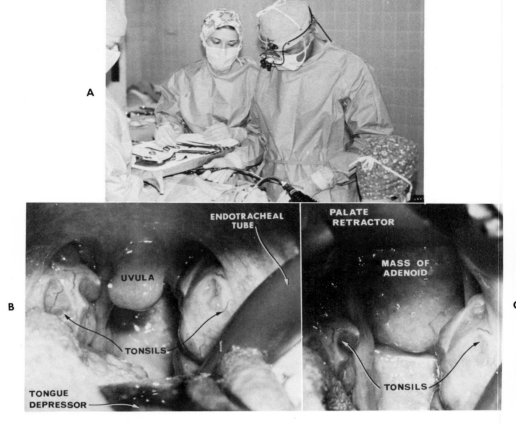

Fig. 17-3. A, Operating room team prepared for tonsillectomy on a child. **B,** Tonsillectomy position. **C,** Adenoid (pharyngeal tonsil) exposed.

PHARYNGEAL TONSIL OR ADENOID

In the infant and young child the pharyngeal tonsil or adenoid is large; during adolescence it undergoes atrophy so that in the adult it is small or even absent. Hypertrophy of the adenoid (with or without infection) causes two chief difficulties: (1) nasal obstruction and (2) obstruction of the eustachian tubes, which predisposes to middle ear infections. Fortunately hearing loss caused by obstruction of the eustachian tube is usually reversible.

Adenoidectomy. Adenoidectomy is an extremely useful operation that helps prevent these problems. The operation is much more useful in the child than in the adult, because children have large and obstructive adenoids, whereas most adults do not. Usually adenoidectomy is done in conjunction with tonsillectomy, but sometimes the adenoid alone is removed. The operation can be done safely at any age. Often it is not possible to

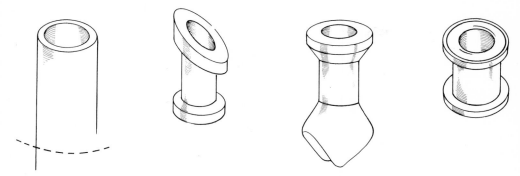

Fig. 17-4. Several different plastic tubes inserted into the tympanic membrane to provide aeration of the middle ear space. The use of these tubes has reduced the need of adenoidectomy. (From Saunders, William H., and Paparella, Michael M.: Atlas of ear surgery, ed. 2, St. Louis, 1971, The C. V. Mosby Co.)

remove all the adenoid—a small percentage remains even though every effort is made to remove all visible and palpable tissue. As a rule, however, this small residual does not matter, since the great bulk of the obstructive lymphoid tissue is removed. In some children, however, especially those with allergy or those who come from families with allergy, there may be rapid regrowth of the adenoid; then a second adenoidectomy is necessary. Radium applications to the nasopharynx, popular thirty years ago, are now seldom used. If radium is considered, it should be reserved for patients who already have had one or more careful adenoidectomies yet continue to have symptoms. There is some evidence that radium applications given many years previously have induced nasopharyngeal carcinoma in later life. The chief reason, however, for the discontinuance of radium application to the nasopharynx is that the efficacy of these applications was uncertain.

The use of polyethylene and other types of plastic or metal aeration tubes placed through the tympanic membrane has also reduced the need for adenoidectomy. These tubes (Fig. 17-4) are inserted into the tympanic membrane, where they remain for weeks or months until extruded spontaneously or removed by the surgeon. The purpose is to provide aeration of the middle ear space, normally done through the eustachian tube whenever the patient yawns or swallows.

Adenoidectomy is done under general anesthesia. Anesthetists use an endotracheal tube with an inflatable cuff to keep blood out of the trachea. A rolled sheet or blanket is placed under the shoulders to extend the head. In the Rose position the surgeon sits at the end of the table, and the patient's head is dropped into his lap. Before the use of endotracheal tubes became common practice, the position of the patient's head was very important, because blood in the throat ran into the trachea. Suction is used throughout the procedure to clear blood from the pharynx.

With a mouth gag in place and the palate retracted the surgeon can look into the nasopharynx. The adenoid appears as a soft mass of tissue with

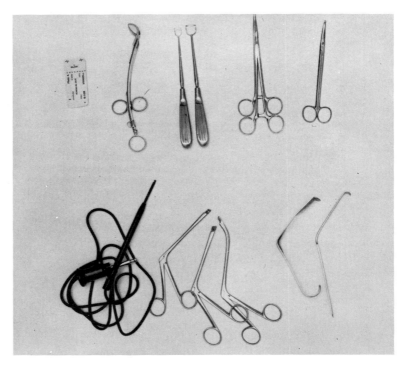

Fig. 17-5. Adenoidectomy instruments. **Top:** No. 1 plain catgut, adenotome, two curettes, two tonsillar hemostats, and dissecting scissors. **Bottom:** Electrocautery (other tips are also used), three punch forceps, and two palate retractors.

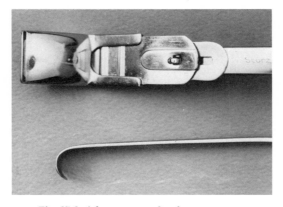

Fig. 17-6. Adenotome and palate retractor.

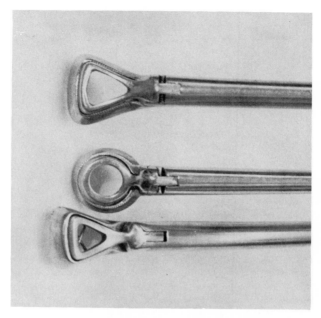

Fig. 17-7. Punch forceps used to bite out residual adenoid after curette or adenotome has removed bulk of tissue.

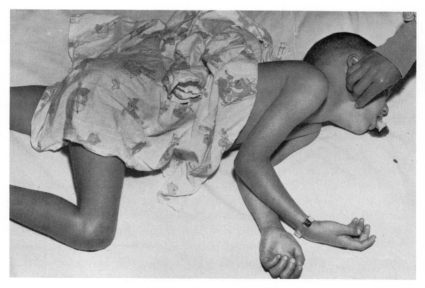

Fig. 17-8. Tonsillectomy, postoperative position. Oral airway in place. Some postoperative bleeding is present. Nurse supports jaw to assist airway.

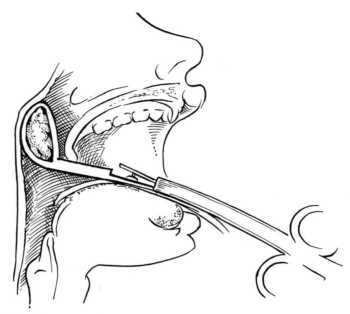

Fig. 17-9. Adenoidectomy. The adenotome is advanced into the nasopharynx, and the major portion of the adenoid is removed. (From Ryan, Robert E., and others: Synopsis of ear, nose, and throat diseases, ed. 3, St. Louis, 1970, The C. V. Mosby Co.)

vertical furrows. It is removed with an adenotome, a curette, and punch forceps (Figs. 17-5, 17-7, 17-9, and 17-10). Special care is given to the region around the eustachian tube.

Bleeding is controlled by packing the nasopharynx with gauze sponges soaked in epinephrine or other hemostatic agent. Sometimes the electrocautery unit is used to control bleeding. In stubborn cases the surgeon may leave a postnasal pack in place, but generally the nasopharynx is expected to be completely dry at the end of the operation. Sutures ordinarily are not used. Even so, the patient may bleed postoperatively, usually in the first hour after anesthesia. If bleeding does not stop spontaneously, a gauze sponge soaked in epinephrine is held for a few minutes in the nasopharynx. It is seldom necessary to take the patient back to the operating room for a second anesthetic.

Immediately after surgery the patient is placed on his side, with his head positioned to allow gravity to assist any possible flow of blood through the nose and mouth (Fig. 17-8). Blood is less likely to be aspirated or swallowed if the patient is kept in this position. Frequent observation of vital signs is essential, and increasing pulse, pallor, or restlessness unrelated to awakening from the general anesthesia should be reported. If postoperative bleeding, which commences soon after the operation, is not discovered, the patient swallows quantities of blood and finally vomits coffee-ground material. By then the pulse is fast and he looks pale. Blood transfusion may be required.

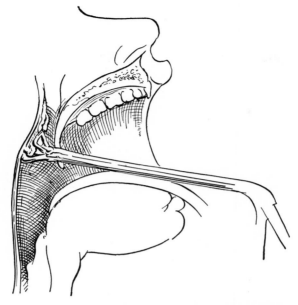

Fig. 17-10. Adenoidectomy. The remaining pieces of lymphoid tissue along the lateral walls of the nasopharynx are removed with biting forceps. (From Ryan, Robert E., and others: Synopsis of ear, nose, and throat diseases, ed. 3, St. Louis, 1970, The C. V. Mosby Co.)

To be safe, the physician or nurse should check the throat an hour after surgery, again that evening, and finally the next morning.

Delayed bleeding may also occur. When it does, it is most frequent on the fifth postoperative day. A child who has gone home from the hospital may seem to be recovering normally when suddenly he has a nosebleed or starts to spit blood. He should be taken at once to the emergency room of the hospital and a blood clot aspirated from the nasopharynx. An epinephrine-soaked tampon can be held in place for a minute or two. Failure to take delayed bleeding seriously can result in major blood loss.

After adenoidectomy the child usually misses a week of school.

There may be a change in the voice because of removal of the large pad of adenoid against which the soft palate formerly could close. With the adenoid out the palate is temporarily too short to approximate the posterior pharyngeal wall, and the patient has a nasal voice. While this clears after several weeks, it is worthwhile warning the parents that nasal voice sometimes occurs after adenoidectomy.

Tonsillectomy. In the *child,* tonsillectomy and adenoidectomy are usually done simultaneously. Sometimes it is the adenoid that has been the major offender and sometimes it is the tonsils.

The tonsil is removed by a combination of sharp and blunt dissection (Figs. 17-11 to 17-14). A No. 12 Bard-Parker blade cuts the mucous membrane around the tonsil, and scissors or blunt dissectors separate the tonsil

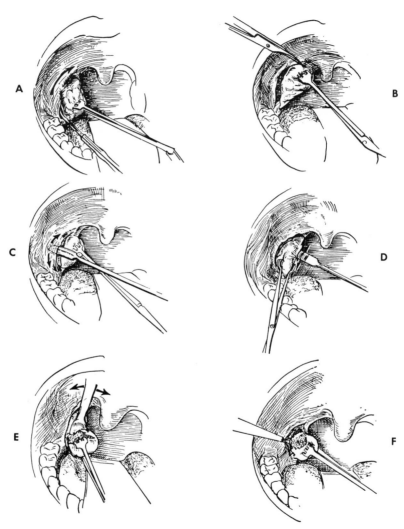

Fig. 17-11. The dissection method of tonsillectomy. **A,** Incision of the mucous membrane along the edge of the anterior pillar. **B,** Extension of the mucosal incision along its superior and posterior attachments. **C,** Separation of the tonsil from the anterior pillar. **D,** Separation of the tonsil from the posterior pillar. **E,** Completion of the dissection along the superior and lateral walls. **F,** Application of the snare for removal of the tonsil. (From Ryan, Robert E., and others: Synopsis of ear, nose, and throat diseases, ed. 3, St. Louis, 1970, The C. V. Mosby Co.)

from its capsule. After the tonsil is removed a pillar retractor exposes the fossa so that bleeders can be identified and grasped with a hemostat. Then a heavy catgut suture, usually No. 1 or No. 2, is tied around the hemostat. The tie can be made in the usual manner or a slip knot, prepared in advance by the nurse, can be used. Instead of using catgut ties some surgeons use the electrocoagulating current to control bleeding.

The nurse's major responsibilities after surgery are maintenance of a patent airway, observation of vital signs, and keeping the patient as quiet as possible. The patient is placed in the side-lying position (Fig. 17-8). If the surgeon is not readily available, the nurse should have no hesitation in looking into the pharynx, using a bright light and tongue blade. This means that the child is turned onto his back (supine) and often restrained. When there is an undue amount of bleeding, the pulse quickens and the child looks pale. Often the blood is swallowed and little or none is seen externally.

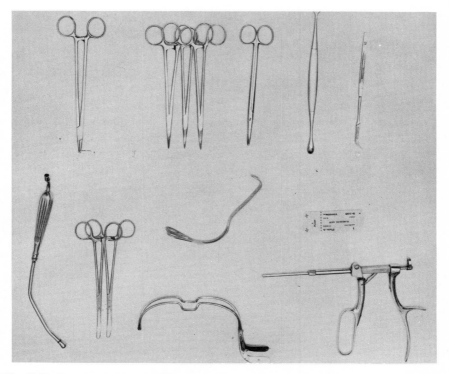

Fig. 17-12. Instruments for tonsillectomy. **Top:** Needle holder and *heavy* round needle (a small needle that could break might never be found in the tonsillar fossa), three tonsillar hemostats, curved dissecting scissors, Hurd pillar retractor (upper end) and blunt dissector (lower end), and No. 12 Bard-Parker blade. **Bottom:** Oral or the tonsil and adenoid sucker (be sure tip is screwed on tight), curved Allis forceps to grasp tonsil (a great many different tonsil-grasping instruments are available), tongue depressor, mouth gag, pack of No. 1 plain catgut, and tonsil snare (many types are in use).

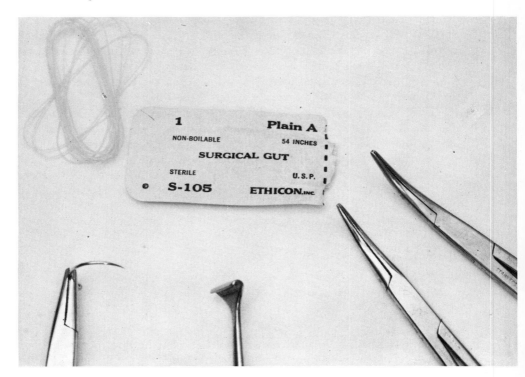

Fig. 17-13. Tonsillar instruments: *heavy* round *needle,* Hurd pillar retractor, and two tonsillar hemostats (note the tapered tips).

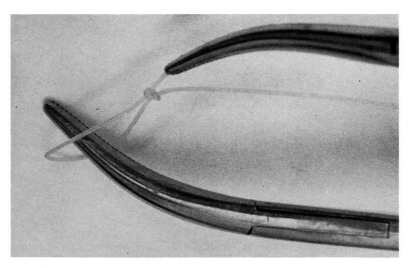

Fig. 17-14. Slip knot tie as used in tonsillar fossa. The nurse prepares the knot in advance. Traction on the hemostat draws the knot tight around the bleeding vessel.

After several hours of swallowing blood, the child vomits quantities of coffee-colored stomach contents.

If bleeding does occur, the patient is instructed to allow blood to run from the mouth. A calm, reassuring manner is necessary to prevent frightening the child.

If the child is fully awake and no symptoms of hemorrhage are present, he is taken from the recovery room to his own hospital room with his parents. Close monitoring of vital signs is required throughout the day of surgery. Analgesics such as acetaminophen (Tylenol) and salicylamide (Liquiprin) are often used. Powdered aspirin in cream and Aspergum are old favorites, although their effectiveness is doubted by some. Dextropropoxyphene (Darvon) also may be prescribed. An ice collar may lessen pain.

Fluids should be encouraged as soon as nausea ceases. There is some indication that having the patient start to swallow in the early postoperative period may decrease his pain by reducing spasms in the pharyngeal muscles. Ice chips may be welcomed. At first swallowing is painful; fluids given one-half hour after the analgesic are taken more easily. A small child can quickly become dehydrated if not taking fluids, for he has had no fluids since the previous evening.

It is important that the patient and his parents understand home care. Giving the mother a printed list of diet instructions is customary but not really necessary, since the patient will not eat what he does not want and anything he wants will not hurt him. In general, however, a bland diet without acid juices (orange or tomato), spices, or excessively hot or cold foods is best. Carbonated beverages are accepted better than milk. Custards, Jell-O, broth, soft-boiled egg, mashed potatoes, and soft milk toasts are acceptable foods. Well-ground hamburger and well-cooked meats should be added as soon as tolerated.

Specific prescription for pain should be given, since the throat remains sore for five to six days. *It is common for the patient to complain of earache,* which is a *referred pain* along a nerve connecting the pharynx and the ear and not caused by an ear infection. Analgesics will control this pain.

The child should be kept quiet and should not overexert himself. He should stay in bed if he feels like it. Quiet play, which can be beneficial in acting out the experience of hospitalization, watching television, and reading should be encouraged. The child is usually kept out of school for a week or until the return checkup with the physician.

Rinsing the mouth with warm salt water (one teaspoon of salt to one pint of water) frequently, in addition to regular toothbrushing, will help reduce odor. A heavy, dirty gray membrane forms in the fossae where the tonsils were removed. This is alarming to the parents if they should look into the child's mouth, and may surprise the nurse if she is not aware that it occurs in all patients who have undergone tonsillectomy. The membrane is the result of a superficial infection of the tonsillar fossae caused by ever-present mouth organisms. It gradually disappears, and healing ordinarily is complete after three or four weeks.

Delayed bleeding, usually on the fifth or sixth day after surgery, *requires a call to the physician*. This bleeding is caused by the separation of a blood clot, which sometimes forms in the tonsillar fossae. Ordinarily the bleeding does not amount to very much, but there have been cases reported in which the patient has bled to death. Similar bleedings can occur in the naso-pharynx after adenoidectomy. While a temperature elevation over 1° F. or persistent and a severe earache should be reported to the physician, it is more than likely that these conditions result from dehydration and from referred pain.

In the *adult*, tonsillectomy usually is done under local anesthesia. If it is also necessary to remove the adenoid, a general anesthesia is given. The patient sits up in an examining chair, or the operating table is broken to simulate a chair. First, the throat is sprayed with a topical anesthetic such as cocaine 5% or tetracaine (Pontocaine) 1%. Then lidocaine hydrochloride (Xylocaine) or other local anesthetic (never cocaine or Pontocaine!) is injected to complete the local anesthesia.

At surgery, the nurse must make absolutely certain of the identity of medications on her table. Solutions commonly employed in the operation are epinephrine, cocaine, saline, and Xylocaine—they all look alike but two (cocaine and epinephrine) can be fatal if injected. Marked medicine glasses are good but are not foolproof. *The doctor himself should be the only one* to draw up solutions to be injected. The use of disposable bottles of Xylocaine, prefilled at the factory, is a good safety measure. These 30 ml. vials are not so large as to be wasteful when discarded after each operation, and the safety factor is inestimable. The same precautions should apply to all operative procedures done under local anesthesia.

After local anesthesia has taken effect, the tonsillectomy proceeds as with the tonsillectomy under general anesthesia. There is the advantage, however, of less bleeding. During the operation some patients become pale and feel faint, and such syncope often is mistaken for a toxic reaction. The nurse should simply lower the patient's head between his knees or help stretch him out on the table.

Postoperatively, the adult characteristically complains more of pain than does the young child. Some adults refuse to eat for as long as several days and sometimes must receive intravenous feeding to prevent dehydration. Ordinarily, however, the patient can take liquids (no acid juices) on the day of surgery and either a liquid or an endentulous diet the next day. Empirin Compound with codeine phosphate No. 3 (½ grain codeine) by mouth or meperidine hydrochloride (Demerol), 100 mg. by injection, may be required in the immediate postoperative period; later, either the same Empirin Compound or aspirin should suffice. Most adults will miss about one week of work after tonsillectomy because of sore throat.

The nurse's chief responsibility as an important member of the operating team is to have available, and in working order, the instruments, suture materials, and other equipment required for that particular procedure. Ear, nose, and throat operations are particularly demanding of the nurse in this respect because the procedures done by the otolaryngologist differ so much from those done by the general surgeon. There are operations on the middle ear that require the most delicate instruments made; operations on the neck that utilize general surgical instruments; operations on the bones of the face and skull that necessitate a knowledge of rongeurs, chisels, and gouges; very special rhinoplasty instruments; and bronchoscopes, laryngoscopes, and esophagoscopes and their respective suction tubes and forceps for biopsy or foreign body extraction. Even the lighting systems are different from those used by the general surgeon, and the nurse must have a detailed working knowledge of the otolaryngologist's headlight if the operating room is to function efficiently.

SUGGESTED READINGS

Bellam, Gwendoline: Tonsillectomy without fear, American Journal of Nursing **51:**244-245, April, 1951.

Boies, L. R.: The tonsil and adenoid problem as seen by the laryngologist, J.A.M.A. **154:**575, 1954.

Dison, Norma: Tonsillectomy—mother view, American Journal of Nursing **69:**1024-1027, May, 1969.

Erickson, Florence: When 6- to 12-year-olds are ill, Nursing Outlook **13:**48-50, July, 1965.

Harlowe, H. D.: Complications following tonsillectomy, Laryngoscope **58:**863, 1948.

Heavenrich, Robert, Erickson, Florence, and Saren, Martin: Viewpoints on children in hospitals, Hospitals **37:**40-52, May 16, 1963.

Mahaffy, Perry R.: The effects of hospitalization on children admitted for tonsillectomy and adenoidectomy, Nursing Research **14:**12-19, Winter, 1965.

Petrillo, Madeline: Preventing hospital trauma in pediatric patients, American Journal of Nursing **68:**1469-1473, July, 1968.

Petrillo, Madeline, and Sanger, Sergay: Emotional care of hospitalized children; an environmental approach, Philadelphia, 1972, J. B. Lippincott Co.

Smith, Margo: Ego support for the child patient, American Journal of Nursing **63:**93-95, Oct., 1963.

HELPFUL BOOKS IN PREPARING CHILDREN FOR HOSPITALIZATION

Clark, Bettina, and Coleman, Lester: Going to the hospital, New York, 1971, Random House, Inc.

Collier, James L.: Danny goes to the hospital, New York, 1970, Grosset and Dunlap.

Rey, Margaret, and Rey, H. A.: Curious George goes to the hospital, New York, 1966, Houghton-Mifflin Co.

Weber, Alfons: Elizabeth gets well, New York, 1970, Thomas Crowell.

CHAPTER EIGHTEEN

Nose and paranasal sinuses—anatomy and physiology

ANATOMY

The supporting structure of the nose is formed by the two nasal bones, the nasal processes of the maxillary bones, the cartilaginous and bony parts of the septum, and the upper and lower lateral nasal cartilages (Fig. 18-1). Variations in the size and shape of the nose are caused, superiorly, by the nasal bones and, inferiorly, by differences in the size and shape of the nasal cartilages. The rudimentary muscles associated with the nose are of little importance.

The *vestibule,* in the anterior part of the nose, is lined with skin containing vibrissae, or nasal hairs. This part of the nose extends a short distance posteriorly, where the skin meets the respiratory mucous membrane. *Cilia* in the mucosa beat in a constant wavelike motion to carry posteriorly mucus and foreign material. In a small area superiorly, there is special *olfactory epithelium* that provides the end organ for the sense of smell.

The nasal *septum* divides the nose into two nasal fossae. Anteriorly the septum is cartilaginous, whereas posteriorly it is bony. The septum, which is usually straight and thin in the child, is rarely so in the adult because it is subject to injury as well as to distortion by the growth process. It acts as a midline supporting structure for the nose but does not otherwise contribute to nasal function. The cartilage of the nasal septum is covered by perichondrium and mucous membrane. It is this sheet of mucoperichondrium that is elevated and separated from the underlying cartilage on both sides when the so-called submucous resection operation is done to remove or straighten deviated parts of the cartilage and bone. The color of the nasal mucous membrane is distinctly redder than that of the oral mucous membrane. In some disease states such as allergic rhinitis, the color becomes pale or slightly bluish.

The lateral walls of the nose contain the ostia or openings of the paranasal sinuses and the nasolacrimal ducts. These openings are small and not seen by the examiner. They provide means of aeration of the sinuses and means by which mucus can drain from the sinuses into the nose. Also on each lateral wall are three turbinate bones covered with thick mucosa. This mucosa is supplied abundantly with blood vessels (especially over the inferior turbinate), which serve to warm and moisten inspired air. The inferior turbinate, the largest, becomes particularly swollen when we have a cold, and it is this structure that vasoconstrictors (nose drops) shrink in providing a better airway. Under each turbinate there is a corresponding meatus. The nasolacrimal duct drains tears from the eye into the inferior meatus; the frontal, maxillary, and anterior ethmoidal sinuses drain into the middle meatus; and the posterior ethmoidal and sphenoid sinuses drain into the superior meatus.

The *blood supply* of the nose comes from both the external and the internal carotid arteries. Rarely, a patient may have severe nosebleeds that cannot be controlled with packing, and then it may be necessary to ligate the external carotid artery in the neck, or one of its branches, the internal maxillary. The anterior and posterior ethmoidal arteries, which derive blood from the internal carotid system, can be ligated through an incision made along the side of the nose near the inner canthus of the eye. The internal carotid itself cannot be ligated safety because it carries the chief blood supply to the brain.

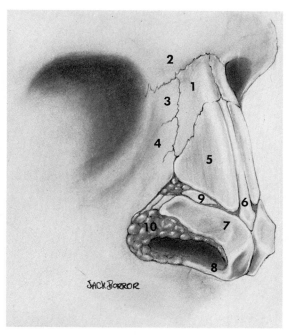

Fig. 18-1. Framework of nose. **1,** Nasal bone; **2,** frontal bone; **3,** lacrimal bone; **4,** maxillary bone; **5,** upper lateral cartilage; **6,** nasal septum; **7,** lower lateral cartilage, lateral crus; **8,** lower lateral cartilage, medial crus; **9,** sesamoid cartilage; **10,** fibrofatty tissue.

None of these vessels, which are deep in the neck or under cover of bone, lend themselves to application of pressure.

The *lymphatic supply* of the nose is important because it leads toward the cavernous sinus within the skull. In spite of antibiotic therapy, thrombosis and infection of the cavernous sinus still remains a very serious disease that may easily cause death. In this connection it may be noted that the nurse is in a good position to instruct the patient in proper nasal hygiene and to discourage the patient from picking at furuncles and other infections about the nose and face and to seek needed medical advice.

There are four *paranasal sinuses* on either side of the head (Fig. 18-2). These are air-filled spaces in the skull that lighten the head but apparently serve no other function. The maxillary sinuses are above the upper teeth and under the eyes, the frontal sinuses are over the eyes, the ethmoid sinuses are between the nose and the orbital cavities, and the sphenoid sinuses are almost in the center of the skull. The mucous membrane of each sinus is continuous with that of the nose, and infections that may start in the nose commonly spread to the paranasal sinuses.

Posteriorly, the nose opens into the nasopharynx through two symmetrical openings called the posterior choanae. This region is examined best by introducing into the mouth a small mirror directed upward toward the nasopharynx.

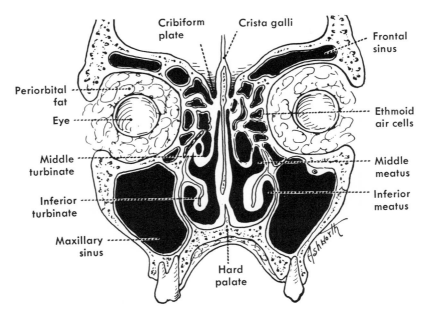

Fig. 18-2. Frontal section showing the paranasal sinuses. (From DeWeese, David D., and Saunders, William H.: Textbook of otolaryngology, ed. 4, St. Louis, 1973, The C. V. Mosby Co.)

PHYSIOLOGY

Medical texts have a tendency to glorify the physiologic functions of the nose. In man, its chief functions are to provide an airway and an organ of smell and to warm and moisten air to prepare it for the lungs.

There are thousands of cilia in the nasal mucosa that beat posteriorly in rhythmic waves to sweep nasal mucus into the nasopharynx, where it is swallowed. Trapped in the mucus are bacteria, dust, and other foreign matter entering the nose. Ciliary motion is influenced by temperature changes, dryness, and application of certain drugs. If ciliary motion is paralyzed either by drugs or drying of the nasal mucosa, there is less resistance to bacterial invasion. Humidification to maintain a relative humidity of 35% to 40% is helpful. Vibrissae, or nasal hairs, serve to catch larger foreign bodies such as lint and dust.

The *olfactory epithelium* contains the sensory end organ for smell and is different histologically from the epithelium of the rest of the nose. It is high in the nose and covers a relatively small area. When air currents cannot reach the olfactory epithelium because of nasal obstruction, there is *anosmia*—loss of the sense of smell. Anosmia may also be the result of skull fracture that passes across the cribriform plate at the roof of the nose. There, filaments of the olfactory nerve pass into the nose to be distributed to the nasal mucous membrane. Also, viral infections are a common cause of anosmia, affecting the olfactory nerve just as they do nerves in other parts of the body. Tumors of the meninges (meningioma) which may form in the olfactory area may also cause anosmia, but rarely do. A perverted sense of smell, called *parosmia,* may follow anosmia; parosmia also may be present temporarily during sinusitis or other upper respiratory infection. The senses of taste and smell are sometimes hard to differentiate, and many things that we think we taste, we actually smell. In some lower animals the olfactory sense is much more highly developed than it is in man; in them the sense of smell is important for survival.

The inferior turbinates, bones with thick vascular mucosa, lie along the lateral walls of the nose and warm inspired air. A part of the inspiratory resistance is provided by the swollen turbinates, which engorge on one side while decongesting on the other at intervals of approximately one-half to two hours, thus shifting the air stream from one nasal passage to the other. During sleep, the dependent side of the nose becomes congested and may cause the individual to turn over.

Just as there is warming of inspired air by the nose, there is also humidification. There are mucous and serous glands in the nasal mucosa that secrete as much as a quart of liquid every day. Most of this moisture is absorbed by the dry air we breathe. From various causes, however, there may be an excess of mucus secreted that cannot be absorbed but is carried posteriorly by nasal cilia. Patients who feel this relatively normal mucus in the pharynx complain of "phlegm" or "catarrh." The appearance of mucus is clear and tenacious, whereas purulent secretions, as in a patient with sinusitis, are white or pus-like. This distinction is important for the examiner to make since many patients who have only an excess of normal mucus complain of "sinus," implying that there is a purulent infection present somewhere in the nose or sinal area.

Although great emphasis is placed on the functions of warming and moistening, one wonders how important these functions really are when considering the patient after laryngectomy. In a laryngectomized patient all air enters the lungs through a tracheostomy and none through the nose, and he has no more lower respiratory infections than anyone else. Of course, after laryngectomy there is a loss of the sense of smell because air no longer reaches the olfactory area.

CHAPTER NINETEEN # Epistaxis (nosebleed)

The cause of most nosebleeds is trauma. Sometimes the trauma is very minor as, for example, that produced by dry air, which causes crusting of the nasal mucosa. Small blood vessels split and bleed. More serious trauma may be inflicted by the nose picker's fingernail or by severe sneezing or coughing. In the posterior part of the nose, where trauma is unlikely to be caused by extrinsic sources, nosebleeds may result from injury to blood vessels by arteriosclerosis or hypertension. It is important to stress trauma as the cause of nosebleeds because all too often the cause mistakenly is thought to be some deficiency in the blood itself. For example, we know that scurvy, the result of insufficient vitamin C, can cause nosebleeds; so can certain conditions caused by lack of vitamin K. In these patients, however, there is bleeding from all parts of the body, not just the nose. Furthermore, these are rare causes of nosebleed. If trauma is not recognized as the usual cause of nosebleed, the patient receives medical treatment for a surgical condition: carbazochrome (Adrenosem), vitamin K, snake venom, or estrogenic substances, none of which has anything to do with treatment of a ruptured blood vessel, are given instead of resorting to local packing and cautery. The chief errors made in the management of nosebleeds are failure to find the exact bleeding site and treating the patient medically for what is really a surgical condition.

ANTERIOR NOSEBLEEDS

Most nosebleeds come from the anterior part of the nasal septum, where there is a plexus of tiny arteries and veins. Sometimes when there is a deflection or protrusion of the anterior part of the nasal septum toward one side of the nose, bleeding is even more likely, because air currents rushing in the nose dry the prominent part and cause crusting. The anterior part of the septum is also a favorite place to start bleeding with the fingernail.

Treatment of anterior nosebleeds is relatively easy (Figs. 19-1 to 19-5). With the patient upright in a chair a strong suction apparatus with an angulated suction tip is used to remove blood clots from the nose. If a suction pump is not available, the patient may hold one side of his nose and blow the bleeding side to remove clots. Immediately a cotton ball soaked in aqueous epinephrine, 1:1,000, is inserted in the bleeding side and pressure applied for several minutes on the side of the nose (the ala). This

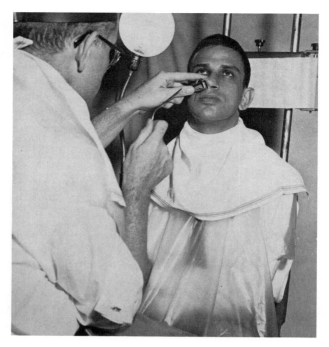

Fig. 19-1. Both the *patient and doctor* are draped for the treatment of nosebleed.

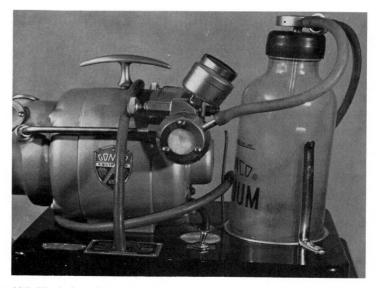

Fig. 19-2. Typical suction pump. Vacuum bottle should be cleaned after each use.

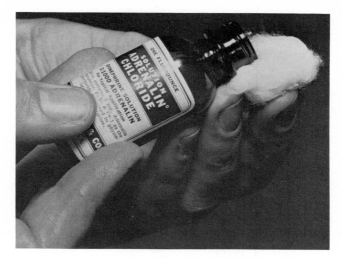

Fig. 19-3. Adrenalin chloride to control anterior nosebleeds until cautery can be applied.

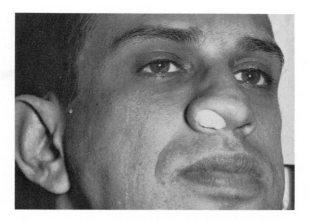

Fig. 19-4. Cotton pack as emergency treatment for nosebleed from the anterior part of the nose.

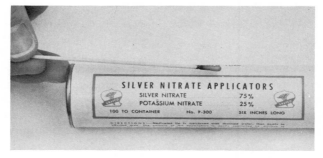

Fig. 19-5. Cautery by silver nitrate is a common method of treating nosebleeds that come from the anterior part of the nasal septum.

routine almost always controls the bleeding. Next, using his head mirror to reflect a bright light and a nasal speculum to open the nostril, the physician locates the *exact* bleeding spot and cauterizes it with a silver nitrate stick or electric cautery. Silver nitrate does not produce very deep cautery, but it coagulates the mucous membrane sufficiently to control most bleeders. Ordinarily, topical anesthesia is unnecessary for silver nitrate cautery. If electric cautery is used, the anterior part of the septum is injected with Xylocaine, 1%. Electric cautery is deeper than silver nitrate cautery. Once bleeding is controlled, no nasal packing is necessary. In those instances in which a severe septal deviation seems to contribute to the bleeding, submucous resection to straighten the septum may be indicated later.

The nurse at times may be able to control anterior nosebleeds. The patient should be placed in a sitting position with his head inclined slightly forward. In this position blood does not flow into the nasopharynx and gag the patient. If a suction machine is not used, the nurse may have the patient blow his nose vigorously to remove blood clots before applying pressure against the ala of the bleeding nostril. The amount of blood lost should be noted and reported, vital signs checked, fear allayed, and the patient kept as quiet as possible. A calm attitude on the part of the nurse will do a great deal in reassuring the apprehensive patient. The nurse herself may feel reassured if she remembers that patients do not die of nosebleeds, although they often faint. Once bleeding is controlled, the patient should be instructed not to blow or pick his nose.

ANTERIOR ETHMOIDAL ARTERY

The second area likely to bleed is high and posterior, where bleeding comes from the anterior ethmoidal artery. Blood runs down the nasal septum from high in the nose, and because the bleeding site cannot be seen and cauterized, packing is used. A piece of petrolatum gauze about as big as a bean is pressed into the crevice between the septum and the middle turbinate. Then additional packing to hold this small piece of gauze in place can be applied. The packing is left two or three days and removed. Ordinarily, there is no further bleeding, but if there is, the pack is replaced.

Rarely, ligation of the anterior ethmoidal artery through an incision along the side of the nose may be necessary. Usually, when this operation is done, it means that packing was not placed correctly.

POSTERIOR NOSEBLEEDS

Bleeding from the posterior part of the nose is more common in the elderly than in young persons. The bleeding here is likely to be severe— sometimes a patient will bleed a pint or even a quart within an hour's time. Because the bleeding is heavy and from far back in the nose, good visualization is not possible. Treatment is not by cautery but by a postnasal pack (Figs. 19-6 and 19-7). A catheter is passed through the nose and pulled out the mouth. Two strings or heavy black sutures already sewn into the pack are tied to the end of the catheter. A third string is attached to the opposite

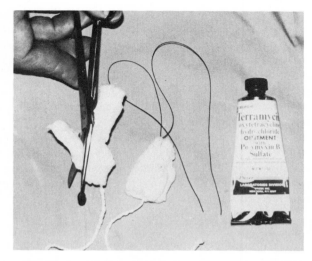

Fig. 19-6. Postnasal pack formed from a vaginal tampon. Note the final shape and the two silk sutures on one end and single string on the other. The antibiotic ointment will lubricate the pack.

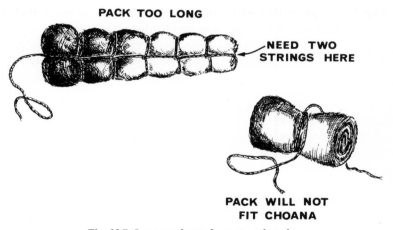

Fig. 19-7. Improperly made postnasal packs.

end of the pack with which it can be withdrawn several days later. Withdrawing the catheter through the nose pulls the strings and the pack into the nasopharynx, where it is seated firmly. The third string dangles in the pharynx. Placing a postnasal pack is distressing; some patients faint. Before the pack is pulled into the nasopharynx it should be well lubricated, *preferably with an antibiotic ointment* such as oxytetracycline (Terramycin) or Neosporin. These ointments inhibit bacterial growth and prevent the pack from developing a foul odor.

The strings pulled out the front of the nose are tied around a gauze but *never around the nasal septum*. Both strings are brought out the same side of the nose. Additional packing is then used anteriorly in the nose. In front, packing is usually ½-inch petrolatum gauze, although gauze impregnated with an antibiotic ointment is preferable to petrolatum.

The postnasal pack is left in place for two or three days and then removed by traction on the string dangling in the pharynx. If the patient continues to bleed, the pack is replaced.

An inflatable, balloon-like postnasal pack can also be obtained, or some physicians use a Foley-type urethral catheter. This balloon, however, does not exert pressure accurately at the bleeding site but merely becomes inflated in the nasopharynx to provide a stabilizing mass against which anterior packing can be placed firmly.

NURSING CARE OF PATIENTS WITH NASAL PACKING

Patients with postnasal packs are usually admitted to the hospital. Those with lesser nosebleeds from the anterior part of the nose are seldom admitted to the hospital. After postnasal packing, roentgenograms will show "clouding" of the maxillary sinus on the side of the pack, because blood is forced into the sinus during the packing procedure. Postnasal packs should be constructed so that they will not occlude the eustachian tube, since if they do, the patient develops serous otitis media on that side, with fullness in the ear and sometimes pain and a minor hearing loss.

The nurse's responsibility in the management of patients with nosebleeds is to have postnasal packs available and to see that the strings are securely attached so that they will not pull off at a crucial time. She must remember that the packing procedure often makes a patient faint and, should he start to faint, that it is important to hold his head so that it does not strike the floor. If the patient seems to be getting weak, lower his head, and usually he will not faint. Even though the patient may faint, there is no likelihood that he will die, because when he faints, his blood pressure falls and the nosebleed stops.

Nosebleeds cause blood to run into the back of the throat so that the patient gags and chokes if he is supine; therefore, the patient is treated while seated upright in a chair.

The nursing care of patients with nasal packing is important. The patient and family are usually concerned that the gauze under the nose ("nasal snuffer") be kept reasonably clean by changing it as often as needed—usually from one to three times on the day of the operation. There always is a little blood leaking from the nose or into the nasopharynx even with packs in place, but this is old blood that the patient has already lost. At first it is bright but later it becomes dark and brownish; the patient needs to be reassured that he is not bleeding anew.

The nurse can explain to the patient that, because his nose is closed by packing, there will be a sucking action in his throat when he swallows but will be relieved as soon as the packing is removed. She may tell the patient that all of his packing is well lubricated and that, while there may be a little bleeding when the packs are removed, there will be no pain. Any temperature elevation should be reported.

Packs are removed with the patient in bed, a large towel tied about his neck, and an emesis basin under his chin where the packing and blood can drop. Some patients become faint whenever there are any manipulative procedures on the body or when they see blood, so that removing packing *in bed* is important.

After the packing is removed, the patient ordinarily can be up and about but remains in the hospital another day or two to make certain that the bleeding does not recur. He should be able to take any ordinary diet. He should expect some minor drainage of old blood from his nose anteriorly and into his throat posteriorly. This may be enough to require the continued use of a nasal snuffer for a day or two. During the next week or so he should avoid blowing his nose and lifting.

Arterial ligations for nosebleed. Ligation of the external carotid controls severe nosebleeds from the posterior part of the nose for which postnasal packing was unsuccessful. An external incision in the neck is used and one or two ligatures placed around the artery.

The internal maxillary artery is a branch of the external carotid artery, and it is through this artery that blood reaches the posterior part of the nose. Instead of ligation of the external carotid, this artery can be ligated by entering the maxillary sinus through a Caldwell-Luc incision (see Fig. 21-6) and then removing the posterior wall of the maxillary sinus. The artery is found in the space just behind the sinus. An operating microscope is used for this operation. Once the artery is identified, two or three metal clips are placed to ligate it. Ligation of this artery may be even more effective than ligation of the external carotid artery, since the blood supply is interrupted nearer the point of bleeding.

The anterior ethmoidal artery provides blood to the upper posterior part of the nose and can be ligated through a curving incision adjacent to the inner canthus of the eye. The periorbital fascia is elevated so that the orbit can be retracted laterally and then the artery is found as it comes through the bone along the side of the nose. A silver clip is placed here and the wound closed.

Arterial ligations, especially ligation of the internal maxillary artery, are used more and more frequently. Some physicians perform such surgery even before attempting to control the bleeding with postnasal packs. They say that discomfort to the patient is less than when postnasal packs are in place. Patients often agree.

HEREDITARY HEMORRHAGIC TELANGIECTASIA

Hereditary hemorrhagic telangiectasia is a disorder causing severe, usually daily, lifelong nosebleeds (Fig. 19-8). These patients, who inherit their disease, have tiny arteriovenous aneurysms, or telangiectasias, in various organs and on most body surfaces (skin, pleura, gastrointestinal

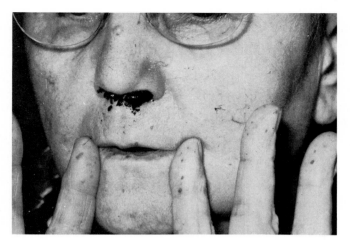

Fig. 19-8. Typical patient with hereditary hemorrhagic telangiectasia. Note nasal obstruction from blood crusts—a lifelong complaint. (From Saunders, William H.: Archives of Otolaryngology 76:245, 1962.)

tract, and ureter). The telangiectasias appear as red spots slightly raised above the surface. On skin or on mucous membranes derived from skin (squamous epithelium) they seldom bleed because the skin and its derivatives are tough and resist bleeding. In the nose, however, with its fragile respiratory epithelium, and in the gastrointestinal tract, where there also is nonsquamous epithelium, hemorrhages are frequent. Some patients with this disease have required 2,000 transfusions during their lifetimes; many have had fifty.

To control epistaxis in patients with hereditary hemorrhagic telangiectasia, an operation called *septal dermoplasty* is done. After removal of mucosa from the anterior one-third of the nose, a split-thickness graft of skin (15/1,000 inch) from the upper thigh is placed on the anterior one-third of the nasal septum, bilaterally, with additional grafts on each lateral wall. Perichondrium under the mucosa is left, and it both nourishes the septal cartilage and serves as a base for the grafts. Nasal packing is placed for five days to hold the grafts. The patient has very little difficulty with nasal discomfort, except that his nasal airway is blocked, but his thigh, from which the split-thickness graft was removed, is sore; loose pajamas and a light gauze dressing over the donor site will be required. The skin grows in the nose, and because it resists trauma, the patient has much less trouble with nosebleeds.

•   •   •

Hemoglobin determinations made at the time a patient is bleeding or just after he has bleed are inaccurate. Hemoconcentration occurs, and it is not until the patient drinks large quantities of water and his blood volume is restored that the hemoglobin determinations reflects a true value. For example, it is not unusual, right after a postnasal pack has been placed, to get a report of 12 grams. The next day, even though the patient has not bled any more, it may be 8 grams.

To help in reestablishing the fluid component of the blood volume, *the nurse* can assist by seeing to it that the patient drinks large quantities of liquids or, if he will not drink, she should call the reduced intake to the physician's attention, and he will order intravenous feedings.

No patient bleeds from both sides of the nose simultaneously unless he has had a severe fracture or unless he has some disease causing generalized bleeding, such as leukemia. Blood does come from both sides of the nose, but it runs from the bleeding side behind the nasal septum and out the *normal* side. This concept is important because it means that in almost all instances it is necessary to pack only one side of the nose.

No special medication is required for the usual patient with epistaxis. Secobarbital (Seconal) is given as a sedative, and morphine or meperidine is given for pain caused by the postnasal pack. Drugs aimed at promoting blood clotting are unnecessary, since this is not a factor in the average nosebleed. The problem is a hole in the blood vessel, and this hole needs to be plugged by packing or cautery.

SUGGESTED READINGS

Chandler, J. R., and Serrins, A. J.: Transantral ligation of the internal maxillary artery for epistaxis, Laryngoscope **75:** 1151, 1965.

Kuhn, A. J., and Hallberg, O. E.: Complications of postnasal packing for epistaxis, Annals of Otology **62:**62, 1955.

Osmun, Paul M.: Nosebleeds, American Journal of Nursing **56:**1411-1413, Nov., 1956.

Saunders, William H.: Practical management of nosebleeds, General Practitioners **17:** 100, 1958.

CHAPTER TWENTY

Nasal obstruction;
nasal injury; septal perforation

OBSTRUCTION

Nasal obstruction is a common and annoying complaint caused by a number of conditions. Some of them are simple mechanical displacements such as might result from a nasal fracture, while others are the result of systemic disorders that cause swelling of the nasal mucous membranes such as occurs with allergic rhinitis or severe hypothyroidism. The *only* way the doctor can identify the cause is by *inspecting the nose,* and this means looking anteriorly with the nasal speculum and posteriorly with a nasopharyngeal mirror. Roentgenographic examination and laboratory tests may assist in some cases.

Hypertrophic adenoid tissue

In infants and young children the cause of nasal obstruction is most likely to be hypertrophic adenoid. Children who have persistent adenoidal obstruction breathe through their mouths, and some eventually may develop a characteristic appearance with broad nose, staring eyes, and open mouth known as adenoid facies. The treatment for this type of nasal obstruction is adenoidectomy.

The nurse in a school setting or in other community service should direct patients with obvious nasal obstruction to a doctor's attention.

Choanal atresia

Choanal atresia is an infrequent congenital condition producing nasal obstruction in which a plate of bone or fibrous tissue blocks one or both of the posterior openings of the nose (the posterior "choanae"). Passage of a small catheter into each side of the nose to see if it appears in the pharynx will demonstrate obstruction, as will an x-ray made with the nose filled with a radiopaque dye—if there is posterior obstruction, the dye remains in the nasal chambers rather than appearing in the throat as it normally would.

The condition can be either unilateral or bilateral. If it is unilateral the infant ordinarily progresses satisfactorily except that there is a collection of mucus in the obstructed side of the nose which cannot drain posteriorly as it normally would. From time to time there is an unexpected dropping out of the mucus. This persists lifelong unless the condition is corrected. In the case of bilateral choanal atresia, the condition may even be incompatible with life since the newborn infant may refuse to breathe through his mouth. In such a case it is necesssary to provide an oral airway that is left taped in place until the choanal atresia can be corrected. Even then the infant has a great deal of difficulty breathing through his mouth and drinking at the same time.

Treatment is surgical and consists of removal of the obstructive partition.

Deformity of the nasal septum

Deformity of the nasal septum is a common cause of nasal obstruction in older children and adults (Fig. 20-1). The nasal septum, which ideally should be thin and straight, is deflected as a result of injury, and it impairs the airway. Almost all young children have a straight nasal septum, but few adults do. Actually, it does not really matter whether the septum is straight so long as it is not obstructive.

When there is enough septal deformity to make the patient complain of nasal obstruction, the condition can be corrected by an operation called *submucous resection*. This is an excellent operation, although its improper use for relief of symptoms such as hearing loss or headache, which are in no way related to the deformed septum, may give it a bad name.

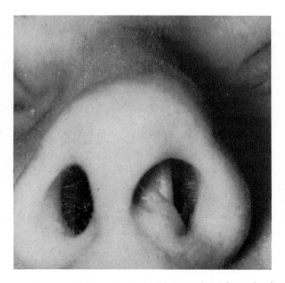

Fig. 20-1. Anterior end of septal cartilage is dislocated and projecting into the nasal vestibule.

The submucous resection operation is done best using local anesthesia. About 0.6 Gm. of cocaine crystals is placed in a medicine glass, and cotton-tipped wire applicators moistened in aqueous epinephrine are dipped in the crystals to form a mixture called cocaine "mud."

The nurse cannot be too careful to make certain that each container on her table is properly marked and that there is never any confusion about which solution or drug the surgeon is using. In this operation, for example, it is common to use cocaine solution, epinephrine, Xylocaine, and saline solution. Injection of either cocaine or epinephrine probably would be fatal, whereas Xylocaine is intended for injection. The surgeon should himself either draw up the solution or at the very least observe the nurse as she does so.

After anesthesia an incision is made on one side of the nasal septum from top to bottom. Working through this incision, the surgeon separates the perichondrium or lining of the cartilage from the cartilage itself. After the cartilaginous and bony parts of the septum are freed of their membranous coverings, obstructive parts of cartilage and bone are removed. There are many variations of the operation: in some the parts removed are discarded, while in others they are straightened and replaced. Packing is placed in both sides of the nose and left for two days to prevent bleeding and to hold the mucoperichondrial flaps together.

Nursing care

Postoperatively, the patient complains that, when he attempts to swallow with his nose packed, there is a sucking action in his throat. This is because the nasal packing does not let air through the nose, and a partial vacuum forms in the throat during swallowing. There is likely to be enough pain for a few hours postoperatively to require meperidine, 100 mg., or morphine, 16 mg., for one or two doses. Sleep may be disturbed because of the packing, and Seconal, 0.1 Gm., may be prescribed before bedtime. A gauze snuffer under the nose is changed by the nurse when it becomes blood soaked. Ordinarily there is little bleeding, perhaps only enough to color the gauze two or three times, but occasionally the nurse must call the surgeon to place additional packing to control greater bleeding. When he does, he will probably want a nasal speculum, bayonet forceps, cotton, and ½-inch petrolatum gauze. Antibiotic ointment (Terramycin) may be added to the petrolatum gauze. Ordinarily nasal packing is used after submucous resection operation does not cause significant obstruction to the ostia of the paranasal sinuses, such as occurs with posterior and anterior nasal packing for nosebleeds. Packs are left in place from twenty-four to forty-eight hours.

Infection is not a problem after the submucous resection operation, probably because of the excellent blood supply of the nose.

The inferior turbinates. The inferior turbinates are sometimes the cause of considerable nasal obstruction, either because the bone of the turbinate is too large and simply juts out into the nasal airway strongly, or because the soft tissue covering the turbinate is hyperplastic or polypoid and redundant. In either case, local surgery on the turbinate bone (submucous resection of the inferior turbinate) or electric fulguration will be effective in restoring an airway. Surgical procedures on the turbinate are apt to be followed by excessive bleeding unless packing is left in place for three or four days.

Tumors as a cause of nasal obstruction

Both *benign and malignant tumors* produce nasal obstruction, either unilateral or bilateral. A carcinoma of the maxillary sinus, for example, may erode through the adjacent nasal wall and block one side of the nose completely. It usually is easily recognized because of its friable, bleeding surface and because of other associated findings of maxillary carcinoma. Carcinoma arising in the ethmoid sinus behaves similarly.

Nasopharyngeal carcinomas can easily obstruct the nose, first one side and then both sides. These tumors tend to metastasize early so that by the time nasal obstruction is advanced, there often is a large mass in the neck.

There is an uncommon benign tumor, seen in young boys almost exclusively, called a *juvenile angiofibroma,* which grows from the periosteum of the bones of the base of the skull and protrudes into the nasopharynx. Eventually it causes obstruction of one or both of the posterior nasal choanae. The other cardinal symptom is bleeding. Treatment is by surgical excision, usually through a transpalatal approach. Irradiation therapy is favored by some.

Choanal polyp has been discussed and is a common cause for obstruction in the posterior nose.

The list of tumors, malignant and benign, that cause nasal obstruction could be extended for several paragraphs, but most of the others are rare.

Nasal allergy

Nasal allergy, a common cause of nasal obstruction, is often seasonal ("hay fever"), or it may be present the year around (perennial allergy). The best treatment for any kind of allergy is to separate the patient from his allergen, but usually this is not practical. An example would be to remove a dog or cat from the house when it is known that animal hair or dander causes the patient's allergic reaction. But usually the problem is not that simple, and the next best measure is to attempt to desensitize the patient to his particular allergen. For some patients a series of shots for desensitization given in anticipation of the hay fever season works very well. The antihistaminic group of drugs also affords relief in allergic rhinitis. The objections that many patients have to antihistaminics are that the medication makes them drowsy or makes their mouths dry.

Finally, when nothing else relieves the nasal obstruction of patients with allergic rhinitis, surgical procedures may be of help. The submucous resection operation will thin and straighten the septum. But in an allergic patient with swollen mucous membranes, it is less effective than in a patient whose only cause for obstruction is a thick, crooked septum.

A procedure that is more effective, although it is not used very often, is submucous resection of the inferior turbinates. The inferior turbinate, the largest of the four turbinal bones in each side of the nose, contains blood spaces, which engorge for the purpose of warming inspired air. In submucous resection only the bone of the turbinate is removed, and the membranous part continues to function. Postoperative care is the same as that for submucous resection of the septum.

Patients with allergic rhinitis frequently have *polyps*—pale, soft, edematous outpocketings of nasal or sinal mucosa that look like skinned white grapes. Polyps, usually present bilaterally, do not originate from the lining of the nose itself but from the mucosa of the sinuses or their ostia and then hang down into the nose to cause obstruction to the airway. A solitary polyp, unless it is very large, usually is not obstructive, but when there are multiple polyps, nasal obstruction may be severe. Polyps also cause anosmia (loss of sense of smell) by preventing air from reaching the olfactory mucosa high in the nose.

Polypectomy is an old and satisfactory procedure. It would give lasting relief were it not there is a strong tendency for nasal polyps to recur after removal. Polypectomy is best done in the hospital, and local anesthesia like that used in the submucous resection operation is adequate. If there are only a few polyps, the doctor may remove them in his office, but the objections to this and similar office procedures are: some patients bleed excessively, some become faint, and some do both. Polyps are removed with an instrument much like a tonsil snare except that it is smaller. No special technique beyond packing is required to control bleeding after polypectomy. Ligatures are not used. A pack of ½-inch gauze, impregnated with an antibiotic ointment such as Terramycin or Neosporin, is left in the nose for a day or two. Packs with these ointments have an advantage compared with packs with petrolatum; the antibiotic ointments inhibit bacterial growth, and odor does not develop even though the packing is left in place several days. In those cases in which simple nasal polypectomy is done two or three times and still there is recurrence, an operation such as intranasal or external ethmoidectomy may be indicated for more complete removal.

Rhinitis medicamentosa

Rhinitis medicamentosa, a very common condition caused by overuse of nose drops, implies a rebound phenomenon in which the patient's nasal mucosa swells worse than ever as soon as the immediate effect of nose drops has worn off; then nothing helps him to breathe freely except more nose drops. Thus a vicious circle is established. Some patients who become addicted to nose drops in this way may use them ten or more times a day for many years. The treatment is simple—the patient must stop using nose drops completely. In two or three weeks he can breathe through his nose again. During the initial period of abstinence a sedative at night such as Seconal, 0.1 Gm., is useful so the patient can sleep even with his obstructed nose. Also, orally administered nasal decongestants such as chlorpheniramine maleate (Ornade Spansules), one capsule twice daily, may help.

Vasomotor rhinitis

Vasomotor rhinitis also causes formation of excessive nasal mucus. The patient's nasal mucosa appears somewhat bluish and swollen and the inferior turbinates, especially, are engorged. The patient and his doctor may suspect a nasal allergy, but testing gives negative results. Such patients often complain of "sinus," meaning they have postnasal discharge ("phlegm") and some nasal obstruction, and often headaches. Whether there is a connection between their headaches and vasomotor rhinitis often is not certain, and in most instances the headache is probably coincidental.

The cause of vasomotor rhinitis is rather unclear. It may result from an unstable autonomic nervous system that permits engorgement of the blood vessels of the nasal mucosa, especially those in the inferior turbinates, and the overproduction of nasal mucus.

Medical treatment with antihistamines is often used but these drugs are more symptomatic than curative, and a patient cannot be expected to use them for years. When all else fails, electrical fulguration of the inferior turbinates or submucous resection of the turbinates may help the nasal obstruction but usually will not reduce excessive nasal mucus.

Other medical causes of nasal obstruction

The causes mentioned in the preceding paragraphs are by far the more important ones. Of course there are patients with uncommon disorders, for example, severe hypothyroidism, who have nasal obstruction; and some drugs such as the rauwolfia group (for reduction of hypertension) produce nasal obstruction. Sinusitis, as such, should *not* cause nasal obstruction, although most laymen think it does.

Foreign body

A nasal foreign body should always be suspected when a child has unilateral nasal obstruction and discharge. Almost anything that a child can put into his nose has been found there; paper wads, erasers, stones, beads, and vegetal foreign bodies are among the more common objects. The 2- or 3-year-old child can be expected to be uncooperative, and restraint is needed to make adequate intranasal inspection possible. The nurse can be of great assistance by correctly wrapping or "mummying" the child in a sheet. She may also need the aid of an assistant to help hold the squirming body for examination. A simple, calm explanation of the purpose of the wrap and the examination may help calm the child. The nurse should ask the parents to leave the room but should reassure the child that he will be with his parents when the examination is complete. The toddler has a strong attachment to his mother and fears abandonment.

The physician needs a suction machine and an angulated nasal suction tip to clear the nose of secretions. Vasoconstrictors such as ephedrine, 1 or 2%, Neo-Synephrine, 1% or topical epinephrine, 1:1,000, instilled into the affected side of the nose provide shrinkage of intranasal membranes and make it easier to locate the foreign body. There are angulated instruments for extraction designed to keep the physician's own hand out of his view.

If there is difficulty in extracting the foreign body, it is best to desist and start again with the patient under general anesthesia.

Septal abscess and septal hematoma, acute causes of nasal obstruction, are discussed later in this chapter.

INJURY OR INFECTION
Fracture

Fractures of the nasal bones or nasal septum are more common than generally supposed. Many are caused by relatively minor injuries such as a fall or being struck by a ball, and in a child they may be unnoticed at the end of the day. Others, especially in the adult, are the result of a more severe blow, as from a fight or automobile accident, and often are associated with other facial trauma (Fig. 20-2). When there is no displacement of the nose and no nasal obstruction, the patient often does not even consult a doctor. In this case it usually does not matter, since if a fracture causes no cosmetic deformity and no obstruction to the airway, there is no disability.

More serious nasal fractures may produce both external deformity and nasal obstruction, and careful reduction is important. Sometimes there are serious facial and skull fractures associated with the nasal fracture. If the patient's general condition is poor, nothing is lost by waiting several days before reducing his nasal fracture. Should ten days go by, however, the nasal bones will have started to unite and reduction becomes difficult.

To reduce many nasal fractures all that is necessary is to press firmly with one or both thumbs on the convex side of the nose (Fig. 20-3). Usually this

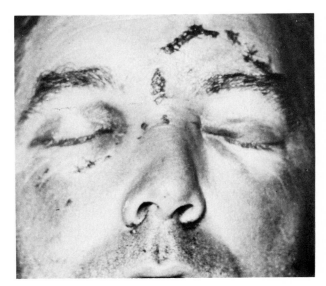

Fig. 20-2. Laterally displaced fracture of nose. Pressure on convex side will restore alignment.

maneuver is easy, and the displaced bones and septum move into their correct position. Ordinarily no anesthetic is needed. The patient's head is placed on a firm support such as a table, with a folded sheet serving as a pad. (Reducing a fracture with the patient upright in a chair invites fainting.) Fractures that cannot be reduced by this technique should be managed in the operating room under local or general anesthesia. Sometimes considerable intranasal manipulation is required to elevate depressed fragments of bone or cartilage. Hematomas forming in the septum require aspiration or drainage.

In treating nasal fractures there is a tendency to disregard the intranasal appearances and concentrate on obtaining a good-looking external nose. This neglect may lead to subsequent impairment of the airway. Associated lacerations must be closed carefully with fine nylon suture such as No. 5-0 Ethilon or Dermalon—monofilamentous threads that give a finer scar than silk or cotton.

Fractures of the maxillary and zygomatic (malar) bones are not as common as nasal fractures but are seen after automobile accidents and fights. The passenger in the right-hand front seat of the automobile is subject to severe facial fractures if the car stops suddenly. As he is thrown forward, his face strikes the dashboard. Nasal fracture, zygomatic fracture, and a loosening of the maxillary bones result. The deformity has been called the "middle third" (of the face) fracture or the "guest passenger" accident.

Uncomplicated zygomatic fractures are easily reduced by means of a small incision just anterior to the ear and above the zygomatic arch, and

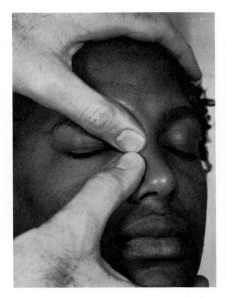

Fig. 20-3. Reduction of simple nasal fracture. Most nasal fractures are simple lateral displacements rather than depressed fractures. Firm pressure on the convex side of the nose pushes it back into position.

then introduction of an elevator deep to the fascia of the temporalis muscle which splits around the zygoma. The elevator is used to pry the zygomatic fracture forward into place. The more severe middle third fractures require interdental wiring, and often several small incisions about the face are needed to wire bones together at the sites of multiple fractures. Nursing care after such an accident becomes extremely important, because with the teeth wired together the patient has great trouble eating, oral hygiene is difficult, and for a time his eyes may be swollen shut.

Padded dashboards and seat belts help greatly in reducing the severity and incidence of these injuries. The lap belt is effective in preventing the rider from being thrown from the car when the door flies open at the moment of impact, but it does nothing to prevent the rider from doubling forward. The face can still strike the dashboard with great force. Additional protection is provided by the shoulder harness. The headrest is also effective in reducing severity of the so-called whiplash injury to the neck, which occurs when a car is struck from behind; the passenger's head is thrown backward, and the neck undergoes great stress, which may cause a number of complaints related to the head and neck.

Blowout fracture. The so-called blowout fracture results when blunt trauma to the orbit suddenly raises the intraorbital pressure and drives orbital fat and muscles through the thin bony floor of the orbit. This means that the orbital contents are hanging into the maxillary sinus. Sometimes there is not a significant depression of the bony fragment, and yet double vision may result from incarceration of the extraocular muscles in the fracture site. Surgical exploration by means of either an orbital or a transsinal approach or both is required if the posttraumatic symptom of diplopia (double vision) is to be prevented (Fig. 20-4).

Mandibular fracture. Mandibular fracture is diagnosed by abnormal occlusion, abnormal mobility with irregularity of the dental arch, and pain on clenching the jaws at the site of the fractures. Careful intraoral inspec-

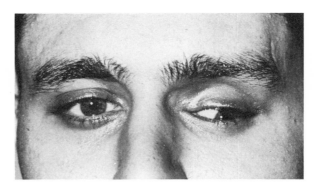

Fig. 20-4. Deformity after untreated fracture of inferior orbital rim and "blowout" fracture. (From DeWeese, David D, and Saunders, William H.: Textbook of otolaryngology, ed. 4, St. Louis, 1973, The C. V. Mosby Co.)

tion and palpation are important. Fractures of the coronoid and condylar processes often must be diagnosed from palpable localized hematoma or point tenderness. Bimanual examination of the retrotonsillar fossa offers further information about the ramus of the mandible. Roentgenograms are invaluable and serve not only as diagnostic aids but also as permanent records of the injury.

Treatment of most mandibular fractures is not difficult if there are teeth in the upper and lower jaws. Then interdental wiring can be used to stabilize the fractured segments until union occurs. In the absence of teeth, fixation may have to be achieved by open reduction and wiring of the fragments or by use of Kirschner wires or metal plate. Generally, the best results are obtained by using the simplest methods because elaborate, complicated appliances may themselves cause complications.

Septal hematoma and septal abscess (Fig. 20-5)

After injury or infection, blood or pus may form between the septal cartilage and its covering membrane of perichondrium. These accumulations separate perichondrium from cartilage, leaving the cartilage without an adequate blood supply. As a result, the cartilage may slough out and the dorsum of the nose drop, causing a saddle nose (Fig. 20-6, *A*). To prevent loss of cartilage, repeated drainage of hematoma or abscess is imperative because the blood or pus often re-forms. In the case of abscess there is additional danger from infection of lymphatic channels leading from the nose to the cavernous sinus within the skull. Infection of the cavernous sinus is associated with a high mortality rate.

Rhinoplasty

Reconstruction of the external nose is called rhinoplasty, an operation done usually for cosmetic reasons. Sometimes the operation is combined with reconstruction of the nasal septum in a patient who also has nasal obstruction. Rhinoplasty is not, or should not, be intended as an operation to improve nasal function; a patient simply does not like his nose and wants it smaller, the tip elevated, a hump removed, or the nose placed more exactly in the midline. To do this is a major procedure involving sawing or chiseling of the nasal bones to free them of their attachments to other bones of the face. It is also necessary to divide and shorten parts of the cartilaginous framework in the tip of the nose and then to reassemble everything for a more attractive centerpiece. The operation is done usually under local anesthesia. (See Fig. 20-6.)

Dressings, which are applied carefully, consist of tape on the skin covered with a metal or hard rubber shield for protection. Postoperatively the patient is placed in Fowler's position to minimize oozing. A patient must necessarily breathe through his mouth, thus requiring measures for preventing drying of the oral mucosa (e.g., sips of water and frequent use of mouthwashes). Postoperatively, black eyes are common. The swelling and ecchymosis around the eyes reach their height within twenty-four to forty-

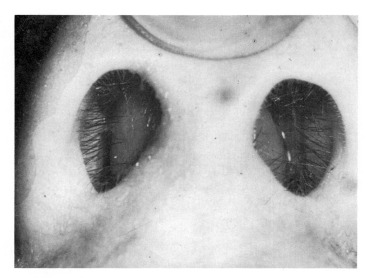

Fig. 20-5. Septal abscess. Note swelling of the septum bilaterally.

eight hours and then gradually disappear, the color changing from dark blue to yellow by the end of the first week. Discoloration is almost completely gone by the end of the second week. Pain is present for a few hours, but usually it is not great. The *nurse's responsibility* is to see that the patient does not remove or pick at the dressing, that he is comfortable, and that instruments are on hand so that the surgeon can change the dressing on the fourth or fifth postoperative day. Surgeons are particular about their rhinoplasty dressings, and no alterations should be made by the nurse without specific orders. Adhesive remover such as chlorothene is useful to cleanse the skin, but great care must be taken to keep these solutions out of the eyes. Mineral oil will also remove tape and causes little or no skin irritation. Many surgeons like to use cotton applicators soaked in hydrogen peroxide to remove dried blood from the rims of the nostrils.

Septal perforation

As the result of nose picking, infection, submucous resection operation, or trauma, a perforation sometimes develops in the nasal septum, usually in the anterior cartilaginous portion. Many perforations are asymptomatic, whereas some cause bleeding and crusting. A small perforation may produce a whistling noise as the patient breathes.

No treatment is needed for perforations that do not cause symptoms. For the perforation that continues to crust and bleed in spite of conservative therapy, a surgical procedure is indicated. Mucoperichondrial flaps can be rotated to cover the perforation or, after denuding mucosa from the surrounding intact septum, skin can be grafted across the hole on each side

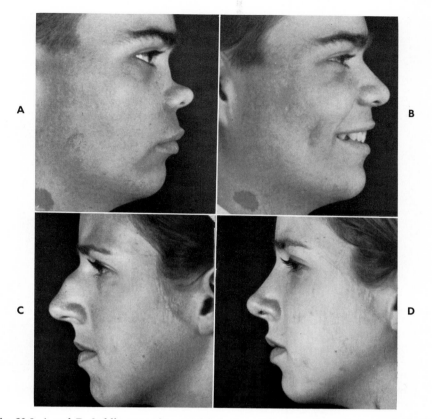

Fig. 20-6. A and **B,** Saddle nose after nasal infection at 8 years of age; it is repaired with silastic nasal implant. **C** and **D,** Nasal convexity and chin retrusion repaired by combined rhinoplasty and chin augmentation. (Courtesy Dr. Trent Smith, Columbus, Ohio.)

of the perforation. Neither method works well in large perforations, but both methods close small holes. The nursing care involved is essentially the same as that for a patient with submucous resection. These patients may have their packs left in place for as long as a week.

Dermabrasion (Fig. 20-7)

After injury in which dirt, grease, or other foreign matter has been ground into the skin, great care must be used to remove all foreign material, or it is incorporated into the healed wound forever. Grease under the skin often produces an unsightly tattoo mark. Dermabrasion is a useful method of removing ground-in debris that cannot be washed or scrubbed off. Sandpaper is fixed to a rapidly rotating wheel and the outer layers of the epithelium planed away. With removal of epithelium the dirt is also removed. Dermabrasion is also of use in patients with pitted skin caused by severe acne.

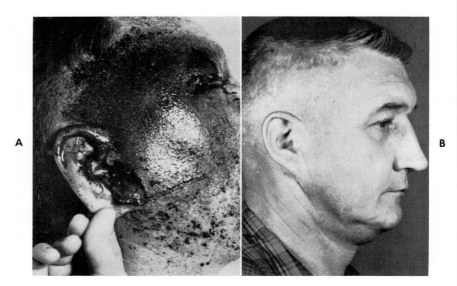

Fig. 20-7. A, Meticulous cleansing and dermabrasion were required to remove impregnated bits of galvanized metal. **B,** Postoperative view of patient 17 years after dermabrasion.

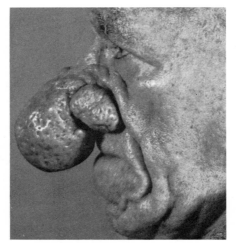

Fig. 20-8. Large rhinophyma.

Rhinophyma (Fig. 20-8)

Rhinophyma is a condition seen in men in which there is a great overgrowth of the normal sebaceous glands in the skin of the nose. Over many years the nose develops a grotesque tip, with redundant masses of thick skin. In spite of the apparent serious deformity, correction is not difficult. With the patient under local anesthesia the surgeon simply cuts away the excessive masses with a razor blade and reshapes the external nasal contour. Bleeding is sometimes rather profuse, but transfusion should not be required. Postoperatively an external petrolatum or rayon gauze dressing protects the nose for a week or ten days. Because the entire thickness of skin of the nose is not removed, the epithelium regenerates promptly, and the final result is a great improvement over the preoperative appearance.

CHAPTER TWENTY-ONE

Sinusitis and related conditions

SINUSITIS

Although less common now than in the preantibiotic era, sinusitis is still a frequent disorder. Actually most patients who complain of sinusitis (or "sinus" as they call it) do not have sinusitis. Instead they have postnasal discharge, nasal obstruction, or headaches, none of which, except postnasal discharge, is ordinarily common to patients with sinusitis. But all are common symptoms of other conditions, including allergic rhinitis, nasal septal deformity, nasal polyposis, and psychologic disorders.

When the otolaryngologist speaks of sinusitis, he implies a suppurative infection in one or more of the paranasal sinuses. Bacteria have infected the mucous membrane of the sinus, producing pus, which drains into the nose. Suppurative sinusitis can be either acute or chronic.

Another form of sinusitis that may or may not be associated with infection and pus is polypoid sinusitis. There is usually an underlying allergic disorder, and polyps, which fill the sinuses, hang out into the nose. These patients have nasal obstruction and postnasal discharge, yet they need not have purulent sinusitis. Still other patients with allergic disorders complain of excessive nasal mucous but no obstruction. They are said to have allergic rhinitis or vasomotor rhinitis.

Clear distinctions are not always possible among the various types of sinusitis because often they overlap, and original causes may be obscure. There is good reason, however, to try to distinguish among the several types of sinusitis because prognosis and treatment differ (Figs. 21-1 and 21-2).

Transillumination of the frontal or maxillary sinuses, done in a dark-room, is a procedure not used as often as it formerly was. Perhaps the reason is more dependence on roentgenograms for diagnosis. A lighted and partially shielded bulb is placed in the mouth, and the patient is asked to close his lips about the bulb. If the maxillary sinuses are normal, light should shine through the palate across the sinal cavities and be seen over the cheeks as a dim red glow. With the light pressed under the floor of the

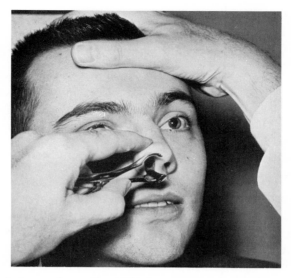

Fig. 21-1. Use of the nasal speculum. This instrument stretches the nasal **alae** so that the examiner can shine light from the headmirror into all parts of the nose. (From Saunders, William H.: Ears, nose, and throat. In Prior, John A., and Silberstein, Jack S.: Physical diagnosis, ed. 4, St. Louis, 1973, The C. V. Mosby Co.)

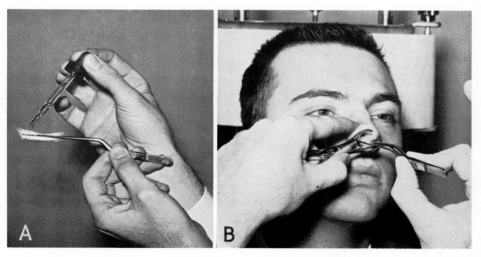

Fig. 21-2. A and B, Placing vasoconstrictor (ephedrine) or topical anesthetic (cocaine or Pontocaine) in the nose. Vasoconstrictors shrink the mucous membrane and make possible better inspection. (From Saunders, William H.: Ears, nose, and throat. In Prior, John A., and Silberstein, Jack S.: Physical diagnosis, ed. 4, St. Louis, 1973, The C. V. Mosby Co.)

frontal sinus, the normal frontal sinus, if it is large enough, will glow dimly in the darkroom.

Roentgenograms of the paranasal sinuses are of great value in establishing a diagnosis of sinusitis, fracture, or neoplastic disease. Ordinarily there is clinical evidence that will make the diagnosis, but roentgenograms sometimes provide the only clue. Furthermore, they define the extent of the disease and indicate involvement of the bony walls. Several different views are necessary to show all four sinuses.

When there is infection of one or more of the sinuses, pus or mucosal thickening produces a cloudy appearance on the x-ray film (Fig. 21-3). Sometimes an air-fluid level is seen in the maxillary or frontal sinus, indicating acute sinusitis with pus partially filling the sinus.

Chronic sinusitis is also seen by rotentgenographic examination, and here one may note increased thickness of the bony walls, thick mucous membranes, and other changes.

Acute suppurative sinusitis

Acute suppurative sinusitis is common; many persons have had it at one time or another because it often accompanies or follows the common cold. There is pain or a sensation of heaviness over the eye or in the cheek, and tenderness to pressure over the maxillary or frontal bone is common (Fig. 21-4). In the case of maxillary sinusitis, the patient may think he has a toothache. When he bends over so that the head is dependent and also

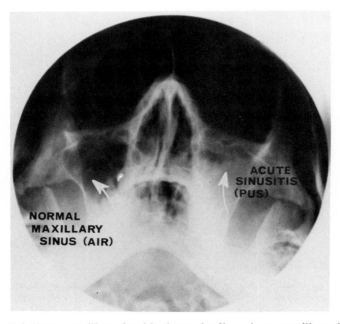

Fig. 21-3. Acute maxillary sinusitis shows clouding of one maxillary sinus.

when he coughs, the pain is worse. This is an infection; therefore, fever and leukocytosis are expected but are not always present, and usually purulent discharge drains from the affected sinus into the nose. If the sinusitis is associated with rhinitis, there is swelling of the nasal mucosa and obstruction to the airway, but sinusitis alone does not cause nasal obstruction.

Most cases of acute suppurative sinusitis clear after several weeks even without treatment. With antibiotic therapy the infection subsides rapidly, provided the drug given is one to which the bacteria will respond. Pain is controlled with analgesics such as codeine, 32 mg., every three hours. The value of nose drops is doubtful, although they often are prescribed. They

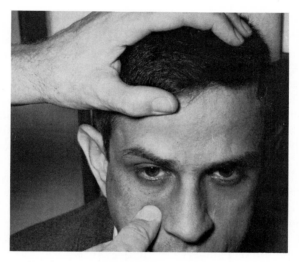

Fig. 21-4. Testing the maxillary sinus for tenderness.

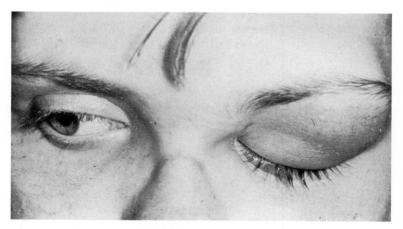

Fig. 21-5. Acute frontal sinusitis with orbital edema.

do shrink or decongest the nasal mucosa, and this gives some symptomatic relief. There is a danger, however, that once started on nose drops, the patient may continue to use them for longer than intended and develop "rhinitis medicamentosa" (see p. 222).

Considering the frequency of acute sinusitis, serious complications such as meningitis, brain abscess, epidural abscess, osteomyelitis, and oribtal cellulitis are uncommon. During the acute stage of sinusitis, manipulative procedures, such as puncturing the sinus to secure better drainage, are avoided because they may make the condition worse and even cause complications (Fig. 21-5).

Chronic suppurative sinusitis

Most patients know what is wrong when they have acute sinusitis, but in the case of chronic sinusitis there is a great deal of misdiagnosis by patient and physician alike. Usually the error is in calling a condition sinusitis that is not. Many persons who have headache, nasal obstruction, or post-nasal discharge are likely to ascribe their symptoms to "sinus," and too often their physician agrees and treats them with antibiotics. There is no improvement because there was no sinusitis in the first place.

Oddly, patients with bona fide chronic purulent sinusitis do not complain as much of their discharge as do patients with mucoid discharge produced by allergic rhinitis or smoking. A few patients with chronic sinusitis have headaches, but the majority have *no headaches or other pain* unless they develop a complication.

Chronic sinusitis begins as acute sinusitis and simply represents an instance in which the acute infection fails to clear. The patient continues with his sinusitis for years or even a lifetime. In general, the antibiotics that do so much for acute sinusitis do little for chronic sinusitis. Operations avoided in the acute stage are often the only worthwhile treatment in the chronic stage. Occasionally, repeated lavage of the maxillary sinus will relieve a purulent process of long standing, but usually, if the disease is really chronic, the physician must remove the lining of the sinus to clear the disease. Sinal operations are done through either an intranasal or an external approach. All are good, time-tested procedures, but they must be used on the right patient. In the past too many patients with headache or nasal discharge of obscure origin had operations for sinusitis. Unfortunately, because they did not have sinusitis in the first place, their symptoms continued, and an operation that was good took the blame for mistakes in diagnosis and judgment.

Dental sinusitis

A special type of maxillary sinusitis occurs when the dentist, in pulling a tooth, breaks off a fragment of root in the maxillary sinus. A particularly foul infection develops, and pus from the sinus often drains into the mouth through the tooth socket (oral-antral fistula) (Fig. 21-6). In most cases an operation is necessary.

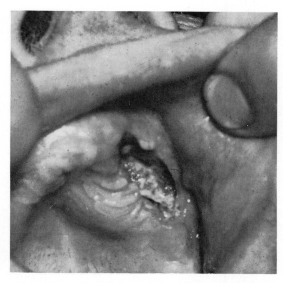

Fig. 21-6. Large oral-antral fistula with granulation tissue protruding from the maxillary sinus.

Swimmers' sinusitis

Swimmers' sinusitis is a special type of sinusitis that comes from forcing infected water into the duct of the frontal sinus during diving or swimming. Swimming and diving in contaminated rivers or lakes are particularly apt to result in this type of infection, as contrasted to swimming in a chlorinated pool. Altogether the infection is not seen very commonly. These patients frequently become very ill and may develop serious complications such as epidural abscess or osteomyelitis.

SINUS OPERATIONS
Antral irrigation

In subacute sinusitis as treatment or in chronic sinusitis for diagnosis, irrigation of the maxillary sinus may be worthwhile. It can be done either by puncturing the thin wall between the inferior meatus with a trocar (Fig. 21-7) or by passing a cannula into the natural ostium of the middle meatus. Sterile physiologic saline solution is then run through tubing connected to the cannula, and if there is pus in the sinus, it runs from the nose into a basin held by the patient. The nurse may have to support the back of the patient's head to hold him steady (he sits upright in a chair), because considerable pressure sometimes must be exerted. There should be no pain, however, if preliminary local anesthesia provided by topical cocaine or Pontocaine is administered carefully.

Maxillary sinus

The Caldwell-Luc operation (Fig. 21-8) is a procedure done on the maxillary sinus through an incision under the upper lip. After elevation of

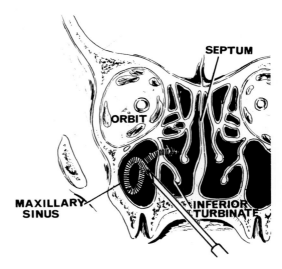

Fig. 21-7. **Large needle** or trocar penetrating thin bone of inferior meatus and irrigating maxillary sinus.

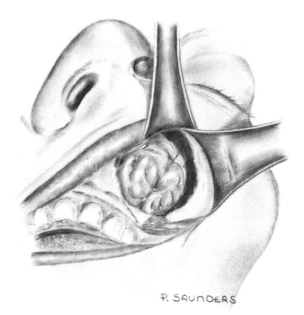

P. SAUNDERS

Fig. 21-8. Caldwell-Luc incision used to expose tumor in maxillary sinus.

periosteum a gouge and mallet are used to make an opening in the anterior wall of the sinus, after which the infected contents of the sinus are stripped out. To promote drainage a large nasoantral "window" is created through the bony wall that separates the nose from the maxillary sinus. This window heals open so that the sinus has a permanent, large opening into the nose for aeration and drainage. The natural ostium or opening of the maxillary sinus is rather highly placed and sometimes quite small. The sinus is packed with gauze stripping lubricated with petrolatum or an antibiotic ointment and one end of the gauze is pulled through the window into the nose. It is removed in forty-eight hours by pulling it from the nose. The same nursing considerations are important here as described for postoperative care of the patient with submucous resection. The packing is removed with the patient sitting upright *in bed,* with a towel tied around his neck and a basin under the chin to catch packing and blood. Bleeding is usually minimal, but bright blood will drip from the nose for ten to twenty minutes.

The incision under the lip is sutured with catgut; these sutures work out by themselves after about ten days. Postoperatively, for a week or two, there may be swelling of the cheek and a black eye. The black eye results because blood readily extravasates into the loose tissue under the eye. Numbness of the upper lip and upper teeth is present for several months, or even permanently, because some nerves to these structures pass through the site of the incision. Ordinarily the Caldwell-Luc operation is not performed on children since they have unerupted teeth near the site of incision.

Nursing care

Nursing care after the Caldwell-Luc operation is important. The patient may want to brush his teeth, and if he does, he must be careful not to abrade the incision above the teeth; since this part may be numb he may need instruction on this point. The nurse may need to employ special soft toothbrushes or sponges to help with oral hygiene. Often the upper lip is so swollen, however, that he cannot brush his teeth for several days. Use of mouthwashes is permitted. The patient should not blow his nose for two weeks once the packing is removed, because blowing could force air from the nose into the maxillary sinus and out the incision. Usually the diet is liquid for several days before advancing to soft foods. The patient ordinarily will avoid chewing on the operated side, but it is a good idea to mention this to him. If he wears an upper denture, the plate should not be worn for ten days to two weeks after surgery since the flange will rub on the suture line.

Ethmoid sinuses

The ethmoidal air cells or ethmoid labyrinth lie between the maxillary sinus below and the frontal sinus above. There may be fifteen or twenty of these small air cells on either side of the head between the inner canthus of the eye and the nose. When nasal polyps are present they frequently find their origin in the ethmoid air cells; as the cells become filled with

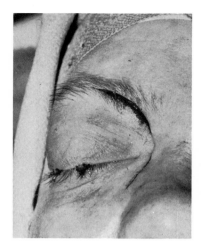

Fig. 21-9. External ethmoidectomy incision through which operations are done on frontal, ethmoid, and sphenoid sinuses.

polyps, the polyps are extruded into the nose where they cause nasal obstruction. Minor infection of the ethmoid sinuses is common with almost every upper respiratory infection (common cold); sometimes a more severe infection occurs causing frank ethmoiditis with pain and swelling along the side of the nose near the inner canthus of the eye. One complication of ethmoiditis is orbital cellulitis or abscess. This condition causes proptosis, loss of vision, and fixation of one eye. Drainage of the orbit is required.

By breaking into the ethmoidal air cells intranasally, a major part of both ethmoid labyrinths can be eviscerated. The ethmoid labyrinth also can be approached *externally* through an incision made in the inner half of the eyebrow downward along the side of the nose (Fig. 21-9). The frontal and sphenoid sinuses can be approached through the same incision. External ethmoidectomy is regarded as more complete and safer than is the intranasal operation because visualization is better.

Frontal sinus

The frontal sinus is usually approached through the incision described for the ethmoidectomy, but sometimes a coronal incision is used and the scalp of the forehead is pulled downward to afford exposure. Care is taken to preserve the nasofrontal duct—the opening from the frontal sinus into the nose. If the duct closes because of scarring, it is likely that a collection of mucus called a *mucocele* may form later in the frontal sinus (Fig. 21-10). Most mucoceles form as a result of chronic sinusitis, not after surgery. An infected mucocele is called a *pyocele*.

The treatment of a mucocele is surgical and consists of removing the lining of the sinus, which is the same as the lining of the mucocele sac. The frontal sinus is the one usually involved. A common procedure is to incise

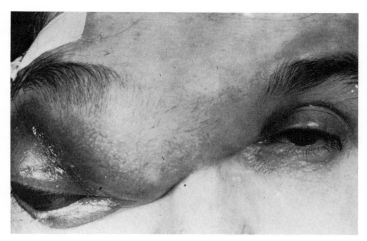

Fig. 21-10. Mucocele of the frontal sinus. Pressure of secretions in the sinus has eroded the bone and displaced the orbit.

through the eyebrow and across the bridge of the nose or to make a coronal incision in the scalp. Then the scalp is raised so as to give access to the bone covering the frontal sinus. By cutting through the outer wall (outer "table") of the frontal sinus on three sides and leaving it hinged below near the eyebrow, the external bony wall of the sinus can be turned downward, exposing the interior of the sinus so that the contents (the mucocele sac) of the sinus can be removed. Some surgeons then fill the sinus with fat (taken from the subcutaneous tissues of the abdominal wall) to obliterate it before returning the bone part ("osteoplastic flap") and suturing the incision.

Nursing care postoperatively consists chiefly of dressing changes and medication for pain. After an external incision, a drain is usually in place, and there is a head dressing to absorb drainage. The drain is removed in forty-eight hours, and the dressing is replaced to hold the scalp firmly against the skull. Sutures may be removed in about one week. Complications of surgery are not common, but the nurse should watch for hematoma; rarely, there may be meningitis with its symptoms of stiff neck, high fever, and headache. Because the head may be shaved or partially shaved for surgery, the patient may be advised preoperatively to shampoo his hair and obtain a wig. Shaving is required for the coronal incision, made across the entire scalp from one ear to the other, but not if the operation is done through a more limited incision through the eyebrow.

Sphenoid sinus

Lying deep in the head, the sphenoid sinuses can be approached either intranasally or externally through the eyebrow incision. Sometimes all four sinuses on one side are operated upon together—the Caldwell-Luc procedure is done on the maxillary sinus, and the external ethmoidectomy incision is used for the frontal, ethmoid, and sphenoid sinuses.

Atrophic rhinitis

Although the exact cause is unknown, atrophic rhinitis seems to be a disease of underprivileged persons and is becoming rare even in that group. Foul green crusts appear in the nose during childhood or adolescence and continue to do so lifelong. There is atrophy of the lateral walls of the nose, especially of the inferior turbinates, so that the nasal airways become larger than normal. The severe crusting, however, tends to produce nasal obstruction, which is one of the symptoms. There is often a bad odor known as *ozena.*

Antibiotics and other medications are of no help in atrophic rhinitis. Patients get relief from crusting and odor by daily snuffing of physiologic saline solution, but improvement is only temporary because the crusts form again overnight.

More permanent relief can be obtained from an operation in which bone chips from the iliac crest are implanted in a pocket created under the periosteum in the lateral walls of the nose. In effect, the nasal chambers are made smaller because the soft tissues of the lateral walls of the nose are moved toward the nasal septum and kept there by bone chips packed between the elevated soft tissues and the bony lateral walls of the nose.

Carcinoma

Malignancy of the paranasal sinuses, a relatively uncommon disease, is most frequent in the maxillary and ethmoid sinuses (Fig. 21-11). When carcinoma begins in the maxillary sinus, there are no early symptoms (Fig. 21-12). The patient may first complain of loosening of the upper teeth, or if

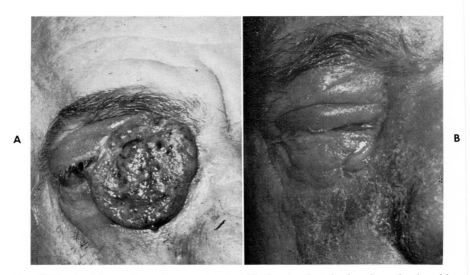

A   B

Fig. 21-11. A, Advanced carcinoma of ethmoid sinuses that broke through the skin. **B,** Same patient immediately after irradiation therapy. Skin reaction will subside.

he wears a denture, he says his upper plate no longer fits; there may be nasal obstruction caused by tumor eroding into the nose; nosebleeds are common; the eye may be displaced by tumor growing through the superior wall of the maxilla. Metastases are late.

Carcinoma of the ethmoid sinuses causes no oral or dental symptoms but displaces the eye outward, blocks one side of the nose because the tumor grows here, disturbs the sense of smell, and often produces nosebleeds. Tearing of the eye is common. Because the eye is displaced the patient may have diplopia (double vision).

Treatment of any type of sinal malignancy is by irradiation therapy, surgery, or a combination of the two. Frequently when surgery is used, the entire upper jaw and even one eye may have to be removed. This is no place for conservative surgical therapy since, if any disease is left behind, there will be a recurrence and an even more heroic operation required the second time. After extensive surgery of the sinal areas for malignancy, split thickness grafts of skin are usually applied to the raw areas. The grafts are packed in place and the packing left for ten days. Postoperatively the deformity in the upper jaw can be managed quite well by a dental prosthesis, which closes off the defect in the mouth. If the eye has been removed, it is better for the patient to wear a patch or to obtain a plastic prosthesis than to have plastic surgery for reconstruction (Fig. 21-13).

The prognosis is never as good as with carcinoma of the larynx, for example, but still is much better than that for carcinoma of the stomach or lung.

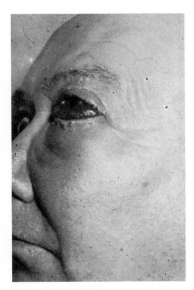

Fig. 21-12. Carcinoma of the maxillary sinus. Note conjunctival **edema** and swelling of the cheek.

The nursing care of postoperative cancer patients with extensive procedures on the paranasal sinuses is complex. Because the operation may well include removal of dura mater and thus cause leakage of cerebrospinal fluid, drugs must be given to prevent meningitis. The best ones are those that pass readily into the cerebrospinal fluid from the bloodstream: sulfadiazine and chloramphenicol. Both drugs, of course, have well-known toxic

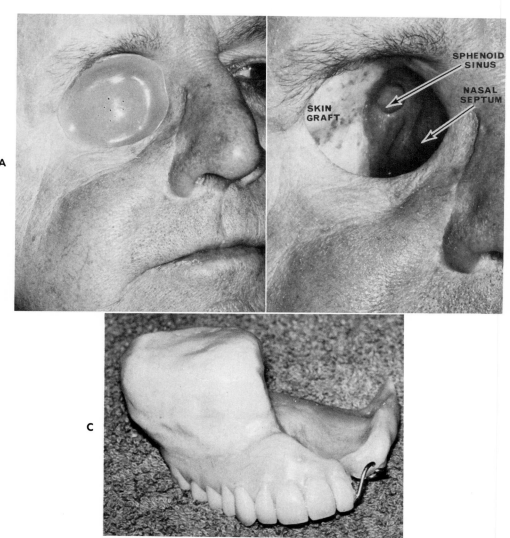

Fig. 21-13. Patient after maxillectomy and orbital exenteration. **A,** Orbital prosthesis in place. Eyeglasses worn over this further improves appearance. **B,** Defect in orbit with skin graft lining the upper and lateral wall of the orbital-maxillary cavity. **C.** Upper denture worn with a large obturator to fill in the defect created by maxillectomy.

effects, but these are relatively infrequent compared to the incidence of meningitis that may occur if they are not used.

The patient may well have trouble eating until a prosthesis can be fitted (Fig. 21-13). Immediately after the operation the palatal defect is grafted and a temporary sponge rubber prosthesis is placed. This sponge rubber fits flush with the remaining opposite half of the palate and permits the patient a reasonable voice and at times permits him to eat a limited diet. Ordinarily, however, a nasogastric feeding tube is inserted to ensure liquid and caloric intake. After margins of the wounds have healed and the skin graft is intact, usually about a week, the sponge rubber is removed and a more permanent prosthesis fitted. Several different prostheses may be needed before a final one fits, because of shrinkage of the cavity as healing progresses.

The nasogastric tube passed at the time of operation tends to rub on the margins of the nasal vestibule, and the nurse should check daily to see that there is not an ulceration. All patients are uncomfortable and require meperdine or codeine and, later, milder analgesics. There is nothing, however, to prevent their early ambulation except that the donor site on the thigh may be painful.

Once the packing is removed from the operative site, the skin grafts require daily care. Crusts must be loosened with saline or hydrogen peroxide and picked off. Bits of excess skin are trimmed with scissors. Small areas of granulation tissue are cauterized with a silver nitrate stick or removed with biting forceps. Instruments are, of course, sterile.

NASAL VESTIBULE
Vestibulitis

The anteriormost part of the nose is called the nasal vestibule (Fig. 21-14). It is skin-lined and contains the nasal hairs or vibrissae. If these hair follicles become infected, there is pain and swelling of the tip of the nose.

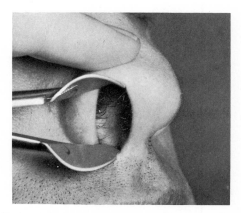

Fig. 21-14. Nasal vestibule. This part of the nose is skin lined and contains vibrissae, or hair, so painful infections of hair follicles and fissures are common here.

Such infections are usually short lived but can be dangerous, since lymphatics from this area drain to the cavernous sinus within the skull. Infection and thrombosis of these blood spaces even in the antibiotic era are extremely dangerous.

One cause of vestibulitis is low humidity. Especially in the winter, when relative humidity is low and most homes are overheated, excessively dry air irritates the nasal vestibule, and infection may follow. Dry air also is responsible for the repeated minor nosebleeds that some persons have during winter months.

Treatment of vestibulitis is by application of hot compresses and incision and drainage of an infected hair follicle if a furuncle forms. Systemic antibiotic therapy may be required in the more severe infections.

Fissures

Fissures in the nasal vestibule are also common. These cracks in the skin are high in the dome of the vestibule and therefore difficult to see. Slow to heal, they may cause pain for weeks or even months. Cautery of granulation tissue in the base of the fissure with silver nitrate and the local use of an antibiotic ointment such as Neosporin or ammoniated mercury ointment, 5% are good local treatments.

SUGGESTED READINGS

Alfaro, V. R., and Krucoff, M. E.: The problems of sinusitis in children, Laryngoscope **69:**750, 1959.

Davidson, F. W.: Antibiotics and sinus infections, Laryngoscope **60:**131, 1950.

Erich, J. B., and Kragh, L. B.: Results of treatment of squamous cell carcinoma of the upper jaw and antrum, American Journal of Surgery **100:**401, 1960.

Gallagher, T. M., and Boles, R.: Symposium; Treatment of malignancies of paranasal sinuses, I, II, and III, Laryngoscope **80:** 924, 1970.

CHAPTER TWENTY-TWO

Larynx—anatomy and physiology; laryngeal paralysis

ANATOMY

The framework of the larynx (pronounced lair'inks) is made of several cartilages held together by muscles and ligaments. It is connected inferiorly with the trachea and above with musculature of the hypopharynx. The cartilaginous framework of the larynx protects the vocal cords and affords a stiffness, which permits an airway. The female larynx is smaller than that of the male, and of course the infant's or child's larynx is smallest of all. (The interior of the larynx is explained in detail on p. 250 under "Soft tissue of larynx.")

Cartilages (Figs. 22-1 to 22-3)

The *thyroid* ("shield-like") cartilage is the largest cartilaginous element in the larynx. Known commonly as the "Adam's apple," the thyroid cartilage, which is more prominent in men than in women, serves to protect the soft inner structures—the false cords, the ventricles, and the true cords. The thyroid cartilage is incomplete posteriorly, this aspect being closed by muscles and ligaments. The *cricoid* ("ring-like") cartilage lies directly under the thyroid cartilage and is the only complete ring in the larynx. Between the cricoid and thyroid cartilages is the cricothyroid space, and at this level the airway is immediately subcutaneous; therefore it is here that an emergency tracheotomy can best be performed. Under the cricoid cartilage are the several rings of the trachea (incomplete posteriorly). The *arytenoid* cartilages articulate with the cricoid and are found posteriorly, behind the protecting thyroid cartilage. The arytenoid cartilages swing in and out (medially and laterally) as if rotating about a fixed point. This action opens and closes the vocal cords, since the posterior end of each cord is attached to one arytenoid cartilage and must move with it. Anteriorly the vocal cords meet in the midline and attach to the inner aspect of the thyroid cartilage. In addition to the three major cartilages of the larynx there are two corniculate cartilages and two cuneiform cartilages.

247

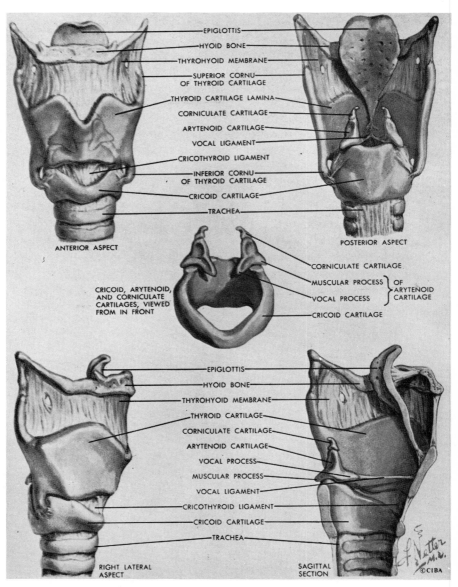

EPIGLOTTIS
HYOID BONE
THYROHYOID MEMBRANE
SUPERIOR CORNU OF THYROID CARTILAGE
THYROID CARTILAGE LAMINA
CORNICULATE CARTILAGE
ARYTENOID CARTILAGE
VOCAL LIGAMENT
CRICOTHYROID LIGAMENT
INFERIOR CORNU OF THYROID CARTILAGE
CRICOID CARTILAGE
TRACHEA

ANTERIOR ASPECT

POSTERIOR ASPECT

CRICOID, ARYTENOID, AND CORNICULATE CARTILAGES, VIEWED FROM IN FRONT

CORNICULATE CARTILAGE
MUSCULAR PROCESS } OF ARYTENOID
VOCAL PROCESS } CARTILAGE
CRICOID CARTILAGE

EPIGLOTTIS
HYOID BONE
THYROHYOID MEMBRANE
THYROID CARTILAGE
CORNICULATE CARTILAGE
ARYTENOID CARTILAGE
VOCAL PROCESS
MUSCULAR PROCESS
VOCAL LIGAMENT
CRICOTHYROID LIGAMENT
CRICOID CARTILAGE
TRACHEA

RIGHT LATERAL ASPECT

SAGITTAL SECTION

Fig. 22-1. Cartilages of the larynx. (Copyright CLINICAL SYMPOSIA, by Frank H. Netter, M.D., published by CIBA Pharmaceutical Co.)

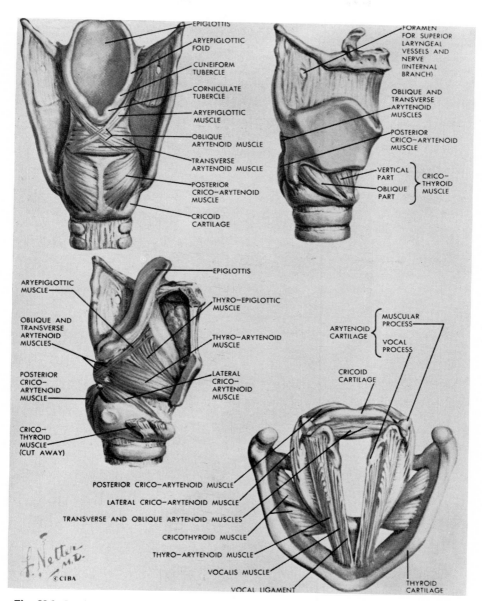

Fig. 22-2. Intrinsic muscles of the larynx. (Copyright CLINICAL SYMPOSIA, by Frank H. Netter, M.D., published by CIBA Pharmaceutical Co.)

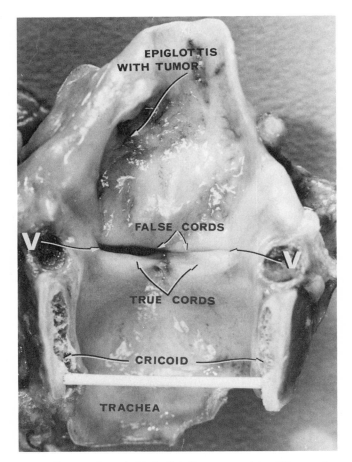

Fig. 22-3. Larynx split open from behind. *V* indicates ventricles. Tissues above true cords are part of the supraglottic larynx. This looks like a supraglottic lesion that could have been treated by horizontal or supraglottic laryngectomy, but tumor had invaded submucosally to one true cord. Postirradiation failure.

Hyoid bone

The hyoid bone lies just above the thyroid cartilage and is joined to it by the thyrohyoid membrane. Not a part of the larynx proper, the hyoid serves to suspend the cartilaginous larynx (Fig. 22-1), and also it affords attachment to many muscles, including some of the tongue.

Soft tissues of the larynx

The mucosa lining the larynx is continuous with that of the hypopharynx above and the trachea below. There is stratified squamous mucosa along the vocal cords, but the rest of the larynx is lined by columnar epithelium. Ligaments and folds of mucous membrane adjoin the cartilages and serve as important landmarks to the examiner.

The true vocal cords, perhaps the best known parts of the larynx, vibrate in order to assist in the production of speech. Anteriorly they are attached to the inner surface of the thyroid cartilage, and posteriorly they are attached to the arytenoid cartilages, which open and close the *glottis* (the space between the true cords) as they move outward and inward; movements of the arytenoid cartilages also help to relax or increase tension in the cords. Thus during quiet respiration the cords are separated so that air can enter and leave the trachea; during phonation the cords meet almost perfectly and vibrate. (See Fig. 23-1, p. 248.)

The vocal cords are folds of mucous membrane covering the underlying thyroarytenoid or vocalis muscles. Above and lateral to the true cords is the laryngeal ventricle, an invagination of mucous membrane forming a pocket just above the cord. As the mucous membrane returns from out of the ventricle, the false cord is formed. In other words, the false cord lies directly above the true cord, and the ventricle of the larynx, ordinarily more of a potential than a real space, lies between the two. The *glottis* is the space between the vocal cords and is the narrowest part of the airway.

Muscles of the larynx that attach it to surrounding bones are called extrinsic; intrinsic muscles join together the various parts of the larynx.

Nerve supply

The entire laryngeal nerve supply comes from the tenth cranial or vagus nerve. Except one, all muscles of the larynx are supplied by the *recurrent laryngeal nerve*. This *motor* nerve branches from the vagus in the neck, dips into the chest, and then courses upward again in the groove between the esophagus and the trachea before entering the larynx at about the cricothyroid level. Because of the long course of this nerve, there are numerous disease processes that may affect it and paralyze the larynx. The *superior laryngeal nerve* affords the entire *sensory* supply of the larynx and also gives motor supply to one muscle, the cricothyroid.

Lymphatic drainage

A knowledge of the lymph drainage from the larynx is important because in carcinoma, metastatic cells spread along lymphatic channels to cervical lymph nodes and grow there. The larynx drains to lymph nodes in the middle and upper cervical chains along the internal jugular vein. Therefore, in performing laryngectomy for carcinoma of the larynx, a neck dissection is often done on one side to remove lymph nodes with possible metastatic involvement. This operation is analogous to the removal of axillary lymph nodes in radical mastectomy for carcinoma of the breast.

Functions of the larynx*

The larynx has many functions. As guardian of the respiratory tract, it keeps us from choking with every swallow of food. Without closure of the

---

*From Saunders, William H.: The larynx, Clinical Symposia **16:**67-69, July, 1964.

glottis, cough would be weak and removal of mucus and foreign matter from the bronchi and lungs less efficient. Also, without the closing or sphincter action of the larynx it would be more difficult to increase intra-abdominal pressure to assist the visceral musculature in such acts as defecation and childbirth.

In addition to these vital functions a most important activity of the larynx is phonation, a faculty that enables us to put most abstract ideas into vocal symbols, thus setting us apart from other members of the animal kingdom.

Physiology of phonation. The sounds we make in speech or song are primarily produced by vibration of the vocal cords, which, like the vibrating reed of an oboe, produces oscillations of pressure in the expired air. The air vibrations thus produced are accentuated or suppressed by the ever-changing resonating qualities of throat and mouth. Thus phonation depends on a delicate coordination of the intrinsic and extrinsic muscle of the larynx with the musculature of the pharynx, soft palate, tongue, and lips.

Nature of sound. Sound waves consist of a rhythmic series of condensations and rarefactions of air. The individual particles move forward and backward. They move forward, propelled by the advance of a vibrating string, for example; then they move backward, following the string in its retreat. The result is a rhythmic series of pressure changes that move away from the source at a constant speed of 1,130 feet per second, or a mile in about five seconds.

This rhythmic motion of air particles may be likened to the movement of the individual stalks in a field of grain, which, as the waves pass across the field, move first in the direction of the wind and then back again, but always maintaining their same relative position with respect to other stalks.

Vocal cords in phonation. The vocal cords produce condensations and rarefaction of air by vibrating laterally, allowing the expired air to escape in little rhythmic puffs. This is best visualized by producing a "raspberry" (a term used in American slang and probably derived from the appearance of the tensed and puckered lips, through which air is being expelled). If one attempts to make a sound in this way, he will quickly notice that the pitch of the sound becomes higher because of a more rapid vibration rate as the tension of the lips is increased. It is by such alterations of lip tension that the musician playing a bugle is able to change the pitch of the tones he produces.

Similarly, changes in pitch of sounds produced by the vocal cords are altered by changes in tension of the laryngeal muscles, to be described later.

The manner in which the cords move to emit the tiny puffs of air cannot, of course, be visualized by the naked eye. However, high-speed motion pictures have shown this very clearly.

Resonating cavities. Everyone has noticed that, as water is poured into a bottle or other container, the pitch rises as the bottle fills. The explanation of this well-known phenomenon is based on the fact that an air-containing cavity will accentuate tones having a certain vibration rate while suppressing others. It is also well known that in a pipe organ the longer pipes resonate the lower notes. Indeed, there is a direct relationship between the length of the cavity or pipe and the *wavelength* of the sounds and an inverse relationship with the *frequency* of vibration. The simplest illustration of the effect of lengthening a resonating cavity or pipe is to be found in a trombone, where the pitch of the tone resonated is lowered by extending the slide.

Mouth and other supralaryngeal structures in phonation. Just as the pitch of the trombone is altered by adjustment of the slide, so the fundamental vibrations produced by the local bands are changed by alterations in the shape and size of the resonating cavities above. These consist of the hypopharynx, pharynx, nasopharynx, and mouth. First, in modifying laryngeal vibration the extrinsic laryngeal muscles, assisted by the muscles that elevate the hyoid bone, cause the larynx to move progressively upward as higher tones are produced. This shortens the posterior pharynx so that higher pitches with shorter wavelengths will be resonated. Second, by changing the position of tongue and lips the relative size of the pharynx and mouth, along with their resonating qualities, can be adjusted. Indeed, in the pronunciation of words used in normal speech the larynx is relatively relaxed, the different sounds being made largely by the tongue and lips, the action of which changes the overtones resonated.

For example, without significant alteration in laryngeal vibration, the "e" of feet is changed to the "aw" of fought, merely by changing the position of the tongue. It is this ability of the soft palate, tongue, teeth, and lips to modify a fundamental vibration that makes it possible for a person whose larynx has been removed to speak intelligibly with a vibrating mechanism known as an electrolarynx, or even with an electric razor held against the neck.

LARYNGEAL PARALYSIS

Laryngeal paralysis may result from disease or injury of either the superior or recurrent laryngeal nerves, or if the vagus nerve itself is affected, both of its branches supplying the larynx will be paralyzed. One need only consider the course of the recurrent laryngeal nerve to think of some of the more common causes of laryngeal paralysis. On the left side the nerve passes under the arch of the aorta and, therefore, may be stretched and paralyzed if the patient has an aortic aneurysm. On the right side the nerve passes under the subclavian artery and may be paralyzed if that vessel is diseased. Certain diseases of the heart that enlarge the atrium, such as mitral stenosis, cause stretching of the left recurrent laryngeal nerve, and the nerve on either side may be affected by bronchial carcinoma, tuberculous scarring of the apex of the lungs, and malignancy anywhere along the course of the nerve as it travels up the neck. Carcinoma of the thyroid gland occasionally interrupts the fibers of the nerve just as they are entering the larynx. One of the more common causes of peripheral laryngeal paralysis is thyroidectomy—the surgeon may cut the recurrent laryngeal nerve.

From a standpoint of symptoms, hoarseness may or may not be present after laryngeal paralysis. *The diagnosis must be made by looking at the larynx*—not by making a guess based on the sound of the patient's voice. If the paralyzed cord rests in the midline and the opposite cord moves sufficiently to approximate it, often there is no hoarseness. On the other

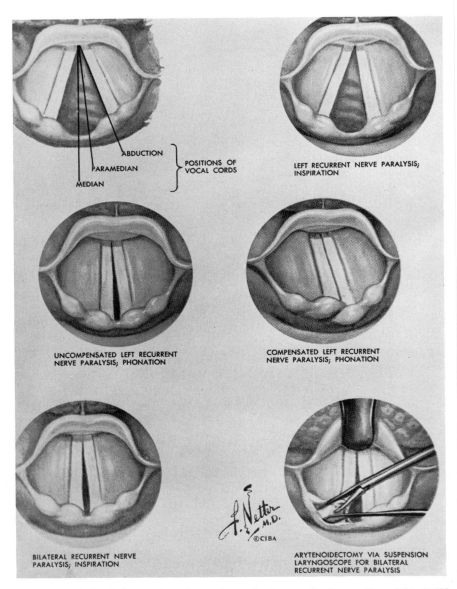

ABDUCTION

PARAMEDIAN } POSITIONS OF VOCAL CORDS

MEDIAN

LEFT RECURRENT NERVE PARALYSIS; INSPIRATION

UNCOMPENSATED LEFT RECURRENT NERVE PARALYSIS; PHONATION

COMPENSATED LEFT RECURRENT NERVE PARALYSIS; PHONATION

BILATERAL RECURRENT NERVE PARALYSIS; INSPIRATION

ARYTENOIDECTOMY VIA SUSPENSION LARYNGOSCOPE FOR BILATERAL RECURRENT NERVE PARALYSIS

Fig. 22-4. Paralysis of the vocal cords as viewed by laryngeal mirror. (Copyright CLIN-ICAL SYMPOSIA, by Frank H. Netter, M.D., published by CIBA Pharmaceutical Co.)

hand, if the paralyzed cord is in the paramedian or partially abducted position, the good cord may not be able to approximate it and there results a hoarse air-spilling voice. There is no shortness of breath when only one cord is paralyzed. Rarely, both recurrent laryngeal nerves are cut at the time of thyroidectomy, and when this happens, the cords usually are paralyzed in the midline. The voice is of fair quality although weak, but the airway is poor. Because the cords are unable to abduct, the very narrow glottic chink will not admit enough air to support any considerable exertion (Fig. 22-4).

In the neck, *carcinoma of the thyroid gland* may cause laryngeal paralysis. If a patient has laryngeal paralysis and a goiter, malignancy of the thyroid gland should be suspected. Usually benign thyroid enlargements do not cause laryngeal paralysis. Carcinoma of the larynx itself eventually produces fixation of one or both vocal cords, but the immobility may be the result of invasion of muscle by carcinoma rather than nerve paralysis.

Laryngeal paralysis may be caused by *neck injuries*. Also, certain metallic poisons (lead) and infectious diseases (diphtheria) cause laryngeal paralysis by producing a neuritis.

Paralysis of the *superior* laryngeal nerve does not appreciably affect the *motor* function of the larynx, since only one muscle is supplied by this nerve, but it does cause a *sensory* paralysis, and secretions sometimes trickle through the larynx into the trachea before the patient realizes that he is aspirating.

Central paralysis. Laryngeal paralyses usually result from peripheral causes, but it is also possible for central nervous system lesions to produce laryngeal paralysis. Each side of the larynx receives a motor supply from both sides of the cerebral cortex. However, the motor areas are so widely separated that it is unusual to see a laryngeal paralysis caused by a cortical lesion. Such lesions would have to be massive (or exactly symmetrical) and ordinarily would be incompatible with life.

Treatment. There is no surgical or medical treatment of value insofar as restoration of normal neural or muscular function is concerned. If both cords are paralyzed and the airway is inadequate, a tracheotomy will restore the airway.

Treatment of bilateral cord paralysis is aimed at restoration of the airway, not at improvement of the voice. One method is to use a transoral approach and to resect one arytenoid cartilage (Fig. 22-4, lower right). This increases the diameter of the posterior part of the glottis sufficiently so that the patient can breathe better. Occasionally the opposite arytenoid is also resected. A second method is through an external approach in which the arytenoid is caught with a suture and pulled and fixed laterally to the thyroid cartilage so that the glottis is spread apart.

A recent method of improving the voice in a patient with unilateral cord paralysis is to inject a small quantity of Teflon into the paralyzed cord. This swells the cord and pushes it toward the midline, where the good cord can approximate it better during phonation. The Teflon remains permanently in place. Of course this does nothing to restore motion to the paralyzed side. The same method is used in other patients who may have lost part of the substance of one or even both cords through surgery or injury.

Hysterical aphonia

Hysterical aphonia is a functional condition that prevents the patient from forcibly adducting the vocal cords for phonation. On inspection of the larynx all parts appear normal but when asked to say "ee," the patient barely makes a sound and the cords fail to approximate normally. Yet when the patient is asked to cough, the cough is sharp and strong, indicating that for purposes other than phonation the cords actually do meet and close strongly. The cause is psychosomatic and may represent, in some patients, a subconscious means of "escape" from an unpleasant duty or situation. Hysterical aphonia is not actually a paralysis. The condition, more common in women than men, usually clears spontaneously after being present for several days or weeks, but then is likely to recur. Treatment is reassurance. Many of these patients would profit from psychotherapy.

CHAPTER TWENTY-THREE   # Larynx—benign conditions

LARYNGEAL EXAMINATION

Indirect or mirror laryngoscopy. The commonest method of examining the larynx is with the patient upright in a chair, using the laryngeal mirror, as illustrated in Fig. 23-1. Indirect laryngoscopy is performed easily and quickly in the doctor's office and serves for most diagnostic purposes. Sometimes therapy is also carried out by this technique, as in removal of tissue for biopsy or excision of a laryngeal polyp. The nurse's responsibility here will be concerned with seeing that the mirrors are clear and not scratched or permanently fogged.

Direct laryngoscopy. Direct laryngoscopy can be carried out with the patient under either local or general anesthesia. Fig. 23-3 shows several laryngoscopes and Fig. 23-2, *A,* shows the patient's and doctor's positions during direct laryngoscopy. When performed under local anesthesia the procedure should be entirely painless, although the patient may find it a little uncomfortable. The nurse can help greatly by offering calm reassurance to the patient that his airway will not be cut off at any time and that there is to be no pain. Adequate preoperative sedation to induce relaxation is important when local anesthesia is used.

Preoperatively the patient is allowed nothing by mouth (NPO), oral hygiene is provided, and all dentures are removed. After a local anesthesia the patient is NPO until he can swallow and the gag reflex has returned. It is best to start fluid with water and observe the patient's ability to swallow without aspirating.

Under general anesthesia the anesthetist may employ an intratracheal tube to ensure the airway; but if the laryngoscopy is to take only a minute or two, a tube may not be required.

Direct laryngoscopy is occasionally used when indirect laryngoscopy was insufficient to provide an adequate view of the larynx, and in most patients in whom a biopsy or other operative intralaryngeal procedure is to be done.

Suspension laryngoscopy is essentially the same as direct laryngoscopy, except that here the laryngoscope is held fixed in place on the patient's chest. In this technique, if desired, an operating microscope can be employed to provide binocular vision and magnification (see Fig. 23-2, *B*).

257

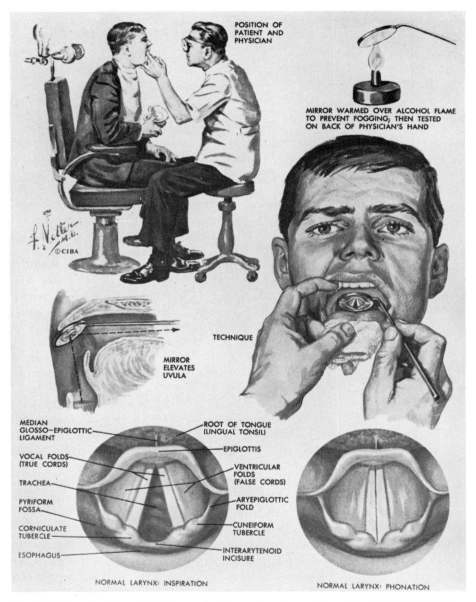

POSITION OF
PATIENT AND
PHYSICIAN

MIRROR WARMED OVER ALCOHOL FLAME
TO PREVENT FOGGING; THEN TESTED
ON BACK OF PHYSICIAN'S HAND

TECHNIQUE

MIRROR
ELEVATES
UVULA

MEDIAN
GLOSSO–EPIGLOTTIC
LIGAMENT

ROOT OF TONGUE
(LINGUAL TONSIL)

VOCAL FOLDS
(TRUE CORDS)

EPIGLOTTIS

TRACHEA

VENTRICULAR
FOLDS
(FALSE CORDS)

PYRIFORM
FOSSA

ARYEPIGLOTTIC
FOLD

CORNICULATE
TUBERCLE

CUNEIFORM
TUBERCLE

ESOPHAGUS

INTERARYTENOID
INCISURE

NORMAL LARYNX: INSPIRATION

NORMAL LARYNX: PHONATION

Fig. 23-1. Examination of the larynx by laryngeal mirror. (Copyright CLINICAL SYM-
POSIA, by Frank H. Netter, M.D., published by CIBA Pharmaceutical Co.)

The nurse is an important member of the laryngoscopy (or endoscopy) team because she must see that all instruments are functioning before the procedure begins—light carriers, suction apparatus, forceps, and so on. It is most distressing for a patient, especially under local anesthesia, to find that lack of preparation has resulted in a prolonged procedure.

Roentgenographic examination. By instilling radiopaque contrast ma-

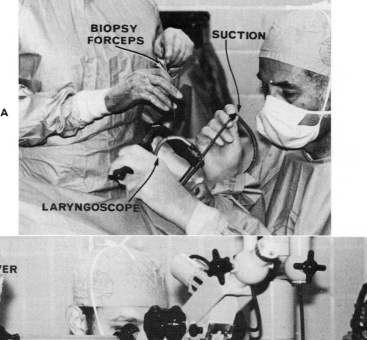

Fig. 23-2. Direct laryngoscopy. **A,** Standard hand-held laryngoscope. **B,** Self-retaining laryngoscope and use of operating microscope for magnification.

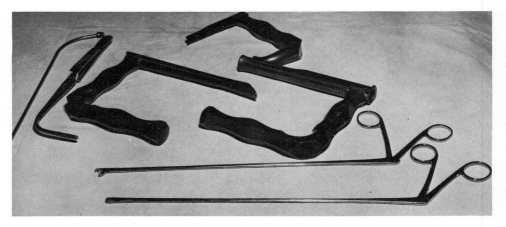

Fig. 23-3. Instruments for direct laryngoscopy. From left: laryngeal sucker, cotton holder (for topical anesthetic), three different laryngoscopes, and two forceps for biopsy.

terial in the larynx (as in a bronchogram) it is possible to obtain clear roentgenograms of the interior of the larynx that will demonstrate normal anatomy as well as tumors, paralysis, and other conditions. This technique is used far less frequently than either indirect or direct laryngoscopy but is of distinct use when indicated. Ordinary laminograms of the larynx without use of contrast material are also useful.

VOCAL NODULES (SPEAKER'S NODES)

Nodules form at the junction of the anterior one third and posterior two thirds of the vocal cords. These nodules are benign growths that result from misuse of the voice, such as might occur in excessive singing or shouting or using the voice outside of one's normal range. The names "singer's nodes," "speaker's nodes," or "preacher's nodes" imply that the nodes occur in individuals who must use their voices excessively.

At first the lesions are likely to appear red and raised above the surface of the vocal cords, but after a time they change into small white bumps that meet and kiss as the cords approximate (Fig. 23-4, *A, center*). Because they are raised, they prop the cords apart, and like any lesion of the true vocal cords that prevents accurate approximation, they produce hoarseness.

Surgical treatment consists of direct laryngoscopy (using either local or general anesthesia) and removal of these small growths with a cupped biting forceps (Fig. 23-3). No more than the nodule itself should be removed, because if muscular tissue is removed, a concavity in one cord, spillage of air during phonation, and a permanent hoarseness are produced. After removal of nodules the patient should observe complete voice rest for several days or, at the most, he should only whisper. In whispering the vocal cords do not quite approximate, and so there is little trauma. The nurse can assist after operation by providing the patient with a "magic" slate on which to write and by hanging a sign over the bed indicating to visitors that the patient is not to talk.

Sometimes vocal nodules are so small as to cause only slight hoarseness or even no hoarseness at all. Unless symptoms warrant, there is no reason to remove them. Their appearance is so characteristic that they can hardly be mistaken for carcinoma or other serious lesions.

The prognosis is good, although if the patient misuses his voice, he may again develop nodules.

LARYNGEAL POLYPS (Figs. 23-4 and 23-5)

Laryngeal polyps may be attached to the vocal cords by either a broad or a narrow base. Some polyps are pedunculated, in which case they may hang under the vocal cord and cause symptoms only intermittently. Most cordal polyps, however, have a broad base so that they interfere permanently with voice production.

A laryngeal polyp looks about like what it usually is—an edematous mass of mucous membrane (Fig. 23-5). As viewed in the laryngeal mirror the polyp seems to flap up and down slightly during inspiration and expiration. Hoarseness is the chief reason for removing a laryngeal polyp.

In heavy smokers polypoid corditis may develop on both cords. The voice becomes deep because the edematous, flabby masses of tissue on the free edges of the cords cannot vibrate properly during phonation. Stripping of the polypoid mucosa from the vocal cords (performed under either local or general anesthesia) permits regeneration of firm mucosa; then if the patient refrains from smoking, he has no further trouble. One must never strip both cords all the way to the anterior commissure (where they meet in the midline), because if the two raw surfaces should grow together, a laryngeal web forms between the cords. Voice rest for seven to ten days postoperatively is customary.

JUVENILE PAPILLOMATOSIS (Fig. 23-4, A)

The cause of juvenile papillomatosis is unknown, but many authorities believe it is a viral infection. These papillomas are multiple and occur in all parts of the larynx, including the epiglottis, true cords, and trachea. Usually found in young boys, they tend to regress after puberty. The symptoms are extreme hoarseness, even aphonia, and sometimes enough impairment of the airways to necessitate a tracheotomy.

Treatment is by biting and stripping off the papillomas through the direct laryngoscope, using cup forceps. The patient is under general anesthesia. There is a strong tendency for papillomas to recur, and some patients have had to have them removed as many as ten or twenty times. Of course, repeated removal is likely to cause trauma to the cords themselves and the resulting voice may be poor.

Recently, other treatments are being used to remove these growths—cryotherapy, laser beams, and ultrasonic techniques, to mention three.

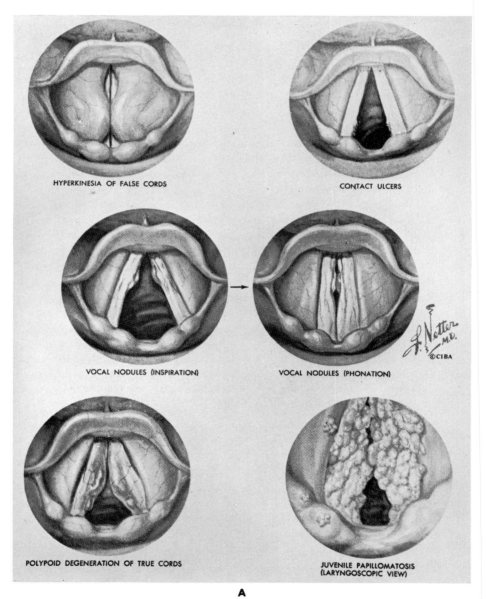

HYPERKINESIA OF FALSE CORDS

CONTACT ULCERS

VOCAL NODULES (INSPIRATION)

VOCAL NODULES (PHONATION)

POLYPOID DEGENERATION OF TRUE CORDS

JUVENILE PAPILLOMATOSIS
(LARYNGOSCOPIC VIEW)

A

Fig. 23-4. Miscellaneous disorders of the larynx. (Copyright CLINICAL SYMPOSIA, by Frank H. Netter, M.D., published by CIBA Pharmaceutical Co.)

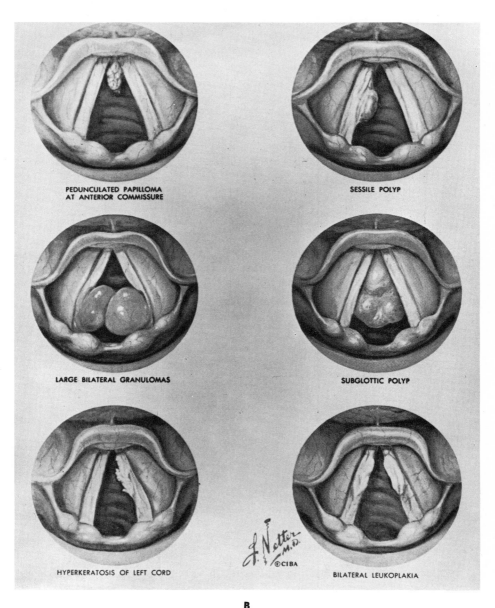

B

Fig. 23-4, cont'd. For legend see opposite page.

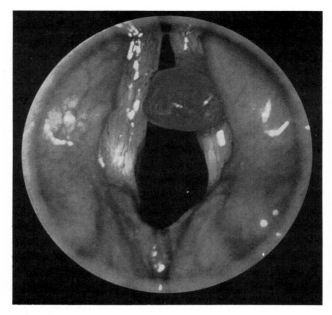

Fig. 23-5. Pedunculated polyp. (Courtesy Dr. Paul Holinger, Chicago, Ill.; from DeWeese, David D., and Saunders, William H.: Textbook of otolaryngology, ed. 4, St. Louis, 1973, The C. V. Mosby Co.)

LARYNGOCELE

Laryngocele results from enlargement or expansion of the laryngeal ventricle, an outpocketing of mucosa reaching upward and outward between the true and false cords. The laryngocele sac may be filled with mucus or air, and by expansion it can compress the larynx to cause hoarseness. It has even become visible externally. Laryngoceles are normal in animals such as apes, who fill their ventricles with air and use them to produce a booming sound. In man the laryngocele either is a congenital anomaly or results from an occupation requiring a blowing effort, such as horn playing or glass blowing. Unless it causes symptoms, surgical treatment is unnecessary.

LEUKOPLAKIA (Fig. 23-4, B)

Leukoplakia means "white plaque." In the larynx, where it is commonly caused by excessive smoking, it appears as a roughness on one or both vocal cords. There is no pain with leukoplakia; hoarseness is the only symptom. Leukoplakia generally is considered a premalignant lesion. Because there is no satisfactory way by physical examination to distinguish leukoplakia from hyperkeratosis, carcinoma in situ, or invasive carcinoma, the white lesions looking like leukoplakia must be stripped from the cords and examined by the pathologist. If the patient has leukoplakia and if he then stops smoking, it is likely that the lesion will not recur.

LARYNGEAL WEB (Fig. 23-6, *upper left*)

Laryngeal web may be congenital or acquired. Rarely, a congenital web is complete and stretches between both vocal cords, a condition incompatible with life. Usually, however, congenital webs are incomplete and join only the anterior parts of the vocal cords to produce a muffled cry. An acquired web results from inflammatory conditions of the larynx or, more commonly, after laryngeal surgery in which mucous membrane is stripped from the anterior aspects of both vocal cords, which then adhere to one another. Treatment is to excise the web and to place between the vocal cords a tantalum or plastic plate to keep the cords separated long enough to permit the mucous membrane to heal; then the plate can be removed.

LARYNGEAL INJURIES

Considering that the cartilages of the larynx are not protected, injury to the larynx is not as common as one might expect. The cause of most laryngeal injuries is high-speed automobile accidents in which the front-seat passenger or driver is thrown forward violently against the dashboard or steering wheel. There is usually laceration of the mucosa on the inside of the larynx, with enough impairment of the airway so that tracheotomy may be required. If the mucosa can be approximated accurately, a fair voice may result, but after severe laryngeal trauma, often the voice remains poor regardless of what is done. Commonly a Portex or other soft plastic tube is placed within the larynx and worn by the patient for two to four months or until an intralaryngeal airway has formed and the lacerated area is epithelialized. The tube is placed after an external incision to split the thyroid cartilage anteriorly in the midline. It is fixed inferiorly to a tracheotomy tube so that it cannot slip up or down.

Nursing care

The chief thing to remember in treating a patient with laryngeal injury is that his airway may become inadequate because of rapidly developing hematoma and edema, even though it seems satisfactory at the time of original examination. Therefore, close watch must be kept on such a patient so that signs of impending asphyxia can be recognized immediately and a tracheotomy performed.

The nurse can be of great importance at this stage, since she may watch for increasing respiratory rate, cyanosis, dyspnea, neck swelling from hematoma, and restlessness. A relaxed manner will do much to calm the patient. Instruments for tracheotomy should be available and endoscopy equipment in working order.

DYSPHONIA PLICA VENTRICULARIS (Fig. 23-4, *upper left*)

In dysphonia plica ventricularis the false cords, which lie just above the true cords, approximate during phonation and thus usurp the action of the true cords and interfere with voice production. During normal phonation

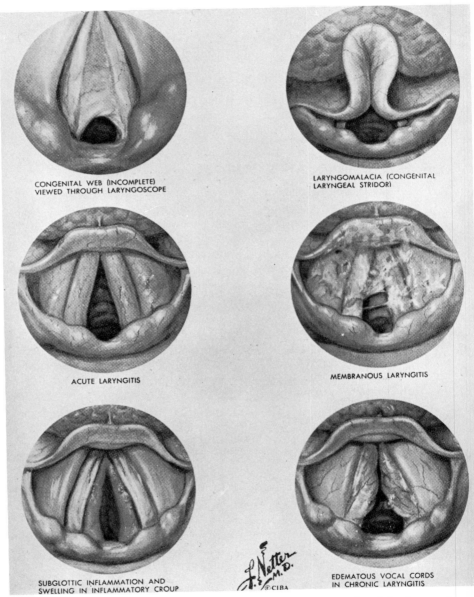

CONGENITAL WEB (INCOMPLETE)
VIEWED THROUGH LARYNGOSCOPE

LARYNGOMALACIA (CONGENITAL
LARYNGEAL STRIDOR)

ACUTE LARYNGITIS

MEMBRANOUS LARYNGITIS

SUBGLOTTIC INFLAMMATION AND
SWELLING IN INFLAMMATORY CROUP

EDEMATOUS VOCAL CORDS
IN CHRONIC LARYNGITIS

Fig. 23-6. Congenital and inflammatory reactions of the larynx as viewed by laryngeal mirror. (Copyright CLINICAL SYMPOSIA, by Frank H. Netter, M.D., published by CIBA Pharmaceutical Co.)

only the true cords vibrate and form the voice. When there is interference with action of the true cords, the false cords may act. The resulting voice breaks and alternates between hoarseness and clarity. Since the condition is inconstant, if the examiner does not look long enough at the larynx, he may fail to appreciate the abnormal action of the false cords and may not recognize dysphonia plica ventricularis as the cause of the patient's hoarseness.

In treatment, if there is any abnormality of the true cord such as vocal nodules or a vocal cord polyp, removal may improve the voice; also, a speech therapist may be able to help.

CONGENITAL LARYNGEAL STRIDOR (Fig. 23-6, *upper right*)

Congenital laryngeal stridor, a common condition, appears shortly after birth and lasts until the child is about 2 years of age; then it disappears spontaneously. The cause is laryngomalacia, involving all structures of the larynx so that during inspiration the epiglottis and other soft structures above the glottis fold and suck into the larynx, partially occluding the airway. Therefore, stridor is present during inspiration but not during expiration. If the baby cries or inspires deeply, he only gets worse. He may become blue but never dies of this condition because when he relaxes he can again breath normally. The parents always need strong reassurance that their baby will not choke; if they can maintain equanimity, their infant does much better.

The chief things to remember about congenital laryngeal stridor are that such a condition exists and that it will improve spontaneously. Diagnosis is made by looking at the larynx with a laryngoscope and noting the furled or omega-shaped epiglottis suck down into the larynx during inspiration. Some surgeons have recommended excising a V-shaped piece of cartilage from the epiglottis, but ordinarily this is not necessary, since the chief symptom of stridor eventually will correct itself.

LARYNGITIS (Fig. 23-6, *left center, lower left*)

Laryngitis exists in both *acute* and *chronic* phases and may be caused by infectious agents, trauma, and other less well-defined causes. Symptoms of acute laryngitis usually are hoarseness and pain and, depending on the etiology, there may be associated systemic symptoms such as fever; cough is also common. Chronic laryngitis is more likely to have hoarseness as its only symptom, although mild pain may also be present.

Infectious and *inflammatory* causes include all of the common upper respiratory diseases produced by bacteria and viruses. Often laryngitis is not an isolated disorder but is a part of a generalized upper respiratory infection such as the common cold or streptococcal sore throat. The cause then is usually rather apparent, and treatment is directed at the entire upper respiratory tract. Occasionally an infection in the lower respiratory tract will produce or be accompanied by laryngitis. Patients with bronchitis and tracheitis may also have laryngitis. A rather classic example of a severe and painful laryngitis, fortunately seldom seen anymore, is tuberculous laryngitis. Here the infection is carried to the larynx from bacteria-laden sputum, which the patient coughs up. The treatment basically is that of the chest disease with symptomatic measures aimed at relief of the laryngeal pain.

Isolated acute or chronic laryngitis also occurs, and in the absence of any apparent associated infection (Fig. 23-3, *lower right*). Specific bacterial infections may attack the larynx, the subglottic area, and the epiglottis.

Acute epiglottitis in the infant is an especially alarming condition since it comes on rapidly and can cause extreme dyspnea and even death if adequate treatment is not immediately instituted. The voice tends to be more thick and muffled than hoarse, and the child may assume a tripod position spontaneously to assist his breathing. The usual organism causing acute epiglottitis is *Haemophilus influenza,* fortunately responsive to ampicillin, the drug of choice. Before this antibiotic can take effect, however, it may be necessary to pass an intratracheal tube or perform a tracheotomy to ensure patency of the airway.

Trauma in the form of vocal abuse and smoking is a common cause of laryngitis, acute and chronic. Everyone is familiar with the hoarseness that follows misuse of the voice at a football game. This acute trauma usually produces symptoms for a few days or a week and then the larynx clears and the voice is again normal. But some persons abuse their voices this severely every day for months or years, and in them the hoarseness is likely to become permanent. They also may have a chronic aching of the throat. Men and women who work in noisy factories sometimes must shout above the noise level to make their instructions heard by other workers, and they are likely to develop chronic laryngitis. Auctioneers have a similar occupational hazard.

Smoking, of course, is a common cause of trauma or irritation to the larynx as well as to the respiratory tract. Some persons tolerate the effect of cigarette smoke much better than others, so that there is considerable variation in laryngeal appearances among smokers. The larynx may appear red overall, or sometimes the true vocal cords become edematous and pale and look polypoid (Fig. 23-2, *lower left*). The patient then develops a very low voice, and women with this type of voice are usually mistaken for men when they talk over the telephone. The treatment is complete cessation of smoking and, if this does not clear the condition, stripping of the vocal cords is done with the patient under local or general anesthesia. This should be followed by a two-week period of complete voice rest.

Cough that is nonproductive is unnecessary and represents another cause of laryngitis. Some patients get into the habit of coughing when they have a respiratory infection and then continue the cough after all infection has cleared. Sometimes this is classified as a psychologic cough, and the patient coughs because he gets attention that he would not otherwise receive.

Nursing care

The nurse can play an important role in the management of laryngitis. She can see to it that the humidity in the hospital room or in the home is high. This is especially important and difficult to achieve in the wintertime. The usual small vaporizer that patients buy and place at the bedside is next to useless. High humidity for the entire room or the entire house is needed. Large commercial units will achieve this, and in severe cases a steam tent or cold mist by mask or tent will be necessary. Probably it is unnecessary to add any medication to the vapor. The nurse should encourage patients to cough if they are actually raising purulent sputum, but if the cough is only a dry, unproductive one, she should discourage cough and see that a sedative is administered at night to give undisturbed sleep. During the daytime cough syrup containing codeine is the best medication.

An important aspect of the care of the person who has laryngitis or who has had surgery on the vocal cords is maintenance of voice rest, a difficult task for most persons. Although carefully instructed not to talk, many persons do talk, almost as much as before their instruction. Relatives and friends should be instructed to help the patient by asking questions that can be answered with a nod of the head. A pad and pencil or magic slate should be available. If there is an intercom system the patient's light at the nurse's station should be marked so that persons answering the intercom will know to tell the patient someone is on the way to his room. Sewing, reading, playing cards, and working puzzles are examples of activities encouraging self-expression that may serve as an alternative to speech.

SUGGESTED READINGS

Becker, W., and others: Atlas of otorhinolaryngology and bronchoesophagology, Philadelphia, 1969, W. B. Saunders Co.

Davidson, F. W.: Inflammatory diseases of the larynx of infants and small children, Annals of Otology **76:**753, 1967.

Reeves, Kathryn R.: Acute epiglottitis: pediatric emergency, American Journal of Nursing **71:**1539-1541, Aug., 1971.

Saunders, W. H.: The larynx, Ciba Clinical Symposia **16:**3, July, Aug., Sept., 1964.

CHAPTER TWENTY-FOUR

Larynx—carcinoma

Squamous cell carcinoma of the larynx, a disease seen much more often in men than in women, is increasing in frequency. One major cause is smoking—most, although certainly not all, patients with carcinoma of the larynx are heavy cigarette smokers. The rising incidence in women is because of their increasing use of tobacco.

SYMPTOMS

Symptoms of laryngeal carcinoma differ, depending on which part of the larynx is affected. Consider the patient fortunate in whom carcinoma begins on the true cord, for he will develop an early symptom—*hoarseness* (Figs. 24-1 and 24-2). This symptom, when taken seriously by both the patient and the physician, permits an early diagnosis and a high percentage of cures. If the symptom is neglected, and all too often it is, the cure rate drops rapidly. Otolaryngologists have a maxim: *Any patient hoarse longer than two weeks must have his larynx examined.* The nurse, of course, can play a significant role in seeing that patients with hoarseness do receive adequate and early examination.

The *glottis* is the space or chink between the true vocal cords (Fig. 23-1). Carcinoma arising on the true vocal cords, therefore, is often called glottic, while carcinoma arising above the level of the true cords (on the epiglottis, for example) is called supraglottic, and carcinoma below the level of the cords, infraglottic. An older terminology referred to lesions of the true cords as "intrinsic" and all other laryngeal lesions as "extrinsic."

Usually there are no early symptoms of supraglottic carcinoma. Lesions of the epiglottis or lateral walls of the hypopharynx are not expected to produce hoarseness, at least not early, since these parts do not function in voice production. The first symptom, although not an early one, may be pain on swallowing such liquids as hot coffee or orange juice. In short, the carcinoma has grown large, is ulcerated, and is painful. Another common way for such a patient first to discover trouble is to note a painless *lump in the neck,* which, of course, represents a metastasis (Fig. 24-1, *lower right*). Carcinoma of the glottic larynx does not metastasize early because the lymphatics leading from the true cords are sparse, whereas from most other parts of the larynx—epiglottis, pyriform recess, arytenoid, and subglottic areas—they are abundant. Sometimes *dysphagia* is the symptom that

270

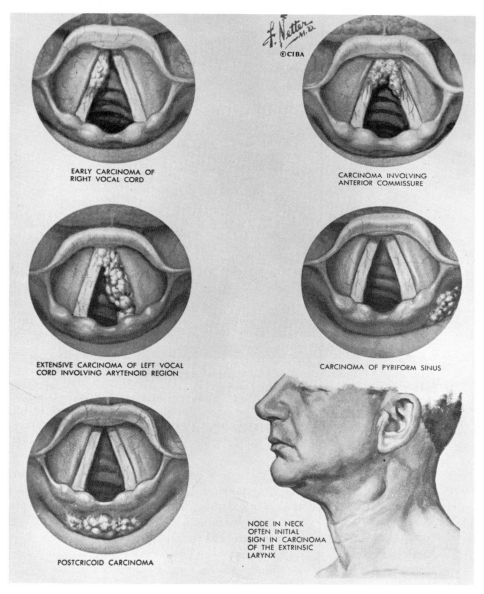

Fig. 24-1. Cancer of the larynx. (Copyright CLINICAL SYMPOSIA, by Frank H. Netter, M.D., published by CIBA Pharmaceutical Co.)

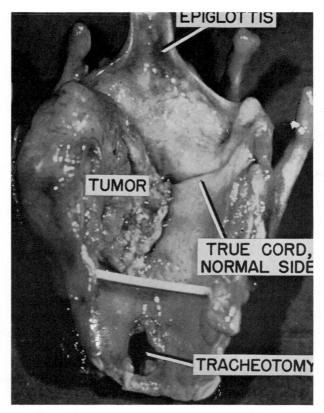

Fig. 24-2. Advanced carcinoma of the larynx that has spread far beyond the confines of the true cord and is actually transglottic since it is present both above and below the level of the true cords. Tracheotomy was required preoperatively because the tumor mass obstructed the airway completely. The larynx has been cut open from behind, and the white stick props it apart. Many surgeons favor a partial course of preoperative irradiation therapy before laryngectomy in advanced tumors like this.

causes the patient to seek a doctor's help. Dysphagia may result because swallowing is painful or simply because there is actual obstruction by a tumorous mass at the esophageal inlet. *Dyspnea* is a very late symptom caused by a tumor growing large enough to obstruct some part of the airway. It is almost always preceded by an earlier symptom, which, had the patient heeded it, would have afforded a much better prognosis.

TREATMENT

The type of treatment required for the patient with carcinoma of the larynx varies, depending upon the exact site of the lesion, its early or advanced stage, presence or absence of regional neck metastases or distant metastases, age, and sometimes the patient's wishes. In general, early lesions of the glottic larynx (true cords) are best treated with irradiation therapy or a limited surgical procedure, while advanced lesions of the glottis or supraglottic or infraglottic larynx are treated surgically. Sometimes a preliminary partial course of irradiation therapy is given before laryngectomy is done. A detailed discussion of several types of surgical procedures and of irradiation therapy follows.

Partial laryngectomy

Partial laryngectomy, applicable to early carcinoma, carries with it a high cure rate. In patients suitable for partial laryngectomy only one vocal cord is diseased, and there is complete mobility of both cords. In short, the malignant process is limited, since it does not invade deeply enough to freeze the laryngeal musculature. The ideal patient for partial laryngectomy has squamous cell carcinoma involving the middle third of one cord but not its posterior attachment to the arytenoid or its anterior attachment at the place where it joins the opposite cord (anterior commissure).

There are several different techniques of partial laryngectomy. The most common is performed through a "laryngofissure"; an incision is made in the midline of the neck, and the thyroid cartilage is split and opened much like a clamshell. The cancer is then excised. Usually this means removal of only the true cord, but sometimes in large lesions the true cord, ventricle, and false cord on one side are removed. A tracheotomy is done to assure a good airway during the immediate postoperative period.

Patients are in the hospital five to seven days. Postoperatively the chief problem (not always present) is difficulty in swallowing for the first three or four days, so that temporary feeding of the patient intravenously or by nasogastric tube may be necessary. Patients need not be placed on absolute "voice rest."

Nursing care. The *nursing care* after partial laryngectomy is of great importance. These patients do have a tracheotomy tube in place and are unable to talk unless the tube is occluded. They experience the usual difficulties associated with the wearing of a tracheotomy tube. Secretions come from around the tube, suctioning is necessary, and there may be a little bleeding from the tracheotomy. Patients need reassurance that the tube is to be in place for only two or three days and not permanently.

Subcutaneous emphysema, in which air dissects under the skin of the neck and face and may even cause enough swelling to close the eyes, is an occasional complication of the laryngofissure operation. It also may occur after any tracheotomy and especially if the skin is closed too tightly around the tracheotomy tube. There is a peculiar crackling sensation as the skin is palpated, and the nurse who recognizes this condition will do well to call it to the surgeon's attention (although there is not much to be done about it except perhaps to remove a suture or two).

These patients do have trouble swallowing for a few days, and the nurse should know that often it is easier for them to take soft foods (such as gelatin, custard, and mashed potatoes) than liquids, because liquids tend to spill over into the trachea and are aspirated, whereas solids enter the esophagus. If there is aspiration of either liquids or solids, the nurse should suction the trachea through the tracheotomy tube. Instructions concerning proper suctioning technique are given in Chapter 26.

In healing, scar tissue fills the defect where the diseased cord was removed. As a rule, the remaining cord approximates or almost approximates the scar, and a fairly good voice results. There is an adequate airway. Although preservation of voice is important, the main consideration is to cure the patient of his cancer. There is a better chance of cure in *early* carcinoma of the glottic larynx (true cord) than in malignant disease of any other visceral organ.

A true *hemilaryngectomy* is sometimes done through the same type of operative approach as the laryngofissure. Here the thyroid cartilage behind the true and false vocal cords (one side only) is also removed. Because this operation is done through a vertical incision it has been called a "vertical laryngectomy," in contrast to the "horizontal laryngectomy" (supraglottic laryngectomy).

Supraglottic laryngectomy

In supraglottic or horizontal laryngectomy, done for carcinoma of the epiglottis and adjacent structures *above* the level of the true vocal cords, the vocal cords themselves are left intact while a horizontal cut passes just above the true cords to remove the diseased tissue. These patients usually have a great deal of difficulty swallowing for the first two or three postoperative weeks because, with the epiglottis and false vocal cords removed, food (especially liquid) tends to spill directly into the trachea. Eventually, however, they do learn how to swallow effectively and do well most of the time. Secretions, however, may still trickle into the larynx and produce annoying cough. The voice is excellent. Supraglottic or horizontal laryngectomy is now more common than total laryngectomy. Usually a unilateral radical neck dissection is done along with supraglottic laryngectomy in order to remove lymph nodes with possible metastases.

Nursing care here is even more important than in vertical laryngectomy. For one thing, most patients with a laryngofissure or vertical laryngectomy have an adequate airway, and tracheotomy is done only as insurance against unusual edema or postoperative hemorrhage. In supraglottic laryngectomy, however, tracheotomy is *mandatory* since none of these patients have an adequate airway. A cuffed tube is used to diminish the aspiration that usually occurs early in the postoperative period. Second, early in the postoperative course the feeding problem of these patients is great and the nurse's assistance and encouragement are most important. Finally, the supraglottic laryngectomy, because it is usually done simultaneously with radical neck dissection, is a much more extensive operation and there are more opportunities for postoperative fistulae, hemorrhage, and infection.

Total laryngectomy

Total laryngectomy is reserved for patients with advanced carcinoma of the true cords, and occasionally for other patients (see Fig. 24-9). Such patients have involvement on both sides of the larynx, fixation of one of the vocal cords, or tumor extending well beyond the true cord. Total laryngectomy used to be more common than it is now because, with the advent of supraglottic laryngectomy (a relatively new procedure), many larynges are saved and rehabilitated that formerly were lost to supraglottic disease.

Preoperative preparation is important, particularly for the patient who will be required postoperatively to face life with a major disability. The nurse along with the surgeon and other members of the health team should evaluate the mental status of the patient. The nurse can assist in assessing the patient's mental and emotional state by noting how he explains what the doctor has told him and how he views the planned surgery. It is important that the nurse spend adequate time with the patient in order for him to develop trust in the nursing staff.

The surgical procedure should be discussed as frankly as possible to avert misunderstanding. Although this is primarily the responsibility of the

Table 2

Structures removed	Structures left	Postoperative condition
Total laryngectomy		
Hyoid bone	Tongue	Loses voice
Entire larynx (epiglottis, false cords, true cords)	Pharyngeal walls	Breathes through tracheostomy
	Lower trachea	No problem swallowing
Cricoid cartilage		
Two or three rings of trachea		
Supraglottic or horizontal laryngectomy		
Hyoid bone	True vocal cords	Normal voice
Epiglottis	Cricoid cartilage	May aspirate occasionally, especially liquids
False vocal cords	Trachea	Normal airway
Vertical (or hemi) laryngectomy		
One true vocal cord	Epiglottis	Hoarse but serviceable voice
False cord	One false cord	
Arytenoid	One true vocal cord	Normal airway
One-half thyroid cartilage	Cricoid	No problem swallowing
Laryngofissure and partial laryngectomy		
One vocal cord	All other structures	Hoarse but serviceable voice; occasionally almost normal voice
		No airway problem
		No swallowing problem
Endoscopic removal of early carcinoma		
Part of one vocal cord	All other structures	May have a normal voice
		No other problems

surgeon, the informed nurse plays a role in interpreting the surgeon's information when necessary. Also she can alleviate worry and misunderstanding, reinforce preoperative teaching, and provide assurance to the patient and family.

Fears expressed by patients prior to laryngectomy are as follows:
1. Fear of the word "cancer" and the implications involved, including fear of mutilation and becoming a social burden
2. Fear of operations in general
3. Fear of loss of voice

Preoperative preparation should include a brief explanation that the patient will breathe through a hole in the neck and when he coughs, secretions will come from this hole. Some means of communication should be planned prior to surgery. The patient should be allowed to make suggestions. Hand signals such as raising one finger to mean need to void and the sign for OK can be used. A picture or word chart can be utilized if the patient is too weak or unable to use a pad and pencil, especially in the immediate postoperative period, when an intravenous needle and tubing may interfere with writing. If the patient is blind or deaf, one must establish how best the patient can communicate, whether by a raised alphabet, by hand signals, or by other means. The signal light or a bell, which may be more satisfying to the patient, must be explained. At any rate *some means of communication must be established* and shared with the staff who will care for the patient immediately after surgery and with his family.

As the ultimate goal after laryngectomy is some form of alaryngeal speech, orientation regarding speech after laryngectomy by the physician, nurse, speech therapist, or a member of the "Lost Chord Club" is of great value. Should the patient be a woman, it may be wise to have a woman visit who has had similar problems and who has adjusted to her limitations.*

Total laryngectomy includes removal of the thyroid cartilage or "Adam's apple," the hyoid bone, the cricoid cartilage, and two or three rings of the trachea. With the larynx removed there is no longer a connection between the trachea below and the pharynx above. The trachea, therefore, is sewed to the skin of the neck with sutures that are removed in a week, and this union forms a permanent tracheostomy (Fig. 24-3) through which the patient breathes the rest of his life; he can no longer inspire through his nose or mouth, but he can eat normally. In fact, he does everything almost as before with one notable exception—there is no voice. Most patients, however, learn so-called esophageal speech, and some use their new voices extremely well (Fig. 24-4).

Postoperative nursing care. Immediately after operation the chief concern is that the airway be maintained. Here the nurse is of paramount importance, and the difference between enlightened, astute nursing care and

---

*Gardner, Warren H.: Adjustment problems of laryngectomized women, Archives of Otolaryngology **83:**57-68, 1966.

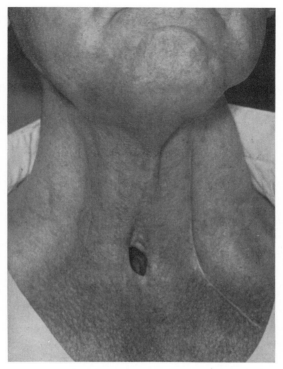

Fig. 24-3. Postoperative laryngeal carcinoma. Note the scars of bilateral radical neck dissections. The patient also had a pneumonectomy for a pulmonary metastasis. He lived four years after the last of his operations. (From DeWeese, David D., and Saunders, William H.: Textbook of otolaryngology, ed. 4, St. Louis, 1973, The C. V. Mosby Co.)

inadequate care may well spell the difference between prompt recovery and prolonged hospitalization, or even between life and death.

Immediately after the operation, especially in the winter months when humidity is low, a cupula over the tracheostomy to deliver moist air is valuable. This device need not be in place all the time. (Lower respiratory infections such as pneumonia or bronchitis are no more common in the healed laryngectomized patients than in normal patients.)

It is customary to have patients wear laryngectomy tubes, usually size 10 or 12, for a week or two postoperatively or at least until the stoma seems to maintain its size. Some doctors, however, believe there is less reaction and a better stoma if the patient wears no tube at any time. Some patients who are overweight tend to have the skin of the neck fold down over the tracheostomy and partially obstruct it. The nurse will note this and call it to the physician's attention so that he can insert a laryngectomy tube, which helps the situation. There often is crusting about the tracheostomy stoma during the first postoperative week. Some of this may be blood and some mucus. In either case the nurse should moisten

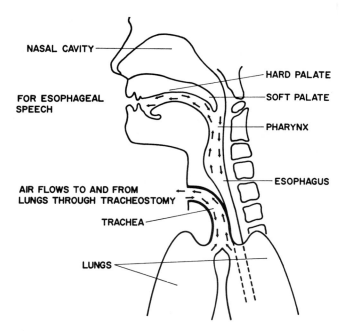

Fig. 24-4. After total laryngectomy. Air for breathing enters through the tracheostomy. The patient must learn to move air in his mouth and throat for alaryngeal speech.

the crusts with sterile normal saline or part saline and part hydrogen peroxide and tease away the crusts. Then application of an ointment such as Borofax or Neosporin will help to prevent additional crusting. If suture ends are too long they also tend to accumulate crusts and the nurse may need to trim these.

The danger of a large plug of blood or mucus obstructing the trachea is not great but it can happen. In that case a physician must be called at once, but if one is not *readily* available, the nurse must herself remove the crust by grasping it with a hemostat and simply pulling it out. Once it is started a little the patient usually expels it with a violent cough.

Later in the postoperative course, contrary to what one might expect, there is very little trouble with crusting and drying of the trachea. Dryness of the tracheal mucosa can be relieved by using a humidifier or by having the patient wear over the tracheostomy a moistened gauze through which he breathes (Fig. 24-5).

After laryngectomy and, more particularly, after laryngectomy and neck dissection, the patient may need help in lifting his head, and a supporting hand behind the patient's head will do much to increase comfort. Postoperatively the patient should be placed in an elevated position of about 30 degrees. The first postoperative night is frightening, not because of pain (which is not great), but because of inability to speak and because of altera-

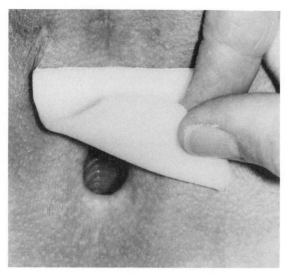

Fig. 24-5. Light-weight tracheostomy shield glued to skin.

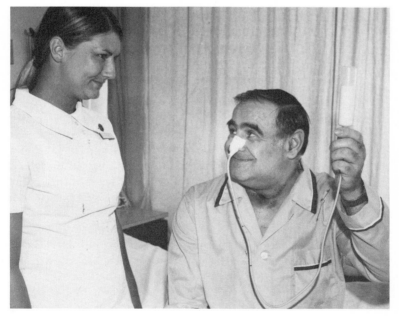

Fig. 24-6. Patient feeding self several days after laryngectomy. Note nasogastric tube securely attached to nose.

tion of the site of intake for air from the nose to the neck. The patient should be in a room close to the nurses' station, where he can be observed closely. It is imperative that he have within reach his signal light or other means of calling for help. His laryngectomy tube (if he wears one), although larger than the tracheotomy tube, may become obstructed. To avoid this the *inner tube* must be removed and cleaned regularly. Suctioning of the trachea is necessary, especially in the early postoperative period. (See Chapter 26.)

On the day of surgery the *feeding tube* is often used as a means of aspirating the stomach to prevent regurgitation. Sometimes a weak constant or intermittent suction is attached to the tube and aspiration carried out in this manner. On the first postoperative day water and skim milk or a low-calorie gastrostomy mixture is put down the tube, and the nurse observes the patient's tolerance. Ordinarily patients after laryngectomy have no particular problem with tube feedings if the strength of the tube feeding is increased gradually. Water in amounts of 50 to 100 ml. should follow the tube feeding.

Tube feedings (Fig. 24-6), started on the first or second postoperative day, are given every two or three hours to avoid gastric distention and nausea. Depending on the size of the nasogastric tube, the gastrostomy formula may run in by gravity alone, or it may be necessary to use a syringe to start the flow. Any vomiting, pain, abdominal distention, or diarrhea must be reported to the surgeon immediately. Nasogastric tubes are always resented by the patient. They pull on his nose and in general are uncomfortable. The nurse can help in knowing how to tape the tube to the nose so that it causes minimal irritation to the nostrils (Fig. 24-7). The use of tincture of benzoin on the skin before tape is applied is worthwhile. The many different types of tape now available usually make it possible to select one that will not cause a skin reaction. The tube should not only be secured at the nose, but also anchored to the face and/or pinned to the gown. When starting to feed the patient, the nurse may want to listen over the stomach through a stethoscope while she simultaneously injects a small quantity of air down the nasogastric tube in order to learn if the tube is actually in the stomach. Usually the physician inserts the nasogastric tube at the time of surgery, but not always. If the tube is inserted later, it must be done gently, since the pharynx and esophagus have just been sutured and must not be traumatized. Most physicians now use a plastic rather than a rubber feeding tube.

Recently there has been a trend toward elimination of the feeding tube and feeding the patient by mouth early in the postoperative course. The reason that tube feedings are used is to prevent breakdown of the pharyngeal suture line, with subsequent fistula formation. With careful attention to suturing and drainage techniques, however, it has been found practical to dispense with the feeding tube and to give the patient regular diet on the second postoperative day; except rarely, fistula does not occur. Even if it does, it probably would have developed in spite of tube feedings for

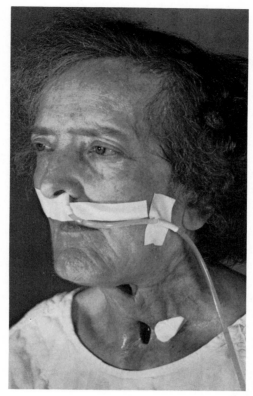

Fig. 24-7. A fistula after laryngectomy (upper hole). The lower hole is the tracheostomy through which the patient breathes. Note also the manner of applying tape to hold the nasogastric tube in place and keep it from rubbing on the nostril. A second strip of tape prevents direct pull on the lip by the weight of the tube.

seven to ten days. As soon as the patient is able, he is encouraged to participate in his own care by helping with tube feedings and care of the laryngectomy tube if present (Fig. 24-6).

Complications. The chief complication of importance after laryngectomy is that of *salivary fistula* formation. There is a breakdown somewhere along the suture line in the pharynx, and salivary secretions, which the patient swallows, leak out the hole and eventually through the overlying skin to produce a pharyngeal-cutaneous fistula. Sometimes the fistulas are small and close in a matter of a few days or a week, but at other times they may become large and require weeks or even months to heal. It is important to observe redness and swelling of the neck, especially near the incisions, in the first few days after laryngectomy, since these signs together with a fever signal the accumulation of secretions beneath the skin and the beginning of a fistula. Once the fistula is established, there is not much anyone can do except to protect the adjacent skin from maceration by the secretions and to see that the secretion from the fistula, which may be profuse, does not run down into the newly established tracheostomy. A large amount of fluid can be lost in this manner and the nurse should monitor fluid intake and output and observe for signs of dehydration. Extra fluid should be given by feeding tube or supplemented by the I.V. route. Fistulas eventually close spontaneously, but until they do the patient must wear a nasogastric feeding tube, since everything he would attempt to eat would leak out the fistula (Fig. 24-7).

Another complication, and a most serious one, is *rupture of the carotid artery*. Ordinarily this complication does not occur after laryngectomy unless that operation is combined with a radical neck dissection, because in laryngectomy alone the carotid artery is not approached in the dissection, whereas in radical neck dissection the common carotid artery is very much within the field of dissection. This dread complication, which fortunately is uncommon, is more likely to occur in a patient who has had a course of irradiation therapy preoperatively than it is in a patient who has never had therapy. It is also much more common in patients with a fistula in whom secretions bathe the carotid artery. The nurse will be told about the danger of a blowout of the carotid by the physician, and she should see to it that someone is always at the bedside who can place pressure on the bleeding site should this become necessary. Continue pressure until help arrives. Pulling the signal cord from the socket is one way of getting help. Even members of the family who are likely to be with the patient and who might be expected to help can be instructed, because recognition of the gushing bleeding and action within a few seconds will be required to save the life of the patient. Sometimes there is a warning or sentinel bleeding of lesser amount, but this cannot be counted on. Treatment is ligation of the common carotid, a procedure that in itself may result in fatality or serious neurologic deficit.

After laryngectomy there is also loss of the sense of smell, since air currents no longer enter the nose to stimulate the olfactory cells. Normal hygienic practices, such as use of deodorants, should be encouraged.

The patient will need to be reminded that, when showering, he must take care not to get water in the tracheostome. Some patients wear a small protective plastic sheet or flap just above the stoma to deflect the shower water. Actually a little water getting into the stoma is harmless except for the coughing it induces.

Occasionally a patient with a fat neck may have enough redundant skin directly above the stoma that when asleep there is interference with the airway as the fold of skin falls over the stoma. In such a case a secondary operation to remove skin and fat may be necessary or the patient may need to wear a laryngectomy tube at night.

Speech after total laryngectomy. Fears are often expressed postoperatively by laryngectomized patients. These can be somewhat eliminated by beginning the rehabilitation program preoperatively and continuing it postoperatively. Laryngectomized patients feel grossly handicapped until they develop an alternative mode of communication. When the ability to speak is impaired, the person may be repeatedly frustrated and experience feelings of doubt about his personal worth; he may become irritable, discouraged, and depressed and ultimately withdraw from those whose fellowship he needs.

The majority of laryngectomized patients can develop alaryngeal, esophageal, or pharyngeal voice without resort to any electronic or mechanical device. They can learn to produce an air change by any of several procedures of intake of air into the esophagus or hypopharynx, the two primary ones being the inhallation method (or aspirate method, involving the sucking back of air with lips open and tongue inactive) and the injection method (the tongue acting as a piston to force the air in the closed mouth backward to be trapped in the esophagus or hypopharynx).* About 75% of laryngectomized patients master some technique of air intake. They learn to use the bolus of air as the energy source and the cricopharyngeal muscle as the vibrator to produce sound, which is shaped in the conventional way by the articulators to form intelligible speech.

Motivation is essential to mastery of alaryngeal speech. It is dependent upon a determination to succeed, a willingness to practice not once or twice a day but constantly, and an effort to cultivate an attitude of relaxation that will permit optimal learning of a new muscular skill through patient application. Personal factors loom larger than any other factors (e.g., age or extent of surgery) in failure to develop alaryngeal speech.

A patient who has not learned alaryngeal speech within sixty to ninety days after surgery may have an artificial larynx prescribed for him. Some surgeons recommend speech aids in the early postoperative period, whereas others fear that electronic aids will induce dependency on the aid. Patients can still learn alaryngeal speech even after temporary or prolonged use of a speech aid.

Various mechanical devices to be used as an artificial larynx are available.† Newer electronic aids allow for naturalness of speech by providing for pitch inflection and volume controls and even the approximating of male and female voices.

The laryngectomized patient may find it helpful to affiliate with a local group of laryngectomees who are organized into "Lost Chord Clubs" or "New Voice Clubs." These clubs provide voice-teaching services, exchange of ideas regarding management of laryngectomy problems, and opportu-

---

*For the nearest competent speech and hearing therapist, write the Executive Secretary of the American Speech and Hearing Association, 1001 Connecticut Ave., N.W., Washington, D. C. The name of the nearest teacher of alaryngeal speech can also be obtained by writing to International Association of Laryngectomees, American Cancer Society, 219 East 42nd St., New York, N. Y. 10017.

†A useful artificial larynx is available at cost from the Bell Telephone Company. Inquiries may be directed to Special Equipment Section, Commercial Department, of the local Bell Telephone Company office.

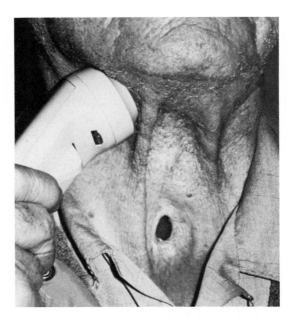

Fig. 24-8. Use of electronic larynx in patient who failed to develop esophageal speech. (From DeWeese, David D., and Saunders, William H.: Textbook of otolaryngology, ed. 4, St. Louis, 1973, The C. V. Mosby Co.)

nities for socal activities. Moral support and encouragement may be derived from associating with others with a like disability who have regained social confidence and emotional security. There are over 175 of these clubs at the present time.* A bimonthly newsletter and other material helpful to the laryngectomized patient are distributed by these clubs. Two guidebooks that will be most helpful are *Your New Voice* and *Helping Words for the Laryngectomee.†*

Radical neck dissection

Although total laryngectomy is an excellent surgical procedure, the incidence of postoperative metastases to the neck (20 to 30%) indicates its relative inadequacy. The same inadequacy points to the need for the technique of simultaneous laryngectomy and radical neck dissection. This technique is always indicated when cervical nodes are palpable at time of initial operation and is usually indicated when, either because of the extent or position of the carcinoma, one suspects the presence of cervical metastases. Lesions arising below or above the true cords and cordal le-

---

*The address of the club closest to the patient's home community may be obtained by writing to International Association of Laryngectomees, 219 East 42nd St., New York, N. Y. 10017.

†Waldrop, William F., and Gould, Marie A.: Your new voice, distributed by the American Cancer Society, Inc., 219 East 42nd St., New York, N. Y. 10017.

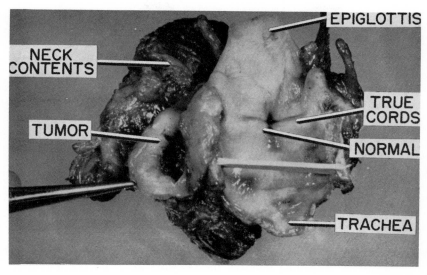

Fig. 24-9. Laryngectomy and neck dissection. The tumor is in pyriform recess. This patient had no early symptoms and was not hoarse because true vocal cords were not affected.

sions with subglottic extension or arytenoid fixation are suited to this method (Fig. 24-9).

Radical neck dissection is also done months or years after laryngectomy, when late metastatic disease appears in one or both sides of the neck. In other patients undergoing neck dissection who do not have laryngeal carcinoma the primary lesion is likely to be in the tongue, tonsil, lip, nasopharynx, or thyroid gland. Neck dissection is done to remove regional metastatic disease in patients with no evidence of remote metastatic spread such as to the lung. Also prerequisite to neck dissection is control of the primary tumor either preoperatively by irradiation therapy or as an integral part of the neck dissection in which the primary lesion and neck contents are removed en bloc. Examples of one-stage procedures for removal of primary and metastatic malignancies are laryngectomy and neck dissection, hemiglossectomy and neck dissection, and hemimandibulectomy and neck dissection (so-called commando operation).

Although the prognosis for five-year survival drops considerably once carcinoma has metastasized to the neck, enough patients are salvaged by radical neck dissection to make the procedure worthwhile.

Nursing care after radical neck dissection is somewhat less demanding than after laryngectomy, since these patients do not have a tracheostomy and can talk and eat normally. Nevertheless there is a constantly recurring problem of hematoma formation under the rather extensive skin flaps that

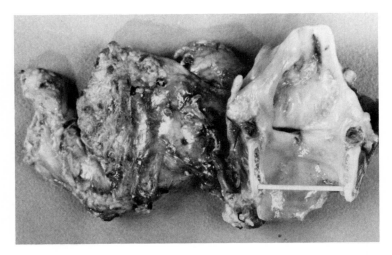

Fig. 24-10. Specimen after total laryngectomy and radical neck dissection.

are formed in this operation. Therefore the nurse has a primary responsibility to see that the Hemovac unit is working efficiently and that there is no swelling which might indicate hematoma (Fig. 24-10).

In this operation there is purposeful resection of the *spinal accessory* or *eleventh cranial nerve,* and loss of this nerve causes atrophy of the large trapezius muscle. In addition the sternocleidomastoid muscle is resected, and loss of these two muscles in the neck results in a *shoulder drop* on one side and aching and pain for several months. (The nurse can explain this to the patient and instruct members of the family in massage, use of liniment, and application of heat as symptomatic measures to reduce pain. She can teach the patient exercises such as crawling up the wall with the fingers of both hands to stretch the arm on the affected side high above the head and thus gradually to replace the function of the lost muscles with other muscles.) Sutures are removed on the fifth to seventh day, and if there is a gap in the long suture line, the nurse should apply tape bridges to pull the skin margins together and reduce the width of the scar.

Dressings and drains. Traditional *drainage methods* have been with Penrose drains and massive neck dressings to absorb blood and provide pressure. Newer and better methods employ closed suction drainage in which a drainage tube from the neck passes to a container, which serves both as suction source and receptacle for blood. One convenient unit is the Hemovac apparatus (Figs. 24-11 to 24-13), which acts as a sterile, portable, and disposable suction apparatus. The nurse should *inspect the bellows frequently* to be certain it is effecting continuous suction. If there is a leak, it may be necessary to attach to constant suction. In this method of drainage the skin remains absolutely dry. Furthermore, there is no need for pressure-type neck dressing, since the drainage tubes, constantly working under

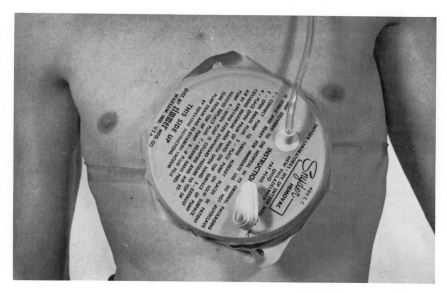

Fig. 24-11. Closed suction-drainage system (Hemovac) for use after laryngectomy or neck dissection. The container has a spring in it that, in pushing the upper and lower lids apart, creates a vacuum when the lids are compressed and the openings are occluded that is transmitted through the plastic tube to a Y adapter. Two smaller plastic tubes with multiple perforations are placed in the wound under the skin flaps and connected to the adapter. This system keeps wound dry, evacuates blood, and sucks skin down tightly so that postoperatively no dressings are needed.

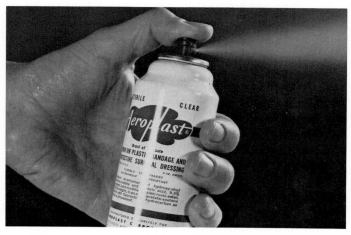

Fig. 24-12. Plastic spray used to seal the incision line against bacterial contamination. With the use of constant suction-drainage (Hemovac) unit, no other neck dressing is required.

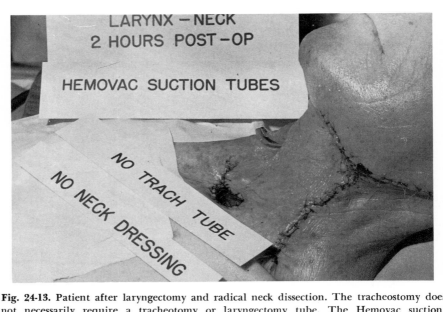

LARYNX — NECK
2 HOURS POST—OP

HEMOVAC SUCTION TUBES

NO TRACH TUBE

NO NECK DRESSING

Fig. 24-13. Patient after laryngectomy and radical neck dissection. The tracheostomy does not necessarily require a tracheotomy or laryngectomy tube. The Hemovac suction-drainage system evacuates blood and by sucking skin flaps down tightly makes pressure dressing unnecessary.

the skin flaps, suck them firmly against the neck. The nurse empties the suction container and reseals it to continue suction. The amount of drainage is recorded. Approximately 70 to 120 ml. of serosanguinous drainage will be recorded for the first day of suction, 30 to 50 ml. the second day, and 0 to 30 ml. the third day.

Irradiation therapy

Also good treatment for carcinoma of the larynx and other malignant conditions about the head and neck is irradiation therapy. Generally the surgeon and the irradiation therapist confer and decide which method of treatment is most applicable to the particular problem at hand. Irradiation therapy is given as a series of treatments, a small dose each day, until the tolerance of skin and other tissue is reached. The tumor, being more sensitive than normal tissue, shrinks and in many instances disappears entirely. The use of irradiation therapy, which is preferable to surgery in many instances, is a special topic requiring authoritative discussion and is therefore not presented here as fully as its importance warrants.

Nursing care during and for a time after irradiation therapy is of considerable importance. Before starting therapy the patient should have it explained to him that, although each treatment is painless, the cumulative effect when the last treatments are given some five to seven weeks later may

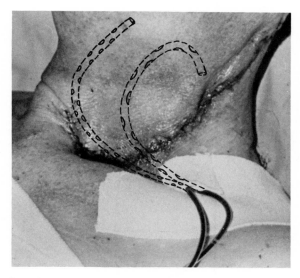

Fig. 24-14. Closed suction drainage tubes under skin after laryngectomy. Note tape firmly securing tubes to skin.

cause severe sore throat, dry ropy secretions in the mouth (if the oral cavity is included in the irradiated field), and malaise. If the patient has a sore throat and feels poorly in general, he often refuses to eat and loses weight. The nurse can do much to assist with oral hygiene, which often breaks down severely during this period, and in observing for weight loss and dehydration. It is important that the patient have adequate fluids and nutrition. Skin care is also important, since the effect of prolonged irradiation therapy on the skin may be that of partial breakdown and even superficial ulceration similar to the mucositis that occurs in the throat. In general, however, the skin of patients undergoing therapy is simply left alone, as creams, powders, and lotions are forbidden by the radiotherapist.

Pedicle grafts

This subject is included with this chapter because sometimes it is necessary to do *even more* than a total laryngectomy in attempting to eradicate carcinoma from the laryngeal area. If, for example, the carcinoma has penetrated anteriorly through the thyroid cartilage and come to invade the overlying skin, then, of course, the skin must be resected along with the larynx. This resection leaves a large defect which must be closed; one of the better methods of closing it is to swing up a so-called pedicle flap from the chest, carrying with it its own blood supply.

There are several well-devised pedicle flaps for use about the head and neck; three of the more commonly used ones are shown in Fig. 24-15. Their use is actually much greater in reconstruction about the oral cavity and face than in association with laryngectomy.

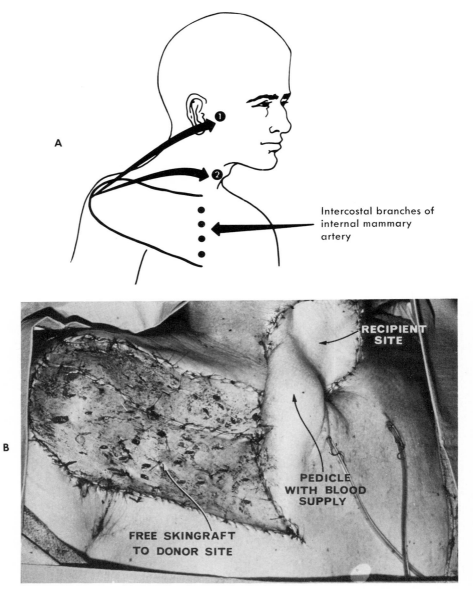

A

Intercostal branches of
internal mammary
artery

B

RECIPIENT
SITE

PEDICLE
WITH BLOOD
SUPPLY

FREE SKINGRAFT
TO DONOR SITE

Fig. 24-15. Three useful pedicle flaps. **A,** Deltopectoral flap which is used to cover skin defects as indicated at *1* and *2* or which also can be used to create a new pharynx and cervical esophagus. In the latter case it is tubed or rolled on itself. **B,** The same type of pedicle graft swung upward to close a defect in anterior neck.

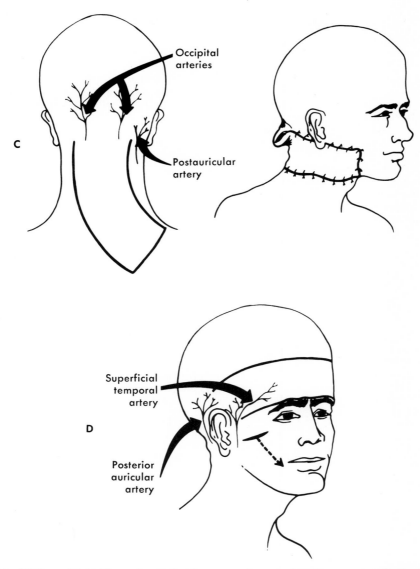

Fig. 24-15, cont'd. C, Nape of neck flap for use as shown or in adjacent areas. **D,** Forehead flap. The far end of the flap, after entire flap is raised along the horizontal lines, is inserted through the lower incision under eye and then pulled into mouth where it serves as lining after removal of tongue or after other major intraoral surgery. The donor site receives a split-thickness graft.

SUGGESTED READINGS

Beattie, Edward J., and Economou, Steven G.: The current status of radical laryngectomy, Nursing Clinics of North America 3:515-518, Sept., 1968.

Flowers, Ann M.: Electronic mechanical aids for the laryngectomized patient, Nursing Clinics of North America 3:529-532, Sept., 1968.

Gardner, Warren H.: Adjustment problems of laryngectomized women, Archives of Otolaryngology 83:57-68, 1966.

Martin, Hayes: Radical neck dissection, Ciba Clinical Symposia 13: Oct., Nov., Dec., 1961.

Martin, Hayes: Rehabilitation of the laryngectomee, Cancer 16:823-841, July, 1963.

Parvulescu, Nina F.: Care of the surgically speechless patient, Nursing Clinics of North America 5:517-525, Sept., 1970.

Pitorak, Elizabeth F.: Laryngectomy, American Journal of Nursing 68:780-786, 1968.

Searey, Laurel: Nursing care of the laryngectomy patient, R.N. 35-41, Oct., 1972.

Sol, Adler: Speech after laryngectomy, American Journal of Nursing 69:2139-2141, Oct., 1969.

Stanley, Lorraine M.: Meeting the psychologic needs of the laryngectomy patient, Nursing Clinics of North America 3:519-528, Sept., 1968.

Sykes, Eleanor M.: No time for silence, American Journal of Nursing 66:1040-1041, May, 1966.

CHAPTER TWENTY-FIVE # Trachea and bronchi

The trachea begins just below the larynx, where its first ring joins the cricoid cartilage above. The cricoid is a complete ring of cartilage, but the cartilaginous rings of the trachea are deficient posteriorly. A membranous partition called the "party wall," which forms the posterior part of the trachea, is also the anterior wall of the esophagus. After entering the chest the trachea divides into the right and left mainstem bronchi from which, in turn, arise the secondary bronchi. The entire bronchial system is likened to a tree with one large trunk, two major branches, and many smaller branches, at the ends of which are leaves corresponding to the air sacs, or alveoli, of the lungs.

Secretions that form in the bronchi are coughed up through the larynx and expectorated or swallowed. When the patient cannot cough efficiently because of paralysis or weakness, secretions accumulate in the chest, and tracheotomy may be necessary to provide easy access to the tracheobronchial tree for suctioning. The entire tracheobronchial tree is lined with ciliated respiratory epithelium, and the cilia beat in a manner that clears the mucous membrane of foreign material and carries it out the larynx.

Diseases of the trachea and bronchi are produced by infection, trauma, neoplasms, and foreign bodies. Methods of diagnosis consist of bronchoscopy and bronchography. *Bronchography* is done by instilling a radiopaque oil such as iodized oil (Lipiodol) into the trachea and letting it drip into the bronchial passages or by having the patient inhale radiopaque oil as a mist. Roentgenograms of the chest can then outline the bronchi because they are coated with dye. These procedures are performed by radiologists, otolaryngologists, and chest physicians.

Bronchoscopic examination. Premedication consisting of an opiate and atropine combined with a barbiturate is usually given about one hour prior to the procedure. If the procedure is scheduled for early in the morning, the patient should not be given any breakfast; a liquid breakfast may be given if he is to be examined late in the morning or early in the afternoon. Solids should be avoided immediately prior to examination to prevent aspiration of partially digested food if nausea or vomiting occurs.

293

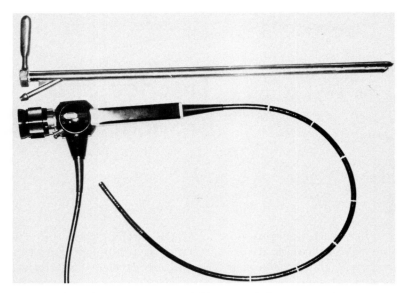

Fig. 25-1. Two bronchoscopes. **Top:** a rigid standard instrument; **bottom:** a flexible fiberoptic bronchoscope.

Adults should be checked for loose crowns and dentures, which should be removed; children should be examined for loose deciduous teeth.

In most cases of endoscopic examination local anesthesia is used, and patients should be informed of this fact. In very young children, those under the age of 2 or 3 years, sometimes no anesthesia is used. General anesthesia increases the element of risk and is unnecessary in most cases. Any of the topical or local anesthetics are potentially dangerous, and the nurse will do well to watch for evidence of reaction to the drugs. Patients may become restless or difficult to communicate with. Convulsive reactions, of course, clearly indicate a toxic reaction. The best treatment for any reaction is the maintenance of an adequate airway and administration of oxygen. Far better than treatment, however, is prevention of the reaction. No more topical anesthetic should be used than is necessary, and great care must be used to identify properly all solutions.

The bronchoscope is a hollow metal tube lighted at its distal end. The light is either a so-called wheat grain bulb, which burns out quickly if the current from the battery box is turned too high, or a fiber optic light. Because bronchoscopy, especially when it is done for the removal of foreign bodies, is dangerous, the nurse must be certain that all parts of the bronchoscope work and that there are spare light bulbs, cords, and light carriers. Light carriers must be matched exactly to the length of the esophagoscope or bronchoscope; there is a number on each light carrier corresponding to a number on the matching bronchoscope. Trouble with the lighting system is common, and although it is merely annoying during routine bronchoscopy, it can contribute to death during attempted extraction of a foreign body.

A newer bronchoscope with great potential is the flexible fiber optic bronchoscope. This instrument is flexible and with a smaller diameter than the rigid metal bronchoscope. It even can be passed through the nose if necessary. Light passes along the fiber optic system even though the instrument curves at some point. Because of its small size and flexible tip, the bronchoscopist using this instrument is able to look further into the smaller bronchi than he ever was able to do with the rigid metal broncho-scope. Tiny forceps at the tip of the bronchoscope can be manipulated to obtain tissue for examination from lesions located in subdivisions of the bronchial tree which were formerly inaccessible. These newer broncho-scopes are vastly more expensive than the older, rigid bronchoscopes and also are subject to breakage. Everyone must use great care in handling them.

The nurse can be of great assistance to the physician during bronchos-copy. In passing forceps or suction she should start the tip of each instru-ment into the bronchoscope. The physician has to hold the bronchoscope in one hand and reach for the forceps with the other, and since the forceps are long, it is difficult for him to place the tip into the relatively small bron-choscope. Additional anesthetic solution that may be needed, usually co-caine 5%, Pontocaine 1%, or Xylocaine 2 or 4%, must be identified clearly. Topical epinephrine, 1:1,000, is used if it is necessary to control bleeding from the mucous membrane. A small piece of cotton or gauze wet with this solution is grasped on the end of a long applicator. The teeth in the applicator grasping the cotton must be securely clamped; if they are not, the cotton might become detached in the bronchus and act as a foreign body. The nurse also must check carefully *before* the operation to make certain that the forceps and suction tube are long enough to pass all the way through the bronchoscope. Bronchoscopes and other endoscopic instru-ments are of different lengths, and it is not uncommon for the physician to be given instruments that are too short for the bronchoscope he is using. Also, the inner diameter of the various instruments is not the same. Forceps intended for large bronchoscopes cannot be passed through small ones. This is particularly true in bronchoscopes designed for infants and children in which the inside diameter may be only 3.5 mm.

Nine times out of ten minor difficulties arising during the performance of an endoscopic procedure could have been prevented by more careful at-tention to preparation of instruments *before the operation began.* There really is no excuse for lack of preparedness during endoscopy, although it is a daily experience in most hospitals.

Postoperative care after endoscopic examination. The best posture for the patient postoperatively is on the side, without a pillow, and with the mouth low. Cough should not be depressed by medication. Atropine in-creases viscosity of secretions and interferes with expulsion of secretions. The cough reflex has been called the "watchdog of the lungs," and no drug should be allowed to lull it to sleep.

After local anesthesia for any part of the upper respiratory tract the patient may aspirate if he drinks too soon afterwards. Usually an hour or two hours should pass before the patient is offered fluids.

CARCINOMA

Carcinoma of the bronchus (bronchogenic carcinoma), a disease affecting middle-aged men much more often than women and one seen with increasing frequency, is almost always associated with smoking. Symptoms are cough, hemoptysis, chest pain, and weight loss. Unfortunately symptoms do not often appear early enough for curative treatment to be possible. The diagnosis, which is often first suspected after a chest roentgenogram, is further demonstrated by bronchography and bronchoscopy. Sometimes a pneumonectomy saves the patient or at least affords palliation. Irradiation therapy usually has little to offer. Local metastases to the mediastinum and distant metastases to bone, liver, and brain come rather early and greatly reduce the prognosis. *The observation that most patients with carcinoma of the bronchus or the larynx are heavy smokers should discourage this habit.* Yearly chest x-ray examinations as part of a regular physical examination do help now and then to pick up an unsuspected case of bronchogenic carcinoma.

OTHER NEOPLASMS

Besides carcinoma there are a few malignant and some benign neoplasms affecting the trachea and bronchi. They are infrequent, however, and the diagnosis is likely to be missed for some time because the symptoms of bleeding or wheezing may be attributed to other causes, and bronchoscopy and bronchography, which might establish the diagnosis, are not done. Asthma, for example, a disease of the bronchi causing wheezing and dyspnea, is sometimes diagnosed when the real cause of the trouble is a laryngeal, tracheal, or bronchial tumor.

FOREIGN BODIES

Foreign bodies in the bronchus or trachea occur chiefly in children. Vegetal foreign bodies such as peanuts are the most common, but small metallic objects are aspirated frequently also. As an example: A child with a peanut in his mouth is running and trips. He inspires deeply, aspirating the peanut through his larynx into the trachea, after which it lodges in one of the bronchi—usually the right, which descends more directly from the trachea than does the left. The child coughs for five or ten minutes and then may stop coughing for several hours or even days. If the foreign body seriously obstructs his airway, there will be dyspnea. A carefully taken history usually will elicit the story of his sudden attack of coughing and choking.

Sometimes a foreign body resides in the bronchus for months or even for years without causing symptoms. Eventually, however, suppuration, cough, or hemoptysis calls attention to the condition, but by then the patient may have forgotten about the original episode of aspiration that caused his trouble. Rarely, pulmonary surgery may be needed to remove a foreign body.

Metallic foreign bodies show on routine roentgenograms, but vegetal foreign bodies and most pieces of glass and plastic do not. Physical examination of the chest may indicate abnormalities in auscultation and percussion because one main bronchus is obstructed while the other is not. Sometimes there is a ball valve action—air can get into the lung but it cannot get out.

Bronchial foreign bodies are extremely serious and should be removed as quickly as possible. The major hazard in removal comes in maintaining a safe airway during extraction.

INFLAMMATION

Inflammatory conditions affecting the trachea and bronchi are often part of an acute generalized respiratory infection caused by viral or bacterial agents. The patient has cough, low-grade fever, and perhaps some chest pain, and he may raise sputum. Usually such infections are self-limited and require only symptomatic treatment.

Infections may also affect the larynx and trachea independently of other parts—laryngotracheitis or laryngotracheobronchitis. In the laryngeal mirror the physician can see the larynx and several tracheal rings, which look red, often with pellets of mucopus lying on the tracheal mucosa. Again, these acute infections ordinarily clear spontaneously, but if the symptoms warrant, antibiotics may be given for several days or a week. Inhalation of steam is comforting, and the patient *must stop smoking*.

CHRONIC BRONCHITIS

Chronic bronchitis is not uncommon. Such patients have a persistent productive cough, and from time to time they may run a low-grade fever. If the terminal bronchioles lose their elastic support because of chronic infection, they dilate and we speak of *bronchiectasis*. In this serious condition there is usually a constant production of purulent secretion from the bronchi that is coughed up through the larynx. It is often associated with chronic sinusitis, and one wonders whether pus from the infected sinuses drained into the bronchi to cause the bronchiectasis or whether there exists a more basic underlying disorder responsible for both conditions. Bronchiectasis, if it is limited to one lobe or even to one lung, may be cured or at least improved by resection of the diseased part. Postural drainage, with the patient hanging over the side of his bed, is also helpful in some cases but can hardly be expected to be curative. Antibiotics are used.

COUGH—A SYMPTOM

Cough, considered as a symptom, deserves a few remarks. There is a condition called *psychogenic cough* in which a patient whose cough starts with laryngitis or bronchitis continues to cough long after the original infection clears. He has a deep, body-racking cough that attracts attention, and he uses this cough, often subconsciously, to continue to attract attention. He develops a sense of proprietorship and speaks rather proudly of "my cough." Thorough examination by roentgenographic methods, bronchoscopy, and laryngoscopy show nothing but the hyperemic effects of coughing on the laryngeal and tracheal mucosa. The patient must be reassured strongly that he has no inflammatory or neoplastic process that should cause cough, and then if cough persists, he should be told about the mechanism responsible for this psychogenic cough. It is a cough that can be suppressed if the patient will try.

As a matter of fact, most coughs that are not productive of sputum can be suppressed by an effort of the will, and therein lies the key to therapy. If the patient will make a strong effort to curb his cough and use it only for the useful purpose of clearing secretions from the chest, he will improve.

Smoking and coughing are directly related. Many patients who cough do so because of the irritant effects of tobacco smoke. In advising a patient about stopping smoking the doctor should tell him to *stop smoking altogether and now* and not tell him to try to "taper off" or to reduce the number of cigarettes to a certain number each day. Many patients will stop smoking if told to do so by an authoritative doctor—they seem to be waiting for someone to order them. There are no effective medications to help the patient stop smoking—he has to want to stop and then he can do it.

Patients with cough from various causes may complain particularly of night cough. A hypnotic such as Seconal, 0.1 Gm., taken at bedtime may keep the patient asleep just enough so that his cough does not disturb and tire him. Of course, neither Seconal nor any other hypnotic should be given over a prolonged period except under exceptional circumstances.

Codeine is the classic medication to suppress the cough reflex. Given as a syrup every two hours, it may help greatly—but, again, it must be used just during the acute stage of an infection or for an equally short time in the patient with annoying night cough or psychogenic cough.

SUGGESTED READINGS

Davidson, F. W.: Chronic sinus and bronchopulmonary disease, Minnesota Medicine **50**:855, 1967.

Richards, L. G.: Vegetal foreign bodies in the bronchi, Annals of Otology **50**:860, 1941.

CHAPTER TWENTY-SIX   # Tracheotomy

Tracheotomy is done for the purposes of (1) improving the airway or (2) providing an easy method of sucking secretions from the trachea and bronchi. Sometimes the operation is done as an emergency, and then it is truly lifesaving. Usually, however, the full operating room team assists, and tracheotomy is an elective, orderly procedure.

Examples of patients with respiratory distress who are helped by tracheotomy are those with advanced carcinomas of the larynx, foreign bodies in the larynx, or severe trauma to the mouth and jaws. There are many other examples.

In another group are patients needing tracheotomy who are unconscious and unable to cough up secretions, for example, patients with head injuries or meningitis. These patients literally drown in their own secretions unless an easy method of aspirating the tracheobronchial tree is available. Suctioning can be done by catheters passed through the mouth or nose, but this technique is difficult and inefficient compared with suctioning through a tracheotomy. Secretions also accumulate in patients who are not unconscious but who are unable to cough effectively because of pain (fractured ribs) or paralysis of muscles of respiration.

EMERGENCY TRACHEOTOMY

Emergency tracheotomy is done only occasionally. The physician uses whatever instruments are at hand. This procedure may have to be performed in the hospital emergency room, in the physician's office, or even in the home or on the street. No effort is made to clean the skin or to administer anesthesia of any kind. A stab incision is made just under the cricoid cartilage (Fig. 26-1), where the airway is immediately subcutaneous and where there are no large vessels. The wound, which usually bleeds only a little, is spread apart with whatever instrument is available—the knife handle or scissors—or by manual retraction. Even a large-bore needle (16- or 18-gauge) has been used. The important thing in emergency tracheotomy is to establish an airway instantly to save the patient's life.

As soon after emergency tracheotomy as practical the patient should be taken to the operating room and a routine or orderly tracheotomy done. If a tracheotomy tube is left for days or weeks in the cricothyroid space (the site for emergency tracheotomy), laryngeal stenosis may result.

299

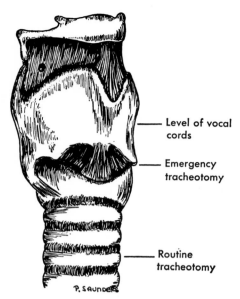

Level of vocal cords

Emergency tracheotomy

Routine tracheotomy

P. SAUNDERS

Fig. 26-1. Levels for tracheotomy. (From DeWeese, David D., and Saunders, William H.: Textbook of otolaryngology, ed. 4, St. Louis, 1973, The C. V. Mosby Co.)

ELECTIVE OR ORDERLY TRACHEOTOMY

In the elective or orderly tracheotomy there is no need for haste. Although the patient needs a better airway or has a chest full of secretions, his immediate condition is good. Sometimes the operation is done with an endotracheal tube in place to avoid disaster should the airway become suddenly worse during operation. The operation is usually done under local anesthesia, but occasionally a general anesthesia is given; in unconscious patients no anesthesia is required (Figs. 26-2 to 26-5).

The neck is cleansed and sterile drapes are applied. A vertical incision is made in the midline from approximately the cricoid cartilage to the suprasternal notch. As soft-tissue and muscle layers are divided, the isthmus of the thyroid gland is exposed. It must be retracted upward or divided between hemostats before the trachea lies exposed. The surgeon cuts through two tracheal rings (usually the third and fourth) and inserts a previously selected tracheotomy tube, the size of which depends upon the age of the patient. In the premature or newborn infant a No. 00 may be the largest that can be inserted. Sizes increase from No. 00 to No. 0 and then from No. 1 to No. 8. A No. 6 tube is the one most used in adults. It provides an adequate airway, yet does not entirely fill the trachea.

A stylet or obturator is used to introduce the tube into the trachea. The stylet fills the end of the outer tube and provides a tapered point so that the advancing end does not tear tissue. Once the tube is in place the stylet is withdrawn immediately, because while it is in place there

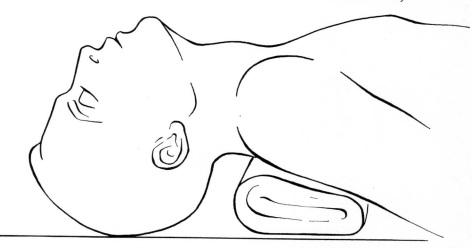

Fig. 26-2. Position for tracheotomy with a roll under the shoulders to extend the neck.

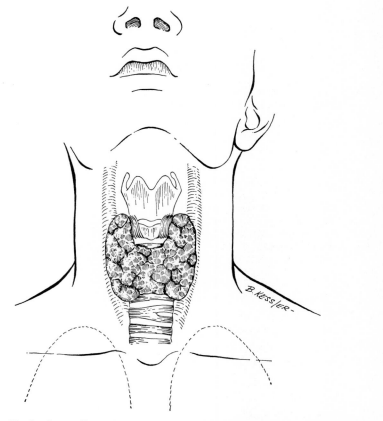

Fig. 26-3. Thyroid gland usually covers the trachea where the incision is to be made.

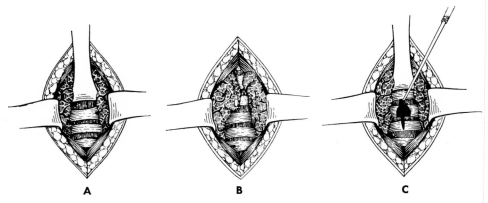

A   **B**   **C**

Fig. 26-4. **A,** Retractor exposing the trachea by drawing the isthmus of the thyroid upward. **B,** Alternate method to that shown in **A** shows the isthmus of the thyroid divided to expose the trachea. **C,** Two tracheal rings are cut and the upper ring is partially resected. The tracheal hook pulls the trachea from the depth of the wound nearer the surface. (From DeWeese, David D., and Saunders, William H.: Textbook of otolaryngology, ed. 4, St. Louis, 1973, The C. V. Mosby Co.)

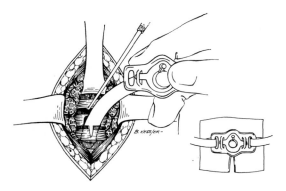

Fig. 26-5. Insertion of the tracheotomy tube with the stylet or obturator in place. The obturator is removed and the inner cannula inserted. Inset shows the tube in place and the ties about the neck. (From DeWeese, David D., and Saunders, William H.: Textbook of otolaryngology, ed. 4, St. Louis, 1973, The C. V. Mosby Co.)

is no airway. The inner cannula is then inserted and locked in place. Gauze tapes previously attached to the outer tube are tied around the neck. These tapes must be adjusted with just the right tension; if they are too tight, the patient finds them uncomfortable, and if too loose, the tracheotomy tube slips out. When tied so that one finger can easily slip under the tape, the tension is about right. If two or three fingers slide under the tape the tracheotomy tube is in danger of coming out if the patient coughs hard (Fig. 26-6). The doctor or nurse puts new ties on the tube every day or two as the old ones become dirty.

The nurse must be completely familiar with tracheotomy tubes, since

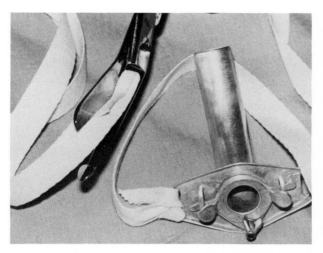

Fig. 26-6. Cutting tracheotomy tapes. Here the inner cannula is in place and the tube is a large one for use after laryngectomy.

she is the one who prepares the tube for the surgeon and also cleans the tube postoperatively. There are three parts to every tracheotomy tube: an outer tube, an inner tube, and a stylet or obturator. After its initial use to introduce the outer tube, the obturator usually is taped to the patient's bed, where it is available for future use should the occasion arise. Should the patient go to surgery, the obturator is sent with his chart. All three parts of the tracheotomy tube fit closely and ordinarily are not interchangeable with parts from other tracheotomy tubes. Until recently tracheotomy tubes were made of silver, and many still are, but an increasing number of plastic tubes are in use today. If the patient is to receive irradiation therapy to the neck, either a plastic tube must be used or the metal tube removed before each treatment.

After operation the outer tube stays in the trachea until the surgeon believes it is safe to remove it for cleansing and inspection of the wound. This might be at forty-eight hours or whenever the tracheotomy channel is established and not likely to collapse if the tube is withdrawn. Ordinarily the nurse does not remove the outer tube unless specifically instructed by the physician because there is sometimes difficulty in replacing it. One mistake is to insert the tube into the soft tissue of the neck rather than into the lumen of the trachea.

The *inner tube* is the province of the nurse. This tube fits the inside of the outer tube snugly, yet loosely enough that it can be removed by light finger traction. The inner tube is removed by the nurse as often as necessary for cleansing. In the immediate postoperative period the inner tube should be removed, inspected, and cleaned every two hours. If this is not done, small amounts or dried blood may cause difficulty in removing the inner cannula. It is by cleansing the inner tube that the airway is maintained. Cleaning is needed more often in a patient whose chest is filled with secretions than in a patient with laryngeal obstruction but no excessive secretions. The best way to clean the inner tube is with hydrogen peroxide and sterile water and a bristle brush. A pipe cleaner is good for small tubes. When clean and dry, there should be no lint left in the tube; by holding the tube to the light and inspecting it from both ends, one can make sure of this point.

Suctioning the tracheotomy tube. In the patient whose chest is filled with secretions, *suctioning must be done frequently*—as often as every five minutes. In other patients suctioning every two or three hours or even once or twice a day may be all that is necessary. In suctioning the aim is to aspirate all secretions that have accumulated in the tracheobronchial tree since the last suctioning and which the patient is unable to cough up himself. This implies a deep passage of the rubber or plastic catheter. The suction should be strong, otherwise thick secretions cannot be pulled from the chest. Sterile physiologic saline solution (without preservative) instilled into the trachea by the tracheotomy tube may help loosen thick secretions. The physician should leave careful orders of the amount to be instilled, usually 1 to 5 cc.

After each suctioning it is important to run sterile normal saline through the aspirator to clean the system. The suction catheter should be discarded after each period of use. Disposable sterile gloves are used. The solutions in bottles used to rinse the catheter and to store the catheter represent sources of infection to the patient. Sterile disposable cups filled with solution to rinse the catheter is an efficient and safe system. *All equipment should be sterile.*

When the catheter is passed down the trachea, the cutoff hole on the

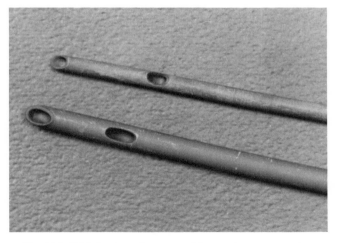

Fig. 26-7. Whistle tip catheters used for tracheotomy suction.

handle of the suction should be *open*. In that way the catheter slides down the trachea easily and does not grab at the walls as it does if the catheter is aspirating on the way down. When the lower limit is reached, the cutoff hole is occluded and secretions rush up the catheter as it is rotated and withdrawn slowly. Patients at first do not like tracheal suctioning because it makes them cough and strain, but with perseverance they become accustomed to the procedure and welcome it, since it helps them breathe much more easily.

Ordinarily a tracheotomy tube does not irritate the trachea. When there is crusting or bleeding from the trachea, it is more likely the effect of dry air on the tracheal lumen than irritation from the tracheotomy tube. In the normal patient the nose warms and moistens air to prepare it for the lower respiratory passages, but in a patient with tracheotomy air enters the trachea without benefit of this previous conditioning. Usually, however, the situation quickly corrects itself and most patients have little trouble. Moisture can be added to the air either by a humidifier (often not efficient) or by having the patient breathe humidified air directly from a cupula fitting over the tracheotomy tube.

For a day or two after tracheotomy, blood may accumulate and crust under the flanges of the tracheotomy tube externally and under the ties used to hold the tube in the neck; later there may be secretions from the trachea that collect here. The nurse should change a gauze dressing placed under the tube as often as necessary to keep the neck clean and comfortable. Sterile gauze squares without cellulose filling cut half way toward the center can be pulled under the tube with a small hemostat or bayonet forceps. Such gauze, however, has the disadvantage that the cut margins are frayed, and bits of gauze enter the wound and may even get into the trachea. Where available, special tracheotomy "pants" with sewn edges are better.

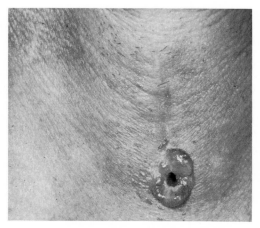

Fig. 26-8. Tracheotomy tube has been removed, but granulation tissue surrounds the stoma. This granulation tissue should be removed, the base cauterized, and the wound pulled together with tape.

Rarely, a patient may develop obstructive plugs of dried mucus in the trachea that actually endanger his airway unless the tracheotomy tube is removed and the plug pulled out with forceps or hemostat. This is usually done by the physician, although the nurse may have to do it in an emergency. Moisture helps prevent these plugs.

When it comes time to close a tracheotomy, all that is necessary is to remove the tube and pull the skin together with several strips of ½-inch tape. The raw edges adhere, and after a few days air no longer escapes (Fig. 26-8). The tape is changed once or twice daily after the skin is cleaned and dried. Rarely, and only in a tracheotomy of long standing, is it necessary to excise the tract and suture the wound.

The airway also can be improved by passing an anesthetist's intratracheal tube through the larynx, but this method is not well suited to long-term care because a tube in the larynx for more than twenty-four hours may cause *permanent laryngeal damage*. Therefore, even though it is sometimes easier to pass an intratracheal tube than to do a tracheotomy, an intratracheal tube should be considered an expedient and removed as soon as possible in favor of a tracheotomy.

Complications. In the *adult* complications of a tracheotomy usually are not serious. There may be *subcutaneous emphysema* if the wound is sutured too tightly about the tracheotomy tube and air can enter the subcutaneous tissues, and sometimes even if the wound is not sutured tightly. This annoyance clears after several days, however, and usually causes no great difficulty. If the nurse notices a crackling sensation under the skin of the neck, chest, or face she should report it to the physician, since he may wish to remove a suture or two.

If the tube is coughed out, it is usually because the ties were not sufficiently tight or because the tube was too short. This can amount to an emergency if it occurs in the first few hours after tracheotomy, because a sufficient tract has not yet been formed between skin and trachea to sustain breathing. The tube must be reinserted at once. The obturator taped to the bed is again used to help guide the tube into the trachea.

Sometimes there is *bleeding* from a thyroid vein or other neck vessel next to the tube, and blood, which runs down into the trachea, is sprayed about with every cough. It can be serious although usually it is not. Local packing with petrolatum gauze is often enough. Sometimes the patient must be taken back to the operating room, where the wound is reopened and the bleeding vessel ligated.

In the *child* any of the foregoing complications can occur and others, too. In almost every instance the complication is more serious, since the relative size of the airway in the child is smaller and there is simply not as much leeway. Infants, of course, have even less tolerance. *Too long a tracheotomy tube* in the infant or young child can easily traverse the entire length of the trachea and the end of the tube come to rest not in the trachea but in one main bronchus—usually the right, since it is more of a direct continuation of the trachea than is the left main bronchus. Then one lung is completely blocked off, and while this is not necessarily an emergency, it does throw an extra burden on the already embarrassed respiratory tract. An x-ray examination of the chest and neck of the patient is a good plan after tracheotomy in the child. Such a film will show the position of the tube and sometimes also will demonstrate *mediastinal emphysema* and *pneumothorax,* both of which are such common complications of tracheotomy in children that they never should be forgotten. Of course these are also changes in breath sounds in each of these conditions, and the nurse will note absence of breath sounds over one side of the chest as compared with the other.

After tracheotomy in infants and children constant nursing attention is advisable since obstruction of the small tubes can cause death quickly, and the patient can do nothing about it. All in all, a nurse skilled in care of patients with tracheotomy may well make the most valuable contribution offered to that patient, since the postoperative care may be more difficult than the operation.

Rather paradoxically, the tracheotomy done to restore an airway may in some cases contribute to physiologic disturbances not present before the operation. Removal of secretions, reduction in the ventilatory dead space, and circumvention of laryngeal and supraglottic obstruction all combine to wash out accumulated carbon dioxide. Sometimes there is profound and abrupt reversal of respiratory acidosis, with resulting arterial hypotension and arrhythmias. The use of a cuffed tracheotomy tube will permit positive-pressure ventilation with oxygen and correct the situation.

The cuffed tube (Fig. 26-9, *A* to *D*). Inflating a cuff about a tracheotomy tube has become a popular method of controlling secretions that trickle down the trachea, and of affording an easy method of positive-pressure breathing. Unfortunately, there are numerous complications that can result from the use of an inflated cuff—such as erosion of the tracheal mucosa (sometimes to the point of producing a tracheoesophageal fistula), stenosis, and infection. Mechanical complications include slippage of the cuff over the end of the tube and a narrowing of the tube during inflation. The cuff, which should be deflated at regular intervals, should be used only when definitely needed. A low-pressure cuff may be used to reduce the risk of some complications.

When the physician inserts a cuffed tube there should be written orders specifically delineating management of the inflation-deflation sequence. To inflate the cuff no more air is injected than is necessary to seal the trachea, and because the diameter of the trachea varies from patient to patient, no exact amount of filling can be specified. The nurse can tell when the cuff is inflated because then she will not hear air escaping from the patient's mouth or from the tracheotomy opening, and the patient loses his voice. There is usually a small pilot balloon which remains inflated as long as the cuff is inflated.

In general, the use of cuffed tubes, valuable as they are, add certain hazards to the patient's management. The nurse will find that in this situation there is no substitute for experience.

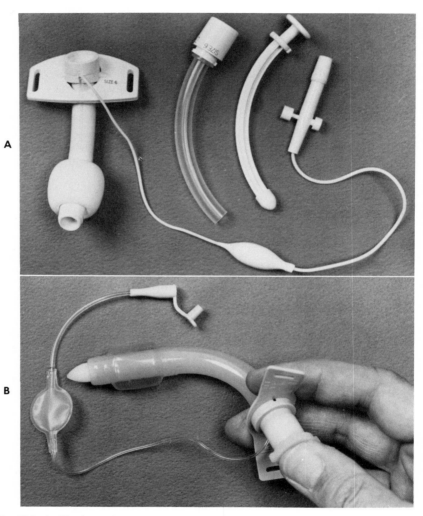

Fig. 26-9. A, Plastic tracheotomy tube with inflatable soft cuff. Note the pilot bag as part of inflating tube attached to outer cannula. The inner cannula and obturator complete the set. This tracheostomy tube has a flexible (moveable) neck plate. **B,** Plastic tracheotomy tube ready for insertion, with stylet or obturator in place. **C,** Metal tracheostomy tube with adaptor for connection to anesthetist's tube or assisted respiration apparatus. The adaptor is attached to inner cannula of a Morsch tracheotomy tube. Small tubing is connected to cuff. **D,** Anesthetist's rubber intratracheal tube with inflated cuff. Note the pilot bag is inflated.

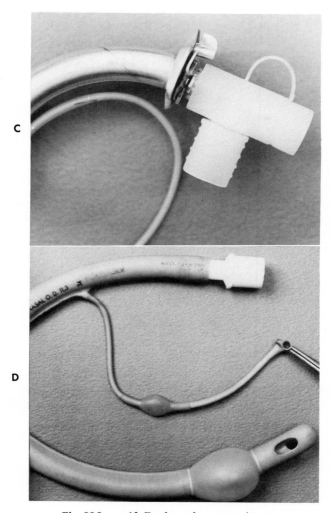

Fig. 26-9, cont'd. For legend see opposite page.

SUGGESTED READINGS

Conner, George H., and others: Tracheostomy, American Journal of Nursing **72:** 68-74, Jan., 1972.

Crocker, Dean: The critically ill child; management of tracheostomy, Pediatrics **46:** 286-296, Aug., 1970.

Jacquette, Germain: To reduce hazards of tracheal suctioning, American Journal of Nursing **71:**2362-2364, Dec., 1971.

Larson, Elaine: Bacterial colonization of tracheal tubes of patients in a surgical intensive care unit, Nursing Research **19:**122-128, March-April, 1970.

Respiratory tract aspiration; programmed instruction, American Journal of Nursing **66:**2483-2510, Nov., 1966.

Sovie, Margaret D., and Isarel, Jacob B.: Use of the cuffed tracheostomy tube, American Journal of Nursing **67:**1854-1856, Sept., 1967.

Totman, Laurence E., and Lehman, Roger H.: Tracheostomy care, American Journal of Nursing **64:**96-99, March, 1964.

Tyler, Martha L.: Artificial airways, Nursing '73, pp. 22-36, Feb., 1973.

White, Helen A.: Tracheostomy care with a cuffed tube, American Journal of Nursing **72:**75-77, Jan., 1972.

CHAPTER TWENTY-SEVEN

Diseases of the esophagus

Esophageal disease may be congenital or acquired, traumatic, neoplastic, or inflammatory. The chief methods of diagnosis are by roentgenographic examination after the swallowing of barium and by direct inspection through the esophagoscope. Usually, roentgenographic examination is made first.

CONGENITAL ABNORMALITIES

Rarely, infants are born with an incomplete esophagus, which ends in a blind pouch not connected with the stomach; there are several other abnormal arrangements associated with congenital esophageal atresia. An infant with such an abnormality may try to eat, but because food cannot reach his stomach, he regurgitates and the overflow spills into the trachea, causing choking and dyspnea. These symptoms should make one suspect the diagnosis. There is additional proof when a small rubber catheter passed into the esophagus fails to enter the stomach. In this instance Lipiodol instilled through the catheter demonstrates that there is a blind pouch or a connection between the esophagus and the trachea (tracheoesophageal fistula). Lipiodol is preferred to barium because, if aspirated, it is easily coughed out of the lungs, whereas barium is hard to cough up and may even result in asphyxia. Postural drainage and coughing also help to clear the tracheobronchial tree of Lipiodol. The nurse can be of great assistance in properly positioning the patient and in offering quiet reassurance.

After esophageal atresia or tracheoesophageal fistula is demonstrated, early surgical correction must be performed if the patient is to live. Such operations are reasonably successful. Postoperatively dilatation of the esophagus may be necessary to prevent stricture.

Another congenital anomaly that may affect the esophagus is the so-called "vascular ring." Large, abnormally placed arteries in the chest that compress the esophagus (and sometimes the trachea and bronchi) cause choking, cyanosis, and dysphagia. Roentgenograms made after the use of Lipiodol show compression of the trachea or esophagus in the region of the aortic arch. Again, surgical treatment may relieve the constriction.

Nursing care in patients with congenital anomalies of the trachea and esophagus is of utmost importance. At best these infants have only a fragile hold on life and often the slightest deviation from the prescribed orders and method of feeding worsens their condition. Hydration may have to be maintained by parenteral means, and careful measurements of intake are essential. Tube feedings, when possible, must be done with extreme care, since regurgitation is common. Accurate observation of weight gain or loss is important.

FOREIGN BODIES

Foreign bodies in the esophagus are fairly common, and almost anything that can be taken into the mouth and swallowed can become lodged in the esophagus (Fig. 27-1). The patient complains that he cannot swallow, he regurgitates, and there is pain in the lower neck or chest. Common esophageal foreign bodies in children include safety pins, coins, and small toys. A child with a foreign body in his mouth or nose should be asked quietly to remove the object and to hand it over. If the child is startled, he may inspire sharply and aspirate the foreign body into the trachea or bronchi. At other times the foreign body is swallowed and may lodge in the esophagus. Similar objects are ingested by psychotic persons attempting suicide. In adults an esophageal foreign body is more likely to be a chicken or pork chop bone or part of a denture. Persons with upper dentures are particularly susceptible to esophageal foreign bodies. The reason is that they cannot feel bones in their mouths as can a person who does not have his palate covered by a denture. With reduced or absent palatal sensation they are likely to swallow meat containing bone. Also persons with dentures may chew their food ineffectively. Most foreign bodies in the esophagus lodge at the level of the cricopharyngeal muscle, and the patient indicates this level by pointing to a spot just above his clavicle. Usually the foreign body is at too low a level to be seen with the laryngeal mirror.

Fish bones, a very common foreign body, ordinarily do not lodge in the esophagus but catch in the palatine tonsil, the lingual tonsil, or some other part of the hypopharynx. Most fish bones as foreign bodies are small and almost translucent so that finding the bone may be difficult. They do not show on a roentgenogram. Often the bone has become dislodged and swallowed by the time the physician sees the patient, yet the patient insists it is still present because of the irritation produced. A careful search of all areas of the pharynx and hypopharynx is necessary, and if no bone is found, the patient is sent home and asked to return the next day if not better.

Roentgenograms demonstrate most metallic foreign bodies and bones. Other foreign bodies that may not appear on ordinary examination can often be demonstrated if the patient is asked to swallow a few strands of cotton coated with thick barium paste. The cotton catches on the foreign body, and because it is coated with radiopaque barium, it is visible. Routine roentgenograms with barium are not used to demonstrate foreign bodies because barium coats the wall of the esophagus as well as the foreign body, and subsequent extraction is rendered more difficult.

Once the foreign body is localized, esophagoscopy is performed with the patient under local or general anesthesia (Fig. 27-2). The foreign body is grasped with suitable forceps and extracted through the esophagoscope. If the foreign body is too large to pass through the esophagoscope, it is held firmly by forceps at the lower end of the esophagoscope, and the esophagoscope and foreign body are withdrawn together. *Removal of esophageal foreign bodies is hazardous* because of the danger of esophageal perforation.

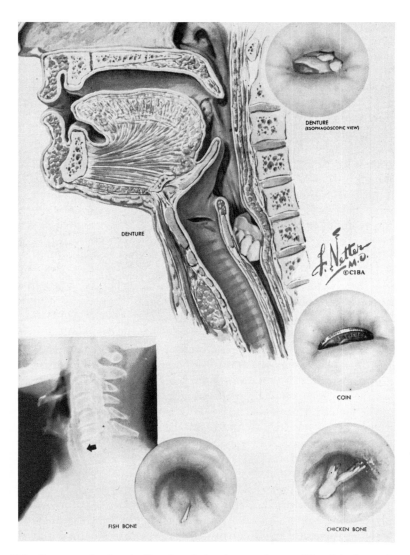

Fig. 27-1. Common foreign bodies found in the esophagus. The fish bone, however, usually catches in the tonsil or base of the tongue and not in the esophagus. (Copyright The CIBA Collection of Medical Illustrations by Frank H. Netter, M.D.)

Foreign bodies in the bronchus are also dangerous because of risk to the airway. The walls of the bronchi and trachea are thick and perforation is not nearly as likely as in the esophagus.

A word about trying to force a foreign body into the stomach by pushing from above with a dilator or other instrument: Don't—it is very dangerous.

In preparing a patient for esophagoscopy, instructions on relaxation are essential. Premedication is ordered an hour prior to examination, or some-

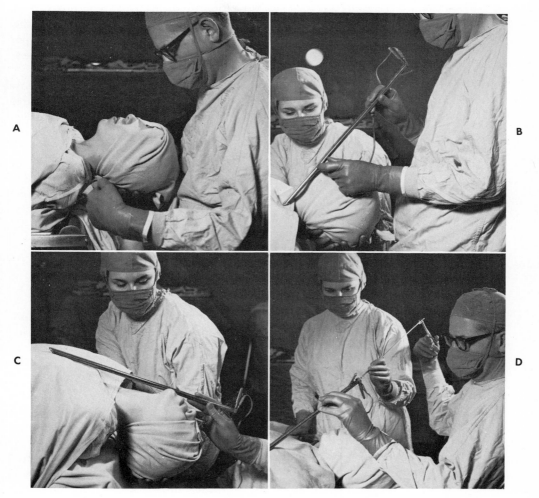

Fig. 27-2. A, Preparation of the patient for esophagoscopy. Note the relationship of the shoulders to the table break. **B,** Initial position. Head is held high, and shoulders must be level with or just beyond the point at which the table breaks. **C,** Final position that will be assumed in esophagoscopy. Head holder raises or lowers the head slowly on direction of the endoscopist. **D,** Demonstrating how the nurse should guide forceps and sucker tips into the endoscopic instruments.

times, especially in patients undergoing a second, third, or fourth examination, no premedication is needed. Esophagoscopy is uncomfortable and causes gagging but is not painful. Analgesics are not required after examination.

Instruments passed by the nurse to the physician for insertion into the esophagoscope should be started by her into the esophagoscope. Otherwise the physician, holding long forceps or an aspirator tip by its handle, will have trouble introducing the tip into the small opening of the esophagoscope. When a biopsy is made, there may be bleeding, which is controlled by the use of cotton or gauze wet with topical epinephrine. The nurse must make sure that the cotton carrier grasps the cotton firmly and that the piece of cotton selected is not too large to pass through the esophagoscope. The same relates to applicators that may be used to apply topical anesthetics (Fig. 27-2, *C*).

The position of the patient on the table is important. For esophagoscopy the head and neck are extended over one end of the table and the head held by an assistant. Therefore the patient is positioned so that when the head piece of the table is dropped, his shoulders come to lie even with or just a little over the edge of the main section of the table.

After esophagoscopy the nurse should report immediately any pain in the back, chest, or shoulder, because such pain may indicate perforation of the esophagus. There should be no fever or chills after esophagoscopy; if there are, perforation is suspected. Patients are not given antibiotics after esophagoscopy. They usually are permitted to eat after six hours.

STRICTURES

Stricture of the esophagus results from ingestion of a caustic or from inflammation in the distal part of the esophagus after repeated regurgitation of acid contents of the stomach. Also, stricture may follow inflammation produced by a foreign body. Most strictures are preventable. Once a stricture has formed, there is tough scar tissue in the esophageal wall, and dilatation is difficult. At times resection of the stricture is necessary to establish a functional lumen.

Probably the most common cause of esophageal stricture is ingestion of lye. This caustic is taken by young children accidentally and by adults bent on suicide. There are usually burns of the lips, tongue, and pharynx, but sometimes the oral cavity is not burned at all and yet the esophagus is burned severely. Because one cannot be certain whether or not the esophagus is burned, it is always best to admit to the hospital a patient who has a history of swallowing lye and then perform esophagoscopy. This policy is best because if the esophagus is burned, stricture almost always forms. Although early treatment of the burn usually prevents stricture, once a stricture forms, treatment is difficult. In those patients in whom esophagoscopy discloses no burn, further treatment is unnecessary.

In the patient with esophageal burn, therapy consists of daily dilatation

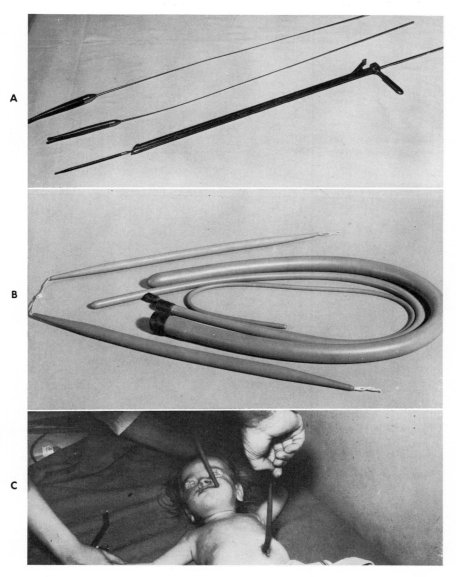

Fig. 27-3. A, Esophagoscope and Jackson dilators used for strictures. **B,** Outer dilators are retrograde dilators; inner three are mercury-filled Hurst dilators. **C,** Retrograde dilatation. These dilators are the same as the retrograde dilators shown in **B.** The dilator is pulled through the gastrostomy, up the esophagus, and out the mouth. Retrograde dilatations may have to be carried out once or twice weekly for a year or more. (Courtesy Dr. Charles S. Giffin, Fort Wayne, Ind.)

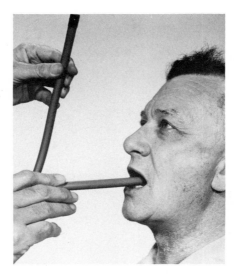

Fig. 27-4. Mercury-filled rubber esophageal dilator of middle size. Almost entire length of tube is passed to reach stomach. (Compare Fig. 27-3, *B*.)

of the esophagus with mercury-filled rubber dilators and the administration of antibiotics and cortisone (Figs. 27-3 and 27-4). Cortisone allows mucous membranes to heal but delays the fibroblastic proliferation leading to stricture. Under this therapy the esophageal mucosa heals in a few weeks. When a second esophagoscopy shows the mucous membrane has regenerated, dilatations and cortisone therapy can be discontinued.

If a lye burn is neglected and stricture forms, it can usually be dilated from above. Sometimes, however, in a severe stricture ordinary methods fail and retrograde dilatations are done. Fusiform dilators linked together like sausages are pulled through a gastrostomy opening into the stomach, up the esophagus, and out the mouth. This treatment is disagreeable but may have to be continued for months or even years. If dilatations fail altogether, the thoracic surgeon may resect the stricture and form a new esophagus using bowel or a part of the stomach rolled into a tube. It is always best to maintain the original esophagus if possible.

Strictures may cause trouble for life because, although liquids and soft foods pass readily, a piece of meat may catch in the stricture and have to be removed through the esophagoscope.

CARDIOSPASM, OR ACHALASIA

Cardiospasm, or achalasia, is a condition probably caused by degeneration in nerve plexuses in the walls of the esophagus, resulting in atrophy of the esophageal mucosa and muscular fibers. In cardiospasm the esophagus dilates greatly, and a roentgenogram of a barium-filled esophagus looks as if the esophagus fills a third of the chest. Food and liquids collect in the greatly dilated esophagus, and before esophagoscopy it is not unusual to aspirate a quart of liquid from such an esophagus. When the patient lies down at night, esophageal contents may regurgitate and be aspirated; these patients, therefore, are likely to develop bronchitis and pneumonia.

The diagnosis of cardiospasm is established by roentgenograms and esophagoscopy. The roentgenogram is characteristic because it shows an enormously dilated esophagus tapering to a point near the stomach. No other condition provides a picture quite like this.

It is well to aspirate the esophagus the night before esophagoscopy. A large tube passed through the nose into the esophagus is connected to the suction apparatus, then aspiration is carried on during the night. If this is not done, the endoscopist must spend a long time aspirating food and liquid. Food that comes from the esophagus in patients with achalasia smells sour, and the entire procedure is unpleasant. After the esophagus is empty, its lower end is inspected to make certain that there is no ulceration or tumor. Then dilatation is carried out, first through the esophagoscope and later with mercury-filled tubes. In a rare case when dilatations fail, the Heller operation is performed: fibrotic tissue and muscle layers around the lower end of the esophagus are split and repaired in a manner that leaves a larger opening into the stomach. Unfortunately this procedure is not always successful.

The nurse can be of great help during esophagoscopy by making certain all instruments are in proper order. The lights on the esophagoscope must work, and there should be substitute lights, light carriers, and light cords.

Medical treatment helps some patients with cardiospasm. Usually belladonna derivatives and sedatives such as phenobarbital are given. The nurse must remember that patients with achalasia, or for that matter patients with esophageal obstruction from any cause, should not take pills. They will lodge above a stricture or, in the case of cardiospasm, they will float around in the dilated esophagus but will never enter the stomach. Therefore, if the physician forgets and orders medication by mouth, the nurse may suggest that it be given parenterally.

NEOPLASMS

Most esophageal neoplasms originate in the esophageal mucosa and are malignant. Occasionally a tumor in the chest or mediastinum compresses the esophagus from without to produce dysphagia, and some of these tumors are benign. The malignant tumors most commonly seen are adenocarcinoma (at the lower end) and squamous cell carcinoma (in the middle and upper thirds).

Symptoms do not arise early, and often the patient's first knowledge of trouble is dysphagia or even complete esophageal obstruction. Naturally, loss of weight follows, with weakness and dehydration. If there is hemorrhage, there may be hematemesis or tarry stools.

Carcinoma of the lower and upper parts of the esophagus is cured now and then after surgical excision, but even in favorable cases the prognosis admittedly is poor (Fig. 27-5). In carcinoma of the middle third any type

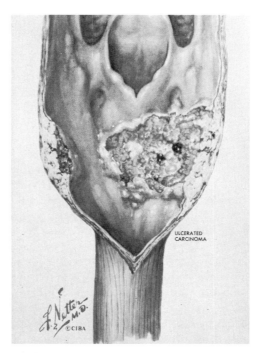

ULCERATED
CARCINOMA

Fig. 27-5. Carcinoma of the upper part of the esophagus. Prognosis is poor with either irradiation therapy or surgical excision. (Copyright The CIBA Collection of Medical Illustrations by Frank H. Netter, M.D.)

of treatment is hopeless; resection or irradiation therapy may give some palliation. For feeding, a gastrostomy often is done, but by the time the patient needs gastrostomy, life usually can be preserved only a few weeks.

There is a special type of upper esophageal tumor called postcricoid carcinoma, occurring chiefly in women. All other malignancies of larynx and esophagus are more common in men. Like globus hystericus, it causes a sensation of a lump in the throat, and for this reason patients suspected of globus hystericus must be investigated carefully. The diagnosis of postcricoid carcinoma is made by mirror laryngoscopy, esophagoscopy, and roentgenography. In all instances a biopsy of the tumor is made before surgical resection or irradiation therapy is carried out.

GLOBUS HYSTERICUS

Globus hystericus is an old name given to a condition in which patients complain of a lump in the throat, which they can neither swallow nor cough up. In demonstrating they point to a level just above the sternum. The cause probably is related to hypertonicity of the inferior constrictor muscle that encircles the lower part of the pharynx. Many of these patients are tense, nervous women who worry about cancer. Characteristically the complaint is worse in the evening than in the morning. Patients say they have no difficulty eating and that they have lost no weight—symptoms one would expect were there an organic obstruction such as carcinoma. The "lump in the throat" does not bother them at mealtime.

There is no abnormality to be found in the physical examination. The vocal cords and all parts of the larynx look normal, and one cannot palpate any lump in the neck. A barium esophagram is expected to be normal. These patients usually improve after a careful physical examination, a barium esophagram, and strong reassurance. The doctor must state with conviction that the patient has no organic disease and particularly that there is no cancer. Globus hystericus is likely to recur anytime the patient is under unaccustomed stress.

DIVERTICULA

Zenker's or pulsion diverticulum occurs in the lower part of the pharynx, where there is a weak spot in the muscular coverings. Gradually over a period of years, the mucous membrane pockets outward and forms a pouch or diverticulum. Some diverticula hold a large quantity of food and actually compress the normal esophageal channel. Instead of entering the esophagus food enters the diverticulum, since its opening is larger than the esophageal lumen. When the patient lies down, liquid regurgitating from the diverticulum runs into the hypopharynx and may be aspirated to produce bronchitis or pneumonia. In an extreme case a patient may even lose weight, because no matter how much he eats, food first fills the diverticulum, which then compresses the esophagus. It may even be necessary for a patient to leave the table and go to the bathroom, where he compresses his neck and squeezes food out of the diverticulum.

Esophageal diverticulectomy, with local or general anesthesia, usually corrects the trouble.

Leaking of the suture line is the chief postoperative complication, and this results in fever and in pain and swelling in the neck. The nurse, therefore, should be watchful for postoperative fever higher than would be expected after this procedure. Patients are usually fed on the first postoperative day, but some surgeons employ a nasogastric feeding tube for several days.

TRACTION DIVERTICULUM

A traction diverticulum occurs in the mid or lower esophagus as the result of scarring associated with tuberculous lymph nodes. Adhesions pull the esophageal wall outward until a small, asymptomatic diverticulum forms. No treatment is required.

VARICES

Esophageal varices may cause hematemesis. They are the result of venous obstruction in the liver or portal system. Communicating veins in the esophagus form varices, which sometimes break and produce severe bleeding. At esophagoscopy these varices are noted bulging into the lumen of the esophagus. Roentgenograms made with barium also show these dilated veins, but failure to demonstrate varices by roentgenographic methods does not mean that they are absent. If possible, the causative factors should be corrected rather than an attempt made to treat the varices locally.

ESOPHAGITIS

Esophagitis is not uncommon. It may result from regurgitation of gastric secretions into the lower part of the esophagus, especially during vomiting of pregnancy. There is a burning sensation. Eventually ulceration develops, but rarely does perforation of the esophagus occur. Treatment is with ant-acids. Sometimes it helps to have the patient sleep partially upright to prevent regurgitation of stomach contents through the lower esophageal sphincter.

SUGGESTED READINGS

Anderson, H. A.: Dysfunction of the esoph-agus, Otolaryngology Clinics of North America, p. 195, 1968.

Cardona, J. C., and Daly, J. F.: Management of corrosive esophagitis; analysis of treat-ment, methods, and results, New York Journal of Medicine **64:**2307, 1964.

DeWeese, David D.: Esophageal dilatation; indications and procedures, Portland Clinic Bulletin **6:**35, 1965.

Goulding, Erna I., and Koop, C. Everett: The newborn; his response to surgery, American Journal of Nursing **65:**84-87, Oct., 1965.

Lewis, Corinne: Nursing care of the neonate requiring surgery for congenital defects, Nursing Clinics of North America **5:** 387, Sept., 1970.

CHAPTER TWENTY-EIGHT # Ear—anatomy and physiology

"A patter of melody faintly traced itself upon the silence. . . . Pongileoni's blowing and the scraping of the anonymous fiddlers had shaken the air in the great hall, had set the glass of the windows looking on to it vibrating; and this in turn had shaken the air in Lord Edward's apartment on the further side. The shaking air rattled Lord Edward's membrana tympani; the interlocked malleus, incus, and the stirrup bones were set in motion so as to agitate the membrane of the oval window and raise an infinitesimal storm in the fluid of the labyrinth. The hairy endings of the auditory nerve shuddered like weeds in a rough sea; a vast number of obscure miracles were performed in the brain, and Lord Edward ecstatically whispered 'Bach'!"

—*Aldous Huxley**

EXTERNAL EAR

The external ear consists of the ear canal and the auricle. The auricle is made of cartilage and skin, except for the lobule, which contains fat but no cartilage (Fig. 28-1). The auricle is particularly subject to frostbite, since it is exposed more than most parts and has very little subcutaneous fat for protection. On the other hand, because of a good blood supply, even if severely lacerated or torn almost from the head, the auricle usually will grow if reattached.

The *auricular muscles* that are important in some lower animals to cock the auricle are also present in man, but in him they are rudimentary and of no use. An occasional person has enough control of these muscles to wiggle his ears.

The *lymphatic* supply of the ear is generous, and in external otitis lymphadenopathy may develop in the periauricular regions behind, under, and in front of the ear. Sometimes postauricular lymphadenopathy is great enough to be mistaken for the subperiosteal abscess of acute mastoiditis.

The *nerve* supply to the external ear is chiefly from the trigeminal (fifth cranial) nerve and from the cervical nerves. The vagus (tenth cranial) nerve gives a branch to the posterior part of the ear canal, and when that part is stimulated, as in removal of wax, many patients cough because the vagus

———

*Huxley, Aldous: Point counter point, New York, 1928, Harper & Row, Publishers.

321

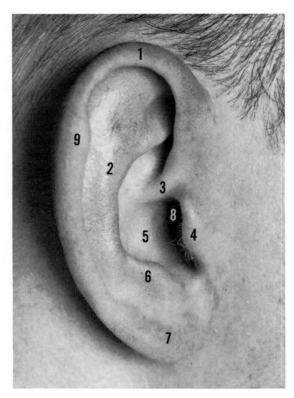

Fig. 28-1. Various landmarks of the auricle. **1,** Helix; **2,** antihelix; **3,** crus of helix; **4,** tragus; **5,** concha; **6,** antitragus; **7,** lobule; **8,** external auditory meatus; **9,** Darwin's tubercle.

nerve also supplies the larynx. Both the external and middle ears have abundant neural anastomoses: the pain of laryngeal disease, for example, frequently is referred to the ear. After tonsillectomy, referred pain almost invariably is present when the patient swallows.

The *temporal bone* contains the most intricate anatomy in the body. It is made up of five separate parts joined together by suture lines. There is the *mastoid* bone, a honeycomb-like collection of air cells lined by mucous membrane that connect with the middle ear; the *squamous* portion, a flat piece of bone superiorly that is often pneumatized; the *tympanic* portion, containing the middle ear and forming a part of the ear canal; the *petrous* bone, extending toward the center of the skull and housing the organs for hearing and equilibrium; and the *zygomatic* portion, extending anteriorly to join the zygoma or malar bone of the cheek. Of these parts, only the tympanic portion and the petrous bone contain elements related to hearing. The better known mastoid bone has no special function, but because its air cells are in continuity with the middle ear, pus from the middle ear may spread to the mastoid and produce infection there (Fig. 28-2).

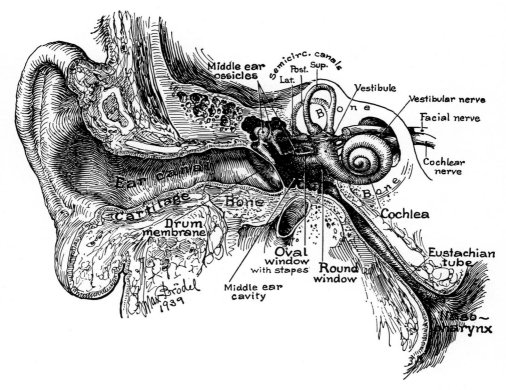

Fig. 28-2. External, middle, and inner ear. (From Brödel, Max: Three unpublished drawings of anatomy of the human ear, Philadelphia, 1946, W. B. Saunders Co.)

The *external auditory canal* provides a channel along which sound travels toward the tympanic membrane or eardrum. The outer part of the canal is lined with skin containing wax and sweat glands as well as hair follicles. In the outer part of the canal there is skin attached to cartilage. The deeper or inner half of the ear canal has a thin squamous epithelium tightly applied to bone. Whereas the outer part of the ear canal is only moderately sensitive, the inner part is exquisitely so. The delicate epithelium of the inner half of the ear canal is easily injured when a person picks his ear to relieve itching. When picking the ear canal causes pain or bleeding, patients usually think they have injured their eardrums, but they seldom have. Squamous epithelium derived from skin covers the outer surface of the eardrum, a fact of some importance—it means that there is no ordinary topical anesthetic that will work on the eardrum.

MIDDLE EAR

The *tympanic membrane* (drumhead or eardrum) stretches across the deepest part of the ear canal and separates the external ear from the middle

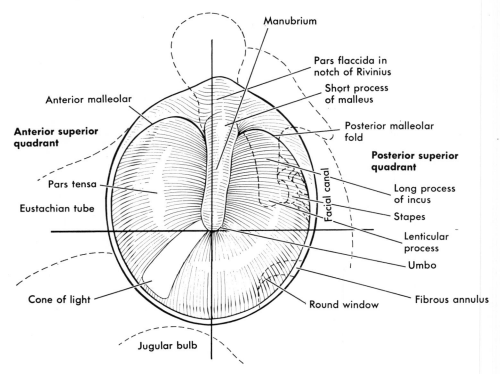

Fig. 28-3. Relationships of important middle ear structures to be considered in myringotomy. Often the incudostapedial joint can be seen dimly through the intact tympanic membrane.

ear. It is about as large as the eraser end of a pencil. Actually it is not as fragile and as easily damaged as most people think; it has three layers that make it rather tough. Its outer lining is squamous epithelium derived from the skin of the ear canal; its inner lining is cuboidal mucosa like that of the middle ear. Between is a tough fibrous layer. Normally the tympanic membrane is slightly cone shaped, with its concavity external. The fibers of the eardrum condense at its margins to form the tympanic *annulus,* a tough ring that fits into the bony *tympanic sulcus.* Both the sulcus and the annulus are incomplete superiorly at the pars flaccida. The normal eardrum is translucent and shiny gray, but in inflammation it becomes pink or dull red; with pus in the middle ear, it looks white; with blood, blue.

The normal eardrum presents certain landmarks, the primary one being the malleus, the first of three tiny middle ear bones that transmit sound from the eardrum to the inner ear. The prominent short process of the malleus stands out superiorly like a tiny knob; extending downward from the short process is the handle or *manubrium; the umbo,* at the end of the handle, is the most retracted part of the eardrum (Fig. 28-3).

The eardrum is of great importance in physical diagnosis because it

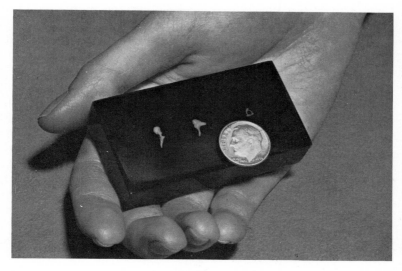

Fig. 28-4. The human malleus, incus, and stapes mounted in a plastic mold. The coin is a dime.

serves as a translucent window through which the examiner may interpret disease processes in the middle ear. Sometimes the eardrum is perforated as a result of injury or infection, and then the examiner actually can see structures in the middle ear that normally are not visible. Besides protecting the middle ear from outside weather and dirt, the eardrum is an important part of the hearing mechanism. This function will be explained later.

The *middle ear,* which lies directly behind the eardrum, is a small air-filled space in the tympanic portion of the temporal bone. In this space are the body's three smallest bones: malleus, incus, and stapes (Fig. 28-4). In it, too, is the *seventh cranial,* or facial, nerve, which controls movements of the face and another nerve, the *chorda tympani,* which provides taste for the anterior two thirds of the tongue.

The middle ear has two exits. One, which is blind, leads posteriorly into the honeycomb of mastoid cells. The other, the eustachian tube, opens into the nasopharynx. The job of the eustachian tube is to equalize air pressure between the middle ear and the throat or pharynx. To feel how it works hold your nose and swallow. You will feel a sensation of pressure in the ear or hear a crack or pop as the tube opens and admits air to the middle ear. Sometimes you must swallow again to relieve the fullness; this time air is escaping from the middle ear, where it has been trapped under slight pressure. Normally our eustachian tubes are closed. Whenever we yawn or swallow, however, the attached palatine muscles open each tube a little and bring air pressure in the middle ear to equilibrium with the outside atmosphere. Such equalization of pressures is especially important during air flight or underwater diving. In severe instances of barotrauma there may be bleeding into the middle ear and even rupture of the eardrum.

The three small bones in the middle ear form a chain that conducts sound from the eardrum across the middle ear to an opening in the inner ear called the oval window. The first bone, the malleus, is attached to the eardrum. It joins the second bone, the incus; an arm of the incus reaches the third and innermost bone, the stapes. The footplate of the stapes, which vibrates in response to sound waves, fits in the oval window. Other parts of the stapes beside the footplate include two legs, a neck, and a head. A tiny tendon attached to the neck of the stapes prevents excessive vibrations and helps to protect the inner ear against intense sound (Fig. 28-5).

The mucosal lining of the middle ear extends into the eustachian tube until it joins with the lining of the nasopharynx. Middle ear mucosa also lines the inner surface of the eardrum—it is entirely separate from the lining on the outer side of the eardrum, which is derived from skin. Later we will see what happens when skin grows through a perforation in the eardrum and lines the middle ear.

There are many important structures close to the middle ear. The seventh cranial, or facial, nerve is enclosed in a bony sheath called the fallopian canal, which runs through the posterior part of the middle ear. In chronic mastoiditis there is sometimes erosion of this bony canal, resulting in facial paralysis. Also the surgeon may injure this nerve at the time of mastoidectomy. The roof of the middle ear is the same as the floor of the middle cranial fossa, and this means that the temporal lobe of the brain with its covering of meninges is only millimeters away from the middle ear and mastoid—thus in otitis media or mastoiditis infection sometimes spreads

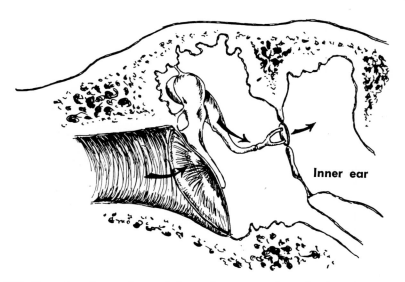

Fig. 28-5. Normal pathway of sound from the ear canal to the inner ear—so-called "ossicular" route. **1,** Malleus; **2,** incus; **3,** stapes.

intracranially. Important vascular channels are also nearby: anteriorly, the internal carotid artery; inferiorly, the bulb of the internal jugular vein; posteriorly, the lateral or sigmoid sinus.

INNER EAR

The inner ear contains the organs of hearing, the cochlea, and the organ of equilibrium, the vestibular labyrinth. Both of these structures are in the petrous portion of the temporal bone, not the mastoid portion. In tiny channels in the bony cochlear and vestibular labyrinths are two separate fluids: perilymph and endolymph. The endolymph, which is contained in a fragile membranous tube, bathes and nourishes the end organs for hearing and equilibrium. This tube of endolymph is surrounded by a larger quantity of perilymph which serves to cushion it. The endolymphatic fluid is contained in a continuous closed system, while the perilymphatic spaces are connected with the subarachnoid space and its cerebrospinal fluid.

The *organ of Corti* in the cochlea serves as the end organ for hearing. From its neuroepithelium project some 24,000 "hair cells." Sound waves, upon entering the cochlea, mechanically bend or distort the hair cells. When this happens, sound, which has been a mechanical force, is converted into an electrochemical impulse, traveling along the acoustic nerve to the temporal cortex of the brain. There it is interpreted as meaningful sound. The hair cells, the most fragile elements in the ear, are subject to injury by *mechanical trauma, oxygen deprivation,* and *the toxic influences of drugs and infection.* As long as a person has normal hair cells, he will have some hearing. The only truly deaf patient is the one whose hair cells no longer function. Stated differently, we may say that a person with no eardrum and no auditory ossicles can still hear *amplified* sound adequately if only the inner ear and its central connections are intact.

PHYSIOLOGY OF HEARING

To understand better how the ear works we must look back millions of years to the time when all animal life was in the sea. Sounds made in the ocean traveled through seawater directly to similar liquids in the inner ears of aquatic animals. These animals had no external or middle ears; theirs was a simple arrangement. Only a membrane separated the sea from the inner ear. Vibration of this membrane produced hearing.

When animals crawled out of the sea to live on land, many adjustments were necessary. For example, the aquatic ear had to be modified if it were to work efficiently in its new environment of air. When sound pressure traveling in air meets water, most of the sound striking the water is absorbed or reflected back into the air. Thus a fisherman in his boat may talk without fear of disturbing the fish, since 99.9% of the sound energy of his voice is absorbed or reflected when it strikes the surface of the lake; only one part in a thousand is transmitted to the water. For that very reason the early land-dwelling animals with their aquatic ears had a hearing problem. The liquids of their inner ear reflected most of the sound energy that originated in their new environment—air. Only 0.1% was effective in producing hearing. To overcome this loss the middle ear evolved.

Two arrangements enable the middle ear to work as it does. First, the middle ear bones are arranged in a lever system, which amplifies sound as it traverses them. The second and more important amplification results from the difference in size between the two parts connected by the chain of ear bones—the relatively large eardrum, which collects sound, and the relatively small footplate of the stapes, which delivers it to the inner ear. The effective area of the eardrum that collects sound pressure is about fourteen times larger than the footplate of the stapes. You can understand how this arrangement works if you recall what would happen if a woman in high heels were to step on your foot. Her entire weight, transmitted to a tiny area, would drive the heel forcibly; if her weight were distributed more widely by a flat shoe, damage would be less. By virtue of the mechanical advantage provided by the lever system and, more importantly, by the differences in the area of the eardrum and the footplate of the stapes, the middle ear regains a great deal of the sound pressure lost in transferring airborne sound pressure to a liquid medium (the inner ear) (Fig. 28-6).

When sound pressure reaches the inner ear, the perilymph and endolymph are agitated. The agitation, in turn, causes a commotion of the hair cells and hearing results.

Sound pressure that stimulates hair cells is delivered through the oval

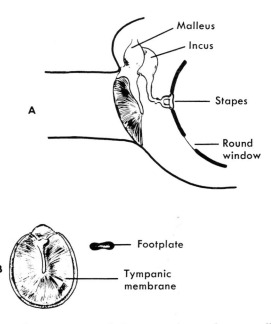

Fig. 28-6. A, The normal arrangement of the tympanic membrane, malleus, and incus for transmitting sound through stapes to the oval window. **B,** Compares area of footplate of stapes with area of tympanic membrane. (From DeWeese, David D., and Saunders, William H.: Textbook of otolaryngology, ed. 4, St. Louis, 1973, The C. V. Mosby Co.)

window into a solid bony chamber, the cochlea. For effective movement of inner ear liquids and stimulation of the hair cells, there must be a second opening for relief of pressure; the round window provides such relief (Fig. 28-7). What would happen if sound pressure were to meet both round and oval window at exactly the same time? The effect would be a cancellation; the ear would hear poorly even if the sound were intense. Experimentally such an arrangement is possible. When two sounds of equal intensity and in the same "phase" are delivered simultaneously to the round and oval window of an experimental animal, there is no hearing.

Under normal circumstances, however, such a thing does not happen. For as the eardrum collects sound energy and transmits it to the oval window, it also shields the round window from sound. By doing so it further increases the discrepancy between the levels of sound pressure delivered to the two windows. In disease, when the eardrum is perforated, some hearing is lost because the eardrum, no longer intact, cannot effectively shield the round window (Figs. 28-8 and 28-9).

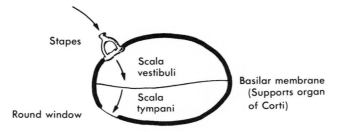

Fig. 28-7. Section through inner ear showing stapes as it fits in oval window and round window. Suspended between the two channels or scalae is the organ of hearing. As sound waves travel from one window to the other the hair cells of the organ of Corti are deflected, producing an electric potential along the auditory nerves. (From DeWeese, David D., and Saunders, William H.: Textbook of otolaryngology, ed. 4, St. Louis, 1973, The C. V. Mosby Co.)

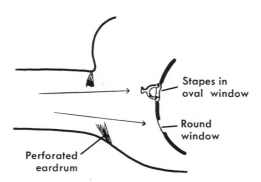

Fig. 28-8. Perforation of drumhead, showing how sound can reach both the oval and round windows at the same time, thereby causing a partial cancellation effect and loss of hearing. (From DeWeese, David D., and Saunders, William H.: Textbook of otolaryngology, ed. 4, St. Louis, 1973, The C. V. Mosby Co.)

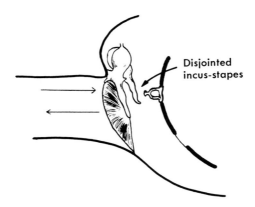

Disjointed
incus-stapes

Fig. 28-9. If the incus were accidentally disconnected from the stapes, sound waves strik-ing the tympanic membrane would not be transmitted effectively to the inner ear, but would be absorbed and reflected from the drumhead and there would be substantial hearing loss. (From DeWeese, David D., and Saunders, William H.: Textbook of oto-laryngology, ed. 4, St. Louis, 1973, The C. V. Mosby Co.)

ORGANS OF BALANCE

The *vestibular portion* of the inner ear is composed of the utricle, sac-cule, and three semicircular canals. Their function is that of maintaining equilibrium. The neural tissue in the vestibular portion of the inner ear, like that of the cochlea, is arranged in groups of cells called cristae, with projecting parts called hair cells. If one turns a patient rapidly in a chair or douches his ear canal with cold water, a current is set up in the endo-lymph and vertigo results. It continues for a minute or two or until there is no longer agitation of the end organ for equilibrium. There may also be nausea and even vomiting if the stimulus is too severe. The three semicir-cular canals in each ear are arranged at right angles to one another so that any movement of the head affects one or more of the canals. Then neural impulses traveling along the vestibular nerve set up reflexes to eye muscles and to muscles of the body to compensate for the change in posi-tion.

For a description of *nystagmus,* which sometimes accompanies vestibular disorder, see Chapter 36, p. 419.

CHAPTER TWENTY-NINE

Diseases of the external ear

INFECTIONS

Infections of the external ear are generally called *external otitis,* although some types of external otitis are not caused by infection but by disorders of the skin such as psoriasis and seborrheic dermatitis. When infection is the cause of external otitis, the causative organism may be either a bacterium or a fungus. Fungal infections are prevalent everywhere but are more common in warm climates than in temperate climates. Too much emphasis has probably been placed on the frequency of fungal infections of the ear canal as compared with bacterial infections. The latter are definitely more common.

External otitis

Acute external otitis is more common in the summer than in the winter, whereas acute otitis media, which is often associated with the common cold and other upper respiratory infections, is more common in the winter. The patient does not always know what started his external otitis. The infection may be the result of abrasion of the ear canal when the patient cleaned the ear, the result of swimming in contaminated water (so-called "swimmer's otitis"), or other known factors. At any rate, bacteria or sometimes fungi invade the epithelium of the ear canal and cause an infection that often becomes exceedingly painful (Fig. 29-1). *Pseudomonas* and other gram-negative organisms are especially common.

Pain is the chief symptom of external otitis, although aural discharge is also annoying. If the ear canal is blocked by the discharge and swelling of the epithelium, there may be partial loss of hearing, a blocked sensation in that ear, and even a little dizziness. If the infection is virulent and spreads to surrounding tissues, there are fever and malaise, and great pain occurs when the auricle or tragus is manipulated (Fig. 29-2). Lymphadenopathy behind the ear, in front of the ear, and under the ear is common. When there is marked adenopathy behind the ear, the ear is pushed forward and the patient may think he has mastoiditis.

The chief differential point between external otitis and otitis media, both of which have symptoms in common, is that *in external otitis movement of the auricle and tragus increases pain greatly,* but in otitis media these manipulations cause no additional pain. Of course, the physician is able to use other signs in the differential diagnosis, such as looking at the eardrum to see whether the patient has a middle ear infection and inspecting the ear canal to see if it is swollen—a sign of external otitis.

The treatment for the *acute* form of external otitis is to relieve pain with analgesics such as aspirin (good only for the mildest stages), codeine

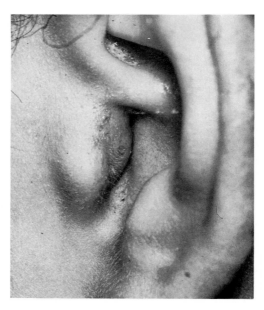

Fig. 29-1. Acute external otitis with furuncle, an extremely painful condition.

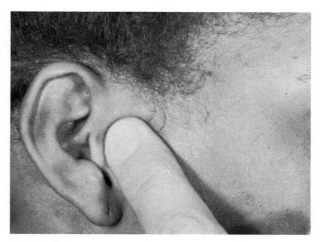

Fig. 29-2. Pressure on the tragus or traction on the auricle increases pain in acute external otitis but not in otitis media.

in dosages of 32 to 64 mg. every three hours, or similar drugs. Heat applied to the ear in the form of hot wet compresses, heating pad, or hot water bottle is often comforting. Whenever heat is applied to any portion of the body, thermal injury must be avoided. Heat is soothing and also exerts a beneficial physiologic effect by inducing hyperemia. Hot compresses need not be sterile, but care must be taken not to transfer infected aural drainage to another patient.

Treatment of the infection necessitates cleansing of the ear canal, although this is often too painful a procedure for the patient to tolerate, and insertion down to the eardrum of an ear wick made of cotton to carry in liquid medication applied to the cotton. In other words, the cotton acts as a wick to permit the medication to enter the ear canal and then to hold it there, which it sometimes cannot do because of swelling. The wick is left in place for twenty-four to forty-eight hours and then removed. If now the canal is less sensitive, and usually it is, it is cleaned. Dead skin, wax, and debris are removed gently from the depths of the canal, and the wick is reinserted for a similar period of time if necessary; if the canal seems patent, ear drops can be used without the wick. Ear drops may be used at room temperature, although if the drops came from a bottle recently in the refrigerator, they may actually cause a mild vertigo (caloric reaction, see p. 417). Introduction of ear drops is simple. The patient tilts his head to one side with the affected ear uppermost; for the adult, the auricle is pulled upward and backward, the solution is dropped into the meatus, without touching it, and the tragus is pressed to drive the fluid inward; for the child, the auricle is drawn downward. Drops tend to run out of the ear canal almost as fast as they are instilled. To ensure that the drops remain in contact with the epithelium, place an ear wick (a wisp of cotton) in the ear canal and then wet it with the ear drops (Fig. 29-3).

The ear drops most useful are a preparation known as Burow's solution and any of several antibiotic preparations, which usually contain polymyxin, sometimes in a solution of cortisone. A common proprietary eardrop with some of these ingredients is Cortisporin. Burow's solution (liquor aluminum subacetate), not an antibiotic, is usually prescribed as Burow's

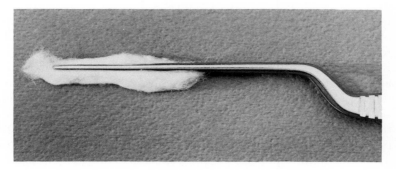

Fig. 29-3. Cotton wick ready for insertion into ear canal in treatment of external otitis. This particular wick is somewhat on the large side.

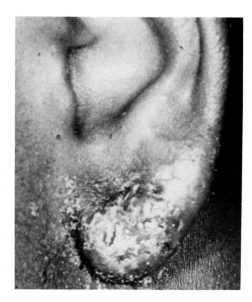

Fig. 29-4. Infection following piercing of ear.

solution, U.S.P., 15 ml. and distilled water 15 ml. Its action is to soothe the inflamed membranes of the ear canal and to exfoliate the outer layers with their collection of bacteria or fungi and debris. Later the desquamated skin can be wiped away.

In many instances, particularly when there is fever and regional cellulitis with lymphadenopathy, systemic antibiotics are required to correct the situation. Almost all cases if left untreated will heal anyway, but the pain and disability may be greatly prolonged. Many patients with acute external otitis who have had other painful conditions say that the pain of external otitis is the worst they ever experienced.

In *chronic external otitis,* pain is not a common symptom as it is in acute external otitis. Instead, there is *itching.* This is not to say that if your ears itch now and then or even all the time that you have chronic external otitis, because some itching of the ear canal seems to be normal in many persons. Aural discharge is common to both the acute and chronic forms of external otitis, although most patients with chronic external otitis seem to have dry scaling ears rather than draining ears. Sometimes the scaliness is visible externally on the auricle or just at the meatus, and it is especially apparent if the patient excoriates the auricle and ear canal to relieve the itching. Associated with many cases of chronic external otitis are various skin disorders such as psoriasis and seborrheic dermatitis. In these instances there may be no infection present but an underlying skin disorder that produces skin changes with scaling, improper wax formation, and itching. The chronic form may go on for years and eventually thicken the skin so much that return to normal, even with treatment, is impossible (Fig. 29-6).

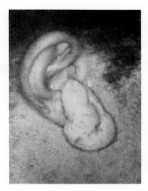

Fig. 29-5. Keloid formation following piercing of ear.

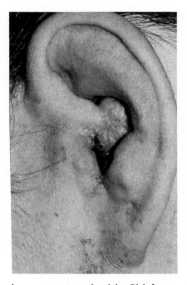

Fig. 29-6. Chronic severe external otitis. Chief symptom is itching.

The *treatment* for the chronic form is often medication prepared as an ointment or cream, in contrast to the acute form in which ointments are avoided. It is a good principle to use wet soaks on skin that is oozing or acutely infected and ointments on skin that is dry and scaly. When the nurse applies wet soaks to any skin surface, she must make provision for the entrance of air if heat is to be allowed to dissipate and maceration of the skin prevented. This is particularly true if the wet compresses are to be continuous. Protection of clothes and linens can be achieved by applying plastic absorptive materials to the pillow, bed surface, or clothing. Wet dressings left exposed to air will dry as the solution evaporates; therefore, the nurse needs to check the dressing frequently.

In other patients with dry external otitis, or when the wet applications

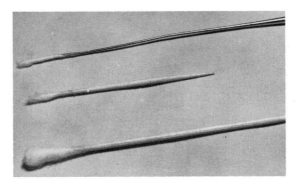

Fig. 29-7. Top: Physician's cotton applicator. Note tuft at end. **Middle:** Toothpick wound with cotton. **Bottom:** The usual commercial applicator (too thick).

have caused a cessation of oozing, ointments are of use. Again, antibiotic ointments are available when needed, and a common one is Neosporin. When itching and not infection is the chief problem, a good ointment to prescribe is one made of 0.9 Gm. each of phenol, salicylic acid, and precipitated sulfur in 30 Gm. of petrolatum. This ointment, applied at first once or twice a day and then less often as symptoms of itching and scaling subside, works well.

Perhaps most important of all is how the patient applies the ointment to the ear canal. No patient does it correctly unless instructed (Fig. 29-7). The commercially prepared cotton applicator such as Q-Tip is too thick and its end too firm to apply ointment effectively deep in the ear canal. The tufted end of a properly prepared applicator is wiped in ointment, and with a twirling motion the applicator is inserted deep into the canal and ointment applied to the outer surface of the eardrum as well as to the deepest part of the ear canal. If the nurse applies the ointment, she should caution the patient not to move the head and she should brace her hand carefully.

Piercing the lobule of the ear to fit an earring ordinarily causes no harm and is easily done. Sometimes, however, an infection may result as in any wound (Fig. 29-4). Then it usually is readily controlled with local or systemic antibiotics. We have seen keloid formation in Negroes after piercing of ears (Fig. 29-5).

CERUMEN (WAX) IN THE CANAL

A certain amount of earwax, or cerumen, is normal and desirable. Some patients who have no earwax find that their ear canals itch and scale excessively. There are variations in the amount and type of cerumen; sometimes it is dry and hard, whereas in other patients it is soft. Ordinarily there is not much difficulty associated with earwax, and one need not think it necessary to clean the ears to remove wax. Occasionally, however, the wax becomes impacted and the physician or nurse must then remove it. Perhaps

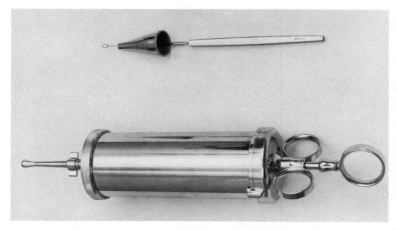

Fig. 29-8. Top: Cerumen spoon used through aural speculum. **Bottom:** Syringe used for irrigation.

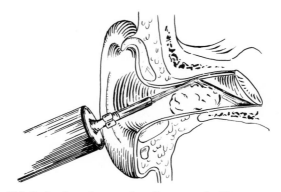

Fig. 29-9. Irrigation of external auditory canal with warm tap water.

the easiest way is with an ear syringe and tap water at body temperature (Fig. 29-8). If water is douched in the ear canal and the water is not at body temperature, the patient will experience vertigo because of a caloric reaction caused by stimulation of the inner ear and its organ of balance.

It is sometimes difficult for a patient to syringe his own ear efficiently, but it is a simple procedure for a nurse or member of the family. Solutions used should be warmed to body temperature. After the syringe is filled and air expelled the patient is seated and his clothing protected. A kidney basin held immediately below his ear and in contact with his skin catches the solution. The head is inclined slightly forward and toward the affected side to prevent the solution from running down the

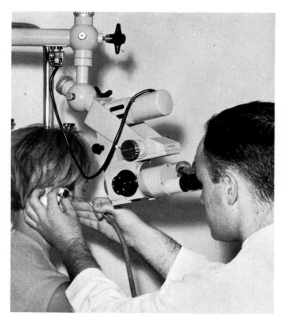

Fig. 29-10. Use of the operating microscope as office equipment. Also note the use of an aural suction tip to remove soft cerumen and pus from the ear canal or the middle ear (in a patient with perforation of the tympanic membrane).

neck. The auricle is pulled upward and backward and the solution injected along the upper wall of the meatus, but the tip of the syringe must not occlude the meatus (Fig. 29-9). After the ear canal is washed it should be dried, preferably with a length of cotton and bayonet forceps.

If irrigation of the canal does not remove the cerumen easily, the physician may use a cerumen spoon to pick it out, or if he is skilled in the use of aural instruments, he may prefer to use the cerumen spoon instead of irrigation (Fig. 29-10).

Rarely, wax is so firmly impacted that neither washing nor use of a cerumen spoon will remove it. Then it is best to give the patient instructions about the use of a bland oily drop, for example, mineral oil, in the ear for several days to further soften the plug of wax. After a few days of using drops the mass of soft wax can be washed out with ease.

Certain proprietary products advertised as cerumenolytic agents should be used cautiously because they sometimes cause an inflammatory reaction.

Too little cerumen may be more annoying to the patient than too much, because the ear canal is dry. There may be scaling and itching. This condition is not readily cured, but it may be improved by the application of suitable ear ointments. Occasionally an inadequacy of cerumen or an abnormal type of cerumen seems to be associated with dermatologic disorders such as seborrheic dermatitis or psoriasis.

FOREIGN BODIES IN THE CANAL

An insect in the ear canal can be a very distressing experience. There is pain and a dreadful noise, which alarms the patient until the insect is killed or removed. The treatment is simple: instill a few drops of any oily substance into the ear canal to smother the insect; then wash it out or remove it with forceps.

Children and mentally retarded adults often put objects in various body orifices, and the ear is one of the common places. Almost anything that will go into the ear canal has been found there. The eraser end of a lead pencil, paper wads, pebbles, and small beans and similar vegetal matter are common examples. Depending on how tightly the foreign body fits the ear canal, the treatment may be removal by irrigation or with forceps. Sometimes, however, particularly in the case of vegetal foreign bodies, water may cause additional swelling of the foreign body and worsen matters. Again, if the foreign body slips deep into the ear canal and passes the isthmus, which is the narrowest part, an operative procedure to widen the canal may be necessary in order to remove the foreign body. Fortunately this situation seldom arises.

The skin over the bony canal of the external auditory canal is very sensitive, is thin, bleeds easily, and forms subepithelial hematomas from minor trauma. Therefore, the removal of a solid foreign body carries a definite risk of additional trauma to the ear if the patient is not completely cooperative or if the removal is difficult. *Whenever the removal is unduly painful, further attempts without anesthesia should not be made.* A child should be hospitalized and the foreign body removed under general anesthesia. It is possible to force a foreign body through the eardrum into the middle ear, with subsequent hearing loss or chronic infection. Trauma to the ear canal, if significant, also may cause stenosis, requiring an operative correction and grafting in order to again obtain a patent external auditory canal.

Hematoma of the epithelium lining the osseous part of the external ear canal is easy to produce inadvertently by wiping too hard with a cotton applicator or other instrument. This epithelium is so delicate that sometimes only the slightest trauma produces a hematoma. On the other hand, the epithelium lining the cartilaginous, or external, half of the ear canal is thick and not as sensitive.

Aural polyps appear in the depth of the ear canal and are almost always covered with purulent discharge. They bleed easily. Larger polyps may present at the external auditory meatus.

The polyp may arise from within the external canal or from the middle ear. It may consist of granulation tissue, or it may be edematous mucosa of the middle ear. Polyps composed of granulation tissue may be partially covered by squamous epithelium, but they still look much redder and bleed more easily than do mucosal polyps. In either case, polyp formation indicates chronicity.

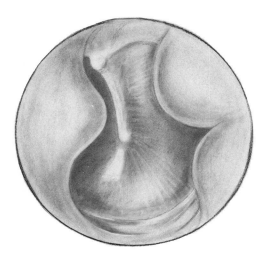

Fig. 29-11. Exostoses, external auditory canal.

The symptoms are a foul purulent discharge (particularly from the polyp composed of granulation tissue) and partial deafness if the polyp arises in the middle ear or obstructs the ear canal. Bleeding sometimes occurs.

Treatment is by removal with a special cup forceps or small snare. In addition, tympanoplasty or mastoidectomy may be required later.

Exostoses in the ear canal arise near the tympanic membrane, where they are attached to the osseous ear canal (Fig. 29-11). They are small, broad-based, bony hard lumps covered with normal epithelium. Often they are multiple, and usually they are bilateral. Some authorities believe that exostoses form because of periosteal irritation resulting from swimming in cold water. Usually they are asymptomatic. Rarely they cause obstruction. Treatment is usually unnecessary.

Sebaceous cysts are common in all parts of the skin. Fig. 29-12 shows a large cyst under the lobule which should be excised.

MALIGNANCY

Cancer of the external ear is not uncommon (Fig. 29-13). Usually the malignancy is a basal cell or squamous cell carcinoma, and the diagnosis is not difficult if only the physician keeps the possibility in mind and does not treat it as a chronic ulcer or skin infection. An ulcer on the auricle is the usual presenting symptom. Early, and even in some late cases, treatment by surgical excision is highly successful. The cosmetic result should be a matter of secondary importance, since the chief aim is to remove all of the tumor at the first attempt. Reconstruction of the auricle can be done later if necessary. Squamous cell carcinoma of the auricle may metastasize to the neck or other parts of the body, although these tumors tend to

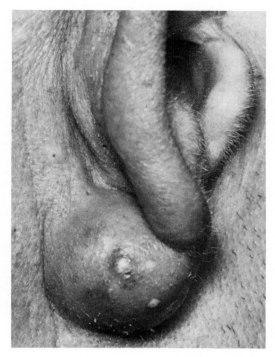

Fig. 29-12. Common site for sebaceous cyst. (From DeWeese, David D., and Saunders, William H.: Textbook of otolaryngology, ed. 4, St. Louis, 1973, The C. V. Mosby Co.)

remain localized for a considerable time. Basal cell carcinomas do not metastasize.

If carcinoma invades the ear canal, and particularly if it invades bone of the ear canal (the deeper part), treatment carries a much poorer prognosis. There are operations to remove the entire temporal bone in cases of carcinoma, with a cure rate of about 25 percent. Irradiation therapy may also cure an occasional patient.

CONGENITAL DEFORMITIES

Absence of the auricle is unusual but is a condition seen often enough to deserve mention. More common than complete absence of the auricle is a partial deformity of the ear, which produces a variable degree of cosmetic deformity in different patients and which may also be associated with an absence of the external auditory meatus (Figs. 29-14 and 29-15). Absence of the meatus, in turn, is frequently associated with a deformity of the middle ear in which one of the tiny ear bones is missing or in which two are fused and therefore useless.

If the auricular malformation is in a girl, probably the best thing to do is nothing but to have the child wear her hair in such a way as to cover the ears. In a boy the situation is, of course, more difficult from the stand-

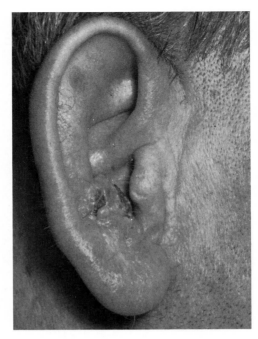

Fig. 29-13. Squamous cell carcinoma of the auricle. Adequate excision should control the disease.

point of trying to hide the deformity, and sometimes attempts are made to reconstruct the auricle. The best that can be said is that the formation of an auricle can be attempted but that it seldom resembles an ear, and often everyone concerned wishes that nothing at all had been tried. Another measure is to fashion an artificial ear that the patient can glue to the side of his head.

Lop ear or outstanding auricle is a congenital condition in which absence of the normal curve of the antihelix causes a cup-shaped auricle as viewed from the front and an auricle that stands far out from the head as seen from behind (Fig. 29-16). The treatment is a surgical procedure in which subcutaneously placed nylon sutures are used to correct the deformity. This is a rather important procedure in the case of some children, who may be teased about their different appearance.

In the case of absence of the external meatus there is always a hearing loss. If the ear canal is missing on just one side of the head, and often that is the case, the opposite ear has good hearing and the patient is not severely handicapped. Occasionally, however, the deformity is bilateral, and then there is severe hearing loss and the patient must either wear a hearing aid or have an operative procedure to restore patency of the ear canal and, if necessary, correct a deformity in the middle ear. These procedures are successful about 50% of the time, and as one might expect, the percentage of success depends on the experience of the surgeon.

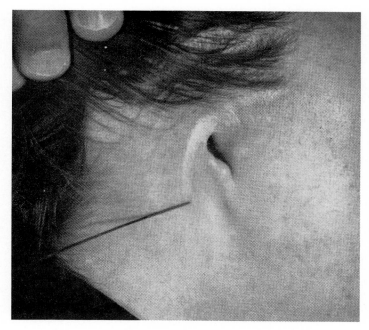

Fig. 29-14. Malformation of the ear caused by arrested development at about the fourth week of embryonic life. Cleftlike opening of the first branchial groove led to a cholesteatoma sac, exteriorized at surgery. Note the curved scar of incision. There is a tiny fistula of the second branchial groove at the tip of the pointer. (From Shambaugh, George E., Jr.: Surgery of the ear, Philadelphia, 1959, W. B. Saunders Co.)

INJURY TO THE CANAL

Injury to the ear is common when a hairpin or other instrument is used to scratch an itchy canal. Hairpins easily abrade the sensitive epithelium in the deeper part of the ear canal and cause bleeding and pain. The patient usually thinks he has perforated his eardrum. Such is rarely the case, however, because the eardrum has three layers and is rather tough and not as fragile as most persons think. On the other hand, the epithelium lining the inner half of the ear canal is thin and very sensitive.

Cauliflower ear occurs when, through trauma or infection, there is destruction of cartilage of the auricle. Wrestlers and boxers may develop this deformity after their ears are injured repeatedly. Blood collects between the cartilage and perichondrium, and if it is not aspirated, the cartilage is deprived of its blood supply and undergoes necrosis. As a rare complication of mastoidectomy, perichondritis and chondritis may develop.

In hematoma of the auricle blood should be aspirated, cotton placed in the creases of the auricle, and a pressure dressing applied. A hematoma may re-form, and repeated aspiration may be necessary (Fig. 29-17).

Lacerations of the auricle are expected to heal well because of the ex-

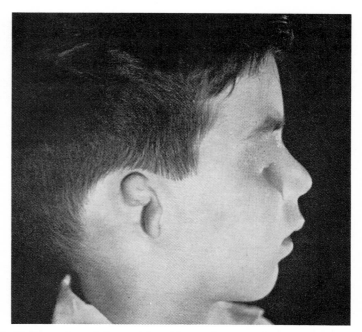

Fig. 29-15. Malformation of the auricle with atresia caused by arrested development at six weeks of embryonic life. (From Shambaugh, George E., Jr.: Surgery of the ear, Philadelphia, 1959, W. B. Saunders Co.)

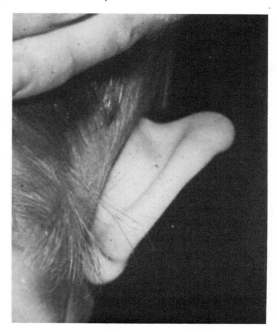

Fig. 29-16. Outstanding auricle or lop ear.

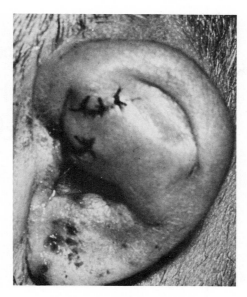

Fig. 29-17. Hematoma after laceration.

cellent blood supply. Even though torn completely from the head, the auricle will sometimes grow if carefully attached. Fine sutures such as No. 5-0 nylon should be used when repairing wounds about the face in order to assure as fine a scar as possible.

Frostbite is likely to affect the ears and the nose, since these parts are exposed and there is little fat under the skin. Blebs form, and if the frostbite is severe, there may be gangrene and loss of the part. Usually, however, except for pain the injury is not serious. Treatment is expectant because the injury is a physical one, not infectious, and once frozen there is not much one can do except to wait and see what the course will be.

CHAPTER THIRTY

Diseases of the middle ear and mastoid; facial paralysis

DISEASES OF THE MIDDLE EAR AND MASTOID

Most of the diseases that affect the middle ear and mastoid are caused by infection. Usually these infections clear spontaneously, but the few that fail to subside may cause the ear to drain pus for years or for a lifetime. They also cause partial loss of hearing. Because the middle ear and mastoid are intimately associated with many important structures, infections of the temporal bone always create a potentially dangerous situation.

Acute otitis media

Acute otitis media often follows an upper respiratory infection such as the common cold or childhood diseases such as measles and scarlet fever. It is the disorder causing "earache" so common during childhood. Bacterial organisms infecting the middle ear cavity almost always reach it via the eustachian tube; infections coming from the bloodstream or through lymphatic channels are much less common. Any of the common pathogenic bacteria may cause otitis media, but the most common are streptococci and pneumococci. Rarely, the tubercle bacillus is the cause. Children and adults with recurrent ear infections should be cautioned against forceful blowing of the nose during colds, since this may drive infected secretions into the middle ear. For this same reason water entering the nose during swimming or diving should be allowed to run out rather than being forcefully expelled.

In infants and children the eustachian tube is shorter and straighter than in adults, and this anatomic variation has been thought to account, in part, for the ease with which children develop otitis media. Probably more important is the mass of adenoid tissue that every child has in the nasopharynx and that few adults have. This lymphoid tissue obstructs the orifice of the eustachian tube, especially when the tissue becomes infected and swells during a cold or other upper respiratory infection.

The chief symptom of acute otitis media is pain. If the eardrum ruptures because of the pressure of pus in the middle ear, aural discharge becomes a symptom while the pain is relieved. There also is partial loss of hearing, but because of earache, the patient usually does not complain much about his hearing loss.

Examination of the eardrum in a patient with acute otitis media shows it to be red and bulging, or if the middle ear contains pus under pressure, it may look white. If it has ruptured, there will be a purulent discharge in the external auditory canal, and when this is removed by wiping or suction, a perforation is visible in the eardrum. Fever, sometimes as high as 104° F., is expected.

Myringotomy is indicated when the eardrum is bulging. This procedure, described on p. 357, is done to relieve pain and to prevent pus from destroying the contents of the middle ear. *After myringotomy the tympanic membrane almost always heals perfectly, and the procedure does not affect hearing.*

The course of acute otitis media is usually toward healing, even without any therapy. With adequate antibiotic therapy almost all patients go on to complete healing, particularly if pus is released by myringotomy. Application of heat may aid in relieving pain either before or after myringotomy. Analgesics such as aspirin or codeine also help. The patient may be acutely ill for several days and his ear drain for several weeks, but eventually the eardrum heals as inflammation resolves. If otitis media is the result of obstruction of the eustachian tube by the adenoid, and in the child it often is, acute otitis media may recur until the adenoid is removed.

Penicillin ordinarily is the antibiotic of choice if the patient is not allergic to that drug, as many are. Other antibiotics such as the tetracyclines are also effective in most instances. Whenever there is uncertainty as to the drug of choice or when a drug selected empirically is not effective, cultures and antibiotic sensitivity studies are indicated to determine the best possible drug. The report from the laboratory ordinarily takes forty-eight hours, however, and one hesitates to delay treatment that long in most cases.

Acute mastoiditis

Acute mastoiditis was a common complication of otitis media before the antibiotic era. It still occurs but less frequently and usually less severely because most patients with acute otitis media receive treatment with antibiotics and are cleared.

Usually in acute mastoiditis the eardrum has ruptured or at least it is bulging. Deep pressure over the mastoid elicits tenderness. A point in differential diagnosis is in order here: In acute external otitis there may be swelling behind the ear and tenderness to superficial pressure because of lymphadenopathy; in acute mastoiditis, if there is not a subperiosteal abscess, deeper pressure is needed to elicit tenderness. When subperiosteal abscess is present, it means that pus has broken through the mastoid cortex and collected under the skin and periosteum behind the ear. X-ray examination of the temporal bone will show a hazy appearance of the affected mastoid.

The treatment for acute mastoiditis is heavy antibiotic therapy—myringotomy may still be indicated. Complications of acute mastoiditis include facial paralysis, meningitis, epidural abscess, brain abscess, and thrombosis of the sigmoid sinus. If acute infection of the middle ear and mastoid fails to clear, chronic otitis media and mastoiditis may ensue.

Surgical treatment of *acute* mastoiditis, formerly common but now done only rarely, is discussed on p. 361.

Chronic suppurative otitis media

Chronic suppurative otitis media is the result of acute otitis media that failed to heal. Of course, most cases of acute otitis media do heal so that chronic otitis media is less common than is acute otitis media (Figs. 30-1 to 30-3). In chronic otitis media there is a perforation in the eardrum through which pus runs more or less continuously. This purulent discharge may continue for months or for life, and part of the eardrum and often some of the middle ear bones are destroyed. The infectious process also extends to the air cells of the mastoid bone, since they are connected directly with the middle ear cavity. Therefore, chronic otitis media and chronic mastoiditis are generally synonymous. Although the treatment for acute otitis media is medical (antibiotics and myringotomy), often surgical treatment is necessary to clear chronic otitis media.

In chronic otitis media usually more than one bacterial organism is found in cultures of pus. Streptococci, staphylococci, proteus, and pseudomonas organisms are most common, and the latter two are often difficult

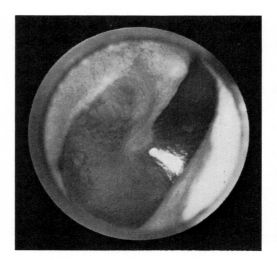

Fig. 30-1. Normal tympanic membrane.

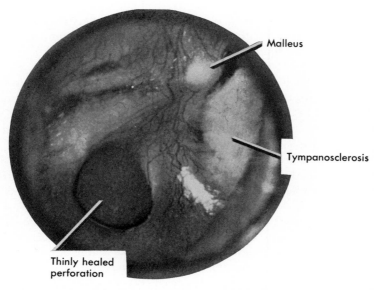

Fig. 30-2. Tympanic membrane with thinly healed perforation and tympanosclerosis.

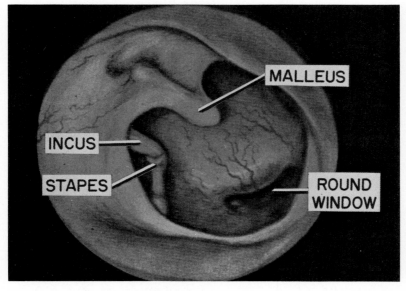

Fig. 30-3. Large perforation showing the incudostapedial joint in the middle ear cavity.

to treat. Recently the antibiotics carbenicillin and gentamicin have been developed and are effective in treatment of infections produced by gram-negative organisms including pseudomonas. Unfortunately, however, patients require hospitalization for parentral therapy when these antibiotics are used. Also, gentamicin is ototoxic. The treatment of acute otitis media with antibiotics is easier, quicker, and more effective than the treatment of chronic otitis media. Cultures are most important in patients with chronic otitis media to make certain of drug choice.

In addition to carefully selected antibiotics, other types of medical treatment for chronic otitis media are sometimes successful—especially when the perforation in the tympanic membrane is large enough to permit treatment of the middle ear cavity. Then irrigations with a solution of vinegar and water *or other irrigant* may wash pus and debris (cholesteatoma) from the middle ear or epitympanum and mastoid and promote healing (Fig. 30-4). Vinegar, half-strength, contains about 2% acetic acid; this medication long has been used against the pseudomonas organism, commonly found in *chronic* purulent otitis media. Patients may be given directions like the following: (1) Mix 1 part of household vinegar and 1 part of boiled and cooled tap water; (2) warm mixture to body temperature—if too hot or too cold, there may be dizziness and nausea; (3) wash ear vigorously with several syringefuls of the mixture; (4) shake water out of ear and dry ear by loosening and teasing out the end of a commercial cotton applicator (Q-Tip); and (5) use ear drops if prescribed. In general, except when irrigations are used as therapy and administered with proper precautions, the ears of patients with tympanic perforations should be *kept dry*. These patients *should not swim* or allower shower water to enter the ear, because

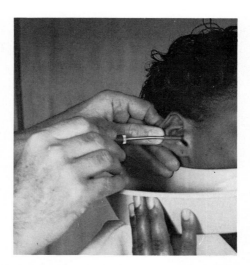

Fig. 30-4. Aural irrigation in chronic otitis media. An overhead can contains normal saline solution at *body temperature,* or equal parts of tap water and household vinegar, or other solution ordered by physician. A pint or more of irrigant is used once or twice a day. The patient does it herself or a family member is instructed.

wetting the middle ear often worsens otitis media or reactivates an infection that had become dormant.

Some otolaryngologists prefer a dry treatment for chronic otitis media. Instead of irrigations they wipe out the ear and blow in powders of various types. It is difficult to see, however, how wiping can improve matters much, for the disease process almost always extends into the mastoid and epitympanum, where no applicator can reach.

Tympanosclerosis is the name given to a special condition occurring in some patients who have had infections in their middle ears. It has nothing to do with a similar-sounding term, otosclerosis, but the two are commonly confused.

In tympanosclerosis there is a deposition of a dense, almost cartilage-like material in the middle or fibrous layer of the eardrum (Fig. 30-2) and about the middle ear bones themselves. This is a nonreactive substance and does no actual harm except that by immobilizing the eardrum and ossicles it reduces hearing. Treatment is to remove the tympanosclerosis during the tympanoplasty procedure. Often deposits of tympanosclerosis cause no symptoms so that no treatment is needed.

Cholesteatoma

Cholesteatoma is a special condition occurring in some patients with chronic otitis media. Skin from the external auditory canal grows through a perforation in the tympanic membrane and lines the middle ear and adjacent mastoid air cells. These spaces normally are lined with mucous membrane, not skin. Dead skin peeling off from this matrix forms a soft white ball called cholesteatoma. Many tympanic perforations are small, and the cholesteatoma is trapped in the middle ear and mastoid. As it enlarges, pressure erosion of bone occurs so that facial paralysis, vertigo, loss of hearing, or even meningitis may result as complications of chronic otitis media. Mastoidectomy is done as often to remove cholesteatoma as to remove granulation tissue and infection. Actually, the conditions usually coexist.

Ordinarily pain is not part of chronic ear infection. When pain is associated with chronic disease of the ear, a complication such as epidural abscess (pus between the bone and dura) should be suspected. Some patients with chronic draining ears become vertiginous; then another complication is suspected, namely, that cholesteatoma has eroded the horizontal semicircular canal.

Tumors

Tumors of the middle ear and mastoid are rare. They are usually squamous cell carcinomas. Symptoms are aural discharge, loss of hearing, deep-seated pain, and eventually facial paralysis. The diagnosis should be suspected in any patient with granulation-like tissue in the ear canal that fails to clear. Radical resection of the temporal bone may be done and while it is only curative in 25% of cases, it is still better than irradiation therapy.

The *glomus jugulare* tumor is a rare growth arising in special tissue normally present in the dome of the jugular bulb just under the floor of the middle ear. These tumors grow slowly but may eventually replace much of the middle ear and mastoid to cause loss of hearing and facial paralysis. Occasionally they metastasize. They bleed so excessively during removal that several units of blood may be lost.

Glomus tympanium is an identical tumor arising in the middle ear (tympanic cavity). These tumors ordinarily are discovered while still small, or since they produce early symptoms of tinnitus and hearing loss. They are relatively easy to remove.

Congenital malformations

Congenital malformations of the middle ear are found sometimes as isolated anomalies and sometimes in association with malformations of other parts of the ear. Occasionally the only abnormality is absence of the incus—the patient has a severe conductive hearing loss. Again, the malleus and incus may be fused and functionless, and in these cases often there is no external auditory canal. Such a major deformity is frequently associated with microtia or even absence of the auricle.

The treatment of congenital deformity of the ear canal and middle ear depends, of course, upon the severity and type of the malformation. If a patient has normal hearing in one ear but no ear canal on the other side, it may be better to rely on the one good ear than to attempt reconstruction of the deformed ear. Reconstructive operations are major procedures, always a little risky, and certainly not always successful. If there is only a conductive hearing loss but a normal external ear and eardrum, exploratory tympanotomy is indicated, since an isolated deformity of the middle ear (such as absence of the incus) often can be corrected.

Serous otitis media

Serous otitis media is a common condition attributed to a number of causes. Unlike purulent otitis media, in which there is pus in the middle ear, in serous otitis the middle ear fluid is a sterile transudate of blood serum. Sometimes the condition lasts only a few days, as when serous otitis results after airplane travel, but at other times it may persist for years and the cause remain obscure.

The ear feels stuffy or blocked, and hearing is reduced. The eardrum looks retracted because with a partial vacuum in the middle ear the greater pressure of the external atmosphere presses it medially (Fig. 30-5). Amber serum in the middle ear changes the color of the eardrum, and if both serum and air are present, the air forms bubbles, which can be seen through the translucent eardrum. At other times there is an air-fluid level with the meniscus of the serum looking like a fine hair.

Treatment is often easy if the cause is mere obstruction of the eustachian tube—inflation of the tube opens it and relieves the obstruction (Fig. 30-6). Unfortunately in some instances the causes are more obscure and the treatment becomes less certain. Some patients have serous otitis for months or even for years despite all types of treatment.

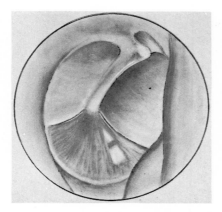

Fig. 30-5. Serous otitis media. Eardrum is retracted because of negative pressure in the middle ear, and there is liquid (blood serum) below and air above. This forms a readily visible air-fluid level.

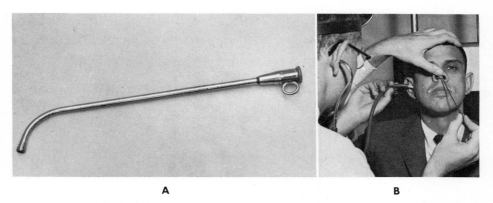

A   B

Fig. 30-6. A, Eustachian catheter. **B,** Introduction of the eustachian catheter. The tip just entering the nose will fall into the eustachian tube orifice. Air is blown through the metal tube into the eustachian tube and middle ear and out the tube again. As the air passes into the middle ear it is heard by the physician if the tube is open.

A relatively new treatment, which now is used commonly, is to open the eardrum as for myringotomy and to insert a small plastic tube or hollow button. This permits aeration of the middle ear even when the eustachian tube is obstructed. These plastic tubes may be left in place indefinitely, although most of them extrude spontaneously. (See p. 360 and Fig. 31-3.)

So-called "glue ear" (Fig. 30-7), a related but different condition, is described in Chapter 31, p. 360.

FACIAL PARALYSIS

Bell's palsy is paralysis of *unknown etiology* affecting the facial nerve (Fig. 30-8). It occurs commonly. In most instances the paralysis recovers

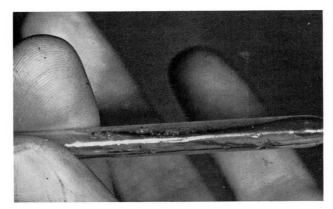

Fig. 30-7. Thick secretions aspirated from the middle ear of a child with adenoidal obstruction of the eustachian tube. So-called "glue ear," which is not the same as serous otitis. (See also pp. 359-360.)

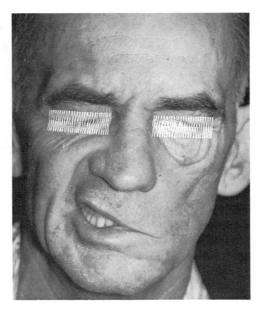

Fig. 30-8. Bell's palsy. Face pulls strongly to the good side.

completely or almost completely, but occasionally there is a failure of return of function, and a significant or even complete paralysis persists on one side. The sooner function returns the better the prognosis for complete recovery. In patients who show no return after one or two months, many authorities have advised decompression of the facial nerve in its bony canal (the fallopian canal). This operation requires mastoidectomy for exposure and then careful removal of the bone sheathing the descending portion of the nerve. More recently, however, the advice has been to treat patients conservatively with cortisone.

The cause of Bell's palsy is not established with certainty, but it is supposed to be related to vascular spasms of arterioles supplying the facial nerve. Another cause is a viral infection. For example, mumps viremia without the customary parotitis is a known cause.

Facial paralysis also occurs from more obvious causes, among which are skull fracture, acute and chronic mastoiditis (especially with cholesteatoma), and central nervous system disease such as brain tumor. Outside the temporal bone, malignant tumors of the parotid gland cause facial paralysis, and a laceration across the cheek can cut peripheral branches of the nerve. The parotidectomy operation is always dangerous because the facial nerve courses through the gland and all branches must be preserved or there will be at least a partial facial paralysis, although this may not be permanent since anastomatic branches from adjacent fibers grow across and reinnervate the face. The most common type of facial paralysis is the peripheral, in which the entire side of the face is paralyzed, including the forehead. When the patient is asked to show his teeth, his mouth pulls strongly toward the good side but the paralyzed side remains immobile. The good eye squeezes shut tightly on command but the paralyzed eyelids do not close. In facial paralysis of the central type the same appearances are present, except that the patient is able to wrinkle his forehead on both sides. The reason has to do with arrangement of neural pathways in the central parts of the facial nerve providing for certain cross-over supply to the forehead. Treatment of facial paralysis depends on its cause. For example, the surgeon may remove a spicule of bone pressing on the nerve after skull fracture or perform mastoidectomy to remove granulation tissue and infection in a patient with mastoiditis.

Nursing care in the patient with facial paralysis is important. Because the patient cannot close his eye completely and does not blink the affected eye at all, the nurse should instruct the patient in the application of eye drops such as Liquifilm, which are designed to keep the eye moist. Also adding to the difficulty is that the lacrimal gland may fail to secrete tears in some patients with facial paralysis, since the parasympathetic nerve supply to the lacrimal gland is derived from the geniculate ganglion of the facial nerve. In advanced cases of corneal drying, permanent damage can occur. The nurse may also need to show the patient how to apply tape across the eye to hold the lids shut or how to apply an eyepad.

Sometimes after operations or trauma to the parotid area, there comes to be a certain misdirection of neural fibers in the healing process that results in so-called *gustatory sweating* or Frey's syndrome. This means that the patient sweats in a localized area of the cheek whenever he eats or thinks about eating. Usually no treatment is necessary but in severe cases an operation on the middle ear to resect the tympanic plexus (from which some of the parasympathetic fibers to this area come) may be required.

CHAPTER THIRTY-ONE

Operations on the middle ear and mastoid— myringotomy, mastoidectomy, and tympanoplasty

Middle ear and mastoid operations are undergoing great change in both concept and technique. Until twenty years ago, emphasis was on elimination of infection, and little attention was paid to restoration of hearing. This is easily understandable if one remembers that in the preantibiotic era, infections that are now controlled by antibiotics or sulfonamide drugs often raged through the patient's middle ear and adjacent mastoid bone, leaving him with a draining ear and a potentially dangerous condition for the remainder of his life. There were no effective medical measures to correct these virulent infections. When otitis media and mastoiditis became established, surgery was needed. Older operations relieved infections but did nothing to reconstruct the ear. Instead, they were intended to spare the patient from further complications and to give him a dry ear.

Antibiotics have provided an effective means of treating acute otitis media and mastoiditis, and consequently there is less opportunity for the development of chronic middle ear and mastoid infections, which may smoulder and eventually, after a period of years, damage vital structures surrounding the middle ear. This is not to say that otitis media and mastoiditis are not still with us—emphatically they are, but the incidence is reduced.

Currently there is great interest in the restoration of hearing by surgical methods. This is possible in four groups of patients: those with middle ears damaged by infection, those with otosclerosis, those with congenital malformations, and those with trauma to the middle ear. With development of the operating microscope we now have an excellent system of illumination and magnification that makes working in the small spaces of the middle ear relatively easy (Fig. 31-1). Operations to improve hearing by reconstructing the sound-conduction pathways in the middle ear are called tympanoplasty, whereas operations for relief of hear-

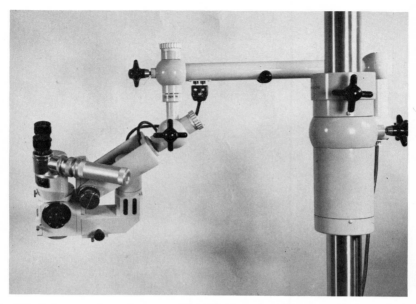

Fig. 31-1. Zeiss operating microscope. Magnification, 4 to 40 power. Entire unit is balanced on a support and moves at the touch of a finger. A metal tube connected to one eyepiece is itself an eyepiece for an observer.

ing loss caused by otosclerosis are the stapes mobilization, stapedectomy, and fenestration operations.

MYRINGOTOMY

Myringotomy is an old and excellent procedure that is done to release pus from the middle ear during acute otitis media. This procedure is often done in the outpatient clinic or physician's office. Smaller incisions (paracentesis) in the eardrum are made to release serum (serous otitis media). Occasionally a myringotomy is done so that the physician can look through the eardrum and inspect the middle ear. Myringotomy, like all surgical procedures for *acute* ear infections, is done less often today than in the years before antibiotics, because infections that usually required drainage often are cured with antibiotics before pus develops. Once a purulent process is established, myringotomy is indicated to evacuate pus. Myringotomy is also a charitable act: An infant may cry all night because of the pressure of pus in his middle ear; then he falls asleep immediately after myringotomy.

Anesthesia. Anesthesia for myringotomy may be local or general. More often than not, no anesthesia is used. Topical anesthesia for the eardrum can be achieved readily by touching a small area of the drumhead lightly with a tightly wound cotton applicator moistened in a saturated solution of phenol. This produces a whitening of a small area of the membrane and instant anesthesia. There is no permanent damage. Common topical anes-

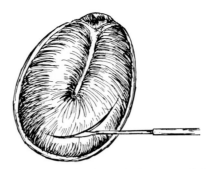

Fig. 31-2. Myringotomy incision made through the posteroinferior part of the eardrum to release pus in acute otitis media. (Compare with Fig. 28-3, p. 324.)

thetics such as cocaine and Pontocaine, which give adequate anesthesia for mucous membranes, have no effect on the eardrum.

Position. For the infant or young child the prone position is best. The patient's arms are extended alongside the body and are held there by a nurse. A sheet is used to mummy the patient. The head is turned on the side. A second attendant presses the head onto a firm table padded with a sheet folded several times—there is no place for pillows. One nurse is usually not enough; it is amazing how much power there is in a 20-pound infant trying to get loose.

There is some difference of opinion about whether parents should remain with the child during operative procedures. Dentists, for example, almost *never* allow parents to remain. Most otolaryngologists prefer not to operate when parents are present. Certainly the parents *should not* be made part of the operative team, for example, to restrain the child. On the other hand, some pediatricians do emphasize the psychologic need for the presence of the parents, saying that there is less trauma.

Incision. A curved incision is made in the posteroinferior part of the tympanic membrane with a *perfectly sharp* myringotomy knife (Fig. 31-2). The sharpness of the blade cannot be overemphasized—there must be no burs at the point. New knives should be used, and dull knives should be discarded or returned to the factory for sharpening. Disposable knives are now available. By checking the sharpness of the blade the nurse can ease the pain of the procedure manyfold.

As soon as the incision is made, pus pours from the middle ear and there is immediate relief of earache. Cotton in the ear canal catches pus and blood. The cotton is changed as needed, and the parents should be warned that pus is infected.

Aftercare. Even though a sweeping incision is made through half of the eardrum, the wound may heal in twenty-four hours, and the myringotomy may have to be repeated next day. Observation is continued until the eardrum returns to normal. The patient, after washing his hands, may insert new pieces of sterile cotton in his ear canal.

Complications. There are surprisingly few complications. To avoid the delicate middle ear bones myringotomy is done in the posteroinferior aspect of the tympanic membrane. A careless incision could dislocate the incus or stapes and result in severe hearing loss. Almost without exception the eardrum heals per primum and quickly. Usually one cannot tell where the incision was made. If, on a rare occasion, a small perforation remains, it may be closed with one of the tympanoplasty techniques.

There is a popular misconception about myringotomy that if the eardrum is cut, hearing is reduced greatly or even lost altogether. Exactly the opposite is true. When pus is left in the middle ear, there may be destruction of the middle ear bones or rupture of the eardrum. *Myringotomy, by releasing pus, saves hearing.* Even if a perforation were to result from myringotomy, little loss of hearing would be expected, since a small hole in the tympanic membrane does not alter hearing appreciably. Laymen often think that without an intact eardrum there can be no hearing, but this is not true.

ADENOIDECTOMY (FOR SEROUS OTITIS)

Although adenoidectomy is described in the discussion on tonsils and adenoids, it is mentioned here to emphasize a procedure of great importance in the restoration and preservation of hearing when hearing loss is caused by obstruction of the eustachian tubes by the adenoid. The condition is common in children. It is less common in adults because in them the adenoid (pharyngeal tonsil) has atrophied. The eustachian tube, which is closed most of the time, opens when we yawn or swallow, admitting air to the middle ear. This equalization of pressures on both sides of the eardrum is necessary for good hearing. When a mass of adenoid obstructs the pharyngeal orifice of the eustachian tube, the small amount of air already present in the middle ear is absorbed into the bloodstream, and since no new air can enter the middle ear via the eustachian tube, a partial vacuum forms. This negative pressure draws serum from the blood vessels of the middle ear mucosa until the serum fills or partially fills the tympanic cavity. The resultant condition is called *serous otitis media*. This fluid is not an exudate such as occurs in purulent otitis media but a sterile transudate. This train of events, which occurs most commonly during a cold, is self-limited. After the cold clears the adenoid regresses and the blocked tube opens. Some children have intermittent hearing loss several times a year caused by serous otitis media.

Treatment is adenoidectomy, a very effective procedure (described on p. 192) for restoring the hearing, especially in children. The nurse has an important postoperative responsibility—it usually is her job to watch for hemorrhage. When these patients bleed, they swallow their blood, and unless someone looks at their throats carefully, bleeding is overlooked. The patient becomes weak, the pulse is fast, and eventually he vomits a stomachful of dark blood.

Actually, although serous otitis media is common in children, serum in

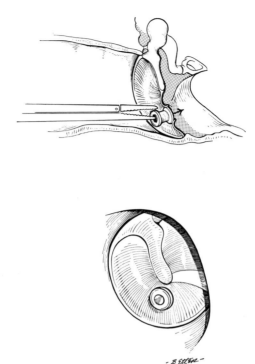

Fig. 31-3. The various plastic tubes to be inserted through the drumhead may be intro-duced with alligator forceps, a special introducer, or on the tip of a myringotomy knife. Where the double-flanged button tube is used, it is best slipped in just as any button is pushed through a buttonhole—edgewise and not full face forward.

the middle ear is less common than an extremely tenacious, semiliquid substance, which has given rise to the term *glue ear*. This middle ear "glue" is so thick that it can be aspirated only with difficulty. Myringotomy is performed just as for serous otitis media, the "glue" is aspirated, and often a small hollow plastic drainage or aerating tube is inserted through the ear-drum and left in place for several weeks or months (Fig. 31-3). These tubes serve as artificial eustachian tubes and permit aeration of the middle ear until the function of the eustachian tube is restored. The same plastic tube is used in the child or adult with serous otitis media.

The poly tube (metal tubes are also available) ordinarily extrudes from the tympanic membrane spontaneously after several weeks or months. Tubes extrude because the surface layer (squamous epithelium) of the tympanic membrane constantly "moves" or migrates from its center to-ward the margins as part of a cleaning process, and as the cells migrate out-ward the tube is carried along. Then the drumhead heals and the tube is free in the ear canal, where it may remain indefinitely or be extruded with wax. Because it is tiny, it usually goes unnoticed by the patient. If the tube does not extrude spontaneously, the doctor may have to remove it (an office procedure). The patient often returns to the doctor's office saying he thinks the tube came out because he is again hard of hearing. This indicates a recurrence of his serous otitis and the need for another tube, or an adenoidectomy, or both.

SIMPLE MASTOIDECTOMY

The mastoid ("breastlike") process is a part of the temporal bone. It has nothing to do with hearing, since other parts of the temporal bone contain the organs of hearing and balance. Visible as a bony prominence directly behind the outer ear, the mastoid is a honeycomb of air cells lined with mucous membrane. Mastoid air cells are not present at birth but develop in early life as a result of ingrowth of epithelium from the middle ear. Because each of the mastoid air cells is in continuity with the middle ear space (tympanic cavity), it is susceptible to any infection that attacks the middle ear. Sometimes, when the infant or young child suffers a middle ear infection (otitis media), the mastoid fails to develop normally. Infections somehow destroy the power of the middle ear mucosa to pneumatize the mastoid. Then instead of a well-pneumatized bone, the mastoid is almost solid—a so-called sclerotic mastoid. The type of mastoid bone, pneumatized or sclerotic, makes no difference to the patient because the mastoid portion of the temporal bone is not concerned with hearing.

Simple mastoidectomy was developed in the nineteenth century. Patients with acute mastoiditis (caused by infection spreading from the middle ear into the adjacent mastoid air cells) were in danger of their lives, since pus bathed vital structures in close contact with the mastoid. An incision was made behind the ear and down to the mastoid bone. In

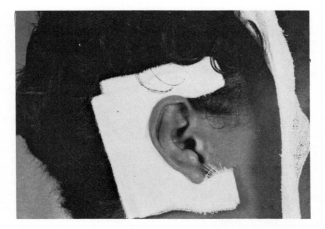

Fig. 31-4. Head dressing after mastoidectomy. It is important to pad the space directly behind the ear because if the ear is pressed tightly against the skull, it becomes painful. The gauze strip will later be used to tie together the several windings of gauze.

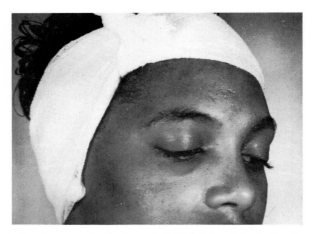

Fig. 31-5. Head dressing completed. Several fluffed 8 by 4 inch dressings were placed over the ear to absorb the drainage before the gauze was wrapped about the head. The common error is in getting the dressing *too low* so that it falls over the eyes—the dressing should be actually in the hair, not across the forehead.

some patients who had a subperiosteal abscess, pus poured out immediately, whereas in others in whom disease had not yet broken through the cortex, pus was found deeper in the mastoid. In either case air cells throughout the entire mastoid bone were infected and filled with pus and unhealthy granulation tissue. In simple mastoidectomy all diseased bone is removed and the mastoid left an empty shell. Nothing, however, is done to other parts of the temporal bone, and the hearing is expected to be unchanged after the operation.

Simple mastoidectomy is seldom done now because antibiotics usually control acute infections of the mastoid. However, in the presence of complications of acute mastoiditis simple mastoidectomy is still advocated. A postauricular incision or, to avoid the possibility of a postauricular fistula, an endaural incision (through the ear canal) can be used.

Postoperative care. After simple mastoidectomy relatively little postoperative care is required. A head dressing is worn (Figs. 31-4 and 31-5) for several days and may be reinforced by the nurse if drainage is noted. Drainage, however, is usually minimal. The initial dressing change is performed by the physician. If a drain has been inserted (Fig. 31-6), it is usually removed in seventy-two hours. Sutures are removed on the fifth or sixth postoperative day.

The defect in the mastoid fills in with granulation tissue, which later changes to scar tissue.

RADICAL MASTOIDECTOMY

Radical mastoidectomy consists of simple mastoidectomy plus an operation on the middle ear (tympanic portion of the temporal bone). This

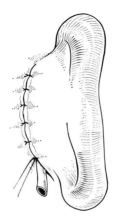

Fig. 31-6. Postauricular incision is sutured, and one Penrose drain is brought out of the lower part of the wound. Such an incision now is commonly used for any type of mastoidectomy and often for tympanoplasty.

operation is used for patients with chronically infected mastoids in contrast to simple mastoidectomy, which is used for patients with acute infections. In other words, patients requiring radical mastoidectomy have passed the stage when merely clearing disease from the mastoid would stop their infection. Unlike simple mastoidectomy, which does not affect hearing, the radical mastoidectomy does affect hearing. Were the operation to be done on a normal ear, which it never is, it would render that ear nonserviceable without the use of a hearing aid. In practice, radical mastoidectomy ordinarily *does not alter hearing appreciably* because by the time the patient needs the operation, hearing is already less than serviceable.

In radical mastoidectomy, after completing the mastoidectomy part of the operation, the surgeon approaches the middle ear and removes remnants of the eardrum, malleus, and incus, but he preserves the stapes and facial nerve. He also removes the posterior wall of the ear canal so that the middle ear and mastoid become one large cavity—easy to inspect and clean postoperatively. Healing occurs as skin grows into the cavity from the external ear canal. Sometimes a procedure called *musculoplasty* is done in conjunction with mastoidectomy. In this technique the mastoid cavity is filled with temporal muscle from above the ear so that postoperatively there is a smaller cavity.

In addition to the granulation tissue and pus commonly found in chronic ear infections, a ball of dead skin called *cholesteatoma* may also appear in the middle ear and mastoid. These spaces are normally lined with mucous membrane. But in chronic otitis media (which is usually synonymous with chronic mastoiditis) skin of the ear canal sometimes grows through a perforation in the eardrum and replaces the mucous membrane of the middle ear and mastoid. When that occurs, there is no easy way for desquamating skin to get out of the mastoid. An expanding ball of this dead skin (cholesteatoma) makes pressure on surrounding structures. Complications may result. Radical mastoidectomy is done probably as often to remove cholesteatoma as to clear infection; frequently the two conditions coexist.

Complications. The most dread complication of radical mastoidectomy is facial paralysis. This complication occurs if there is damage to the facial nerve in its course through the temporal bone. Normally the nerve is enclosed in a bony covering, the fallopian canal, but sometimes, either as a result of disease or because of a natural dehiscence, the nerve lies bare; then it is even more susceptible to injury. Postoperatively the nurse is instructed to watch the face for paralysis (on the same side as the operation, of course). In facial paralysis the patient closes one eye but not the other, he wrinkles his forehead on one side only, and his mouth pulls strongly to the good side when he tries to smile or show his teeth.

If the stapes bone, the innermost of the three middle ear bones, is dislodged from the oval window, there is a good chance that the patient will lose all hearing in that ear because of damage to the inner ear, which lies just on the other side of the footplate of the stapes. With severe inner ear damage even a hearing aid will not help. In the usual case when there is no trauma to the stapes or cochlea, radical mastoidectomy leaves the patient with hearing that is serviceable if a hearing aid is worn.

Postoperative care. At completion of the operation the mastoid cavity is packed—usually with a long strip of ½-inch gauze generously greased with petrolatum or, better, with an antibiotic ointment such as Neosporin or Terramycin. The packing is removed on the fourth or fifth postoperative day. Usually removal of packing is not painful, but a sensitive patient may appreciate the previous administration of meperidine (Demerol) or other analgesic. After the packing is removed there is a little bleeding, but it lasts only a short time. The patient is instructed how to place an untouched part of a cotton ball in the ear canal to absorb serum and other secretions.

While packing was still in the ear, a head dressing was in place (Figs. 31-4 and 31-5). This dressing must have gauze or cotton behind the ear, because if the ear is pressed hard against the head, there is pain. Another common mistake is applying the mastoid dressing *too low;* it soon falls over the eyes.

Dizziness or vertigo may be present for several days after radical mastoidectomy because of stimulation of the inner ear. The nurse should warn the patient to be careful about getting out of bed unassisted until it is clear that dizziness is not great enough to cause falling. She may need to assist him to the toilet for a day or two. Antiemetic drugs, sometimes prescribed, probably help some patients.

Unlike patients with simple mastoidectomy who require relatively little postoperative care, after radical mastoidectomy patients must be seen regularly (every week or two) for six or eight weeks or until the cavities are dry. After that the cavities should be inspected and cleaned once or twice yearly. Otherwise the skin that lines the cavities tends to become infected, and the ear may start to drain again.

Actually, radical mastoidectomy is now done rarely because the newer technique of tympanoplasty has supplanted this operation. Therefore the rather lengthy discussion of the radical mastoidectomy is somewhat of historical interest. The procedure was done frequently in the past, however, and many patients still require care to their cavities.

TYMPANOPLASTY

Tympanoplasty is the general name given to a group of operative procedures designed to restore hearing in patients with middle ear or conductive-type hearing loss. Usually such a patient has had a middle ear infection that left him with perforation of the tympanic membrane or necrosis of one of the middle ear bones. In congenital conditions a middle ear bone may be missing. After an injury, such as a slap on the ear, there may be dislocation of the incus. Tympanoplasty is used in all of these conditions and in others. Theoretically improvement of hearing is possible in any patient with loss of hearing who has a normal inner ear.

Tympanoplasty differs basically from mastoidectomy because in tympanoplasty it is sought to correct hearing loss, whereas in mastoidectomy the effort is to correct infection even with sacrifice of hearing. Tympanoplasty preferably is not done in an infected ear; mastoidectomy is done almost exclusively in infected ears in an effort to convert a dangerous ear into a safe ear and a draining ear into a dry ear. Tympanoplasty is often combined with mastoidectomy, either simple or radical.

Tympanoplasty operations have been performed for about twenty years. Different methods and materials are still being introduced in a search for the most successful techniques. For best results these operations should be done on clean, dry ears. If an ear is not free of infection, the operation must include removal of all infected tissue to make sure that the fascia grafts and various artificial prostheses that are used do not become infected and slough out.

Techniques. The simplest tympanoplasty is called myringoplasty, or type I tympanoplasty, and is a procedure performed to close a perforation in the eardrum that resulted from trauma or infection. One of the earlier procedures was to denude the remaining part of the eardrum by stripping the outer layer of squamous epithelium from the middle fibrous layer and then placing a skin graft from behind the ear onto the raw surface. The graft grew and, by bridging across the perforation, closed it. More recently epithelium from the ear canal has been used instead of postauricular skin because it is thinner and contains fewer glands. Sometimes the graft from the ear canal is handled as a free graft, whereas at other times it is left attached to a pedicle for better blood supply. Now skin is seldom used as a grafting material.

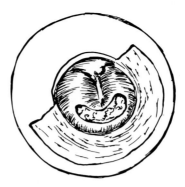

Fig. 31-7. Central perforation of the tympanic membrane. Epithelium has been removed from the ear canal and outer surface of the tympanic membrane.

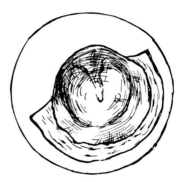

Fig. 31-8. Fascia from the temporalis area has been placed as a graft over the denuded tympanic membrane that suffered a perforation.

The most favored method of repairing a perforation is to use a *fascia graft* placed either on the outside or inside of the eardrum. Such a graft grows on the undersurface of the eardrum even though there is little denuded surface to afford a blood supply. Apparently it picks up sufficient nourishment from the mucosal layer to support it. Before the fascia is inserted through the perforation and placed against the inside of the eardrum, bits of Gelfoam soaked in saline solution are packed in the tympanic cavity to form a bed for the fascia and hold it against the eardrum. The Gelfoam is absorbed later. After several weeks the graft is well attached to the margins of the perforation, and the patient hears better. He also benefits because with the middle ear sealed, infection is less likely (Figs. 31-7 and 31-8).

The most popular tissue used for grafting is fascia stripped from the temporal muscle. A small piece of fascia can be removed easily and kept in a press, which stretches and thins the fascia, making it much easier to handle. The fascia is stretched over the defect in the eardrum and up onto the denuded adjacent walls of the ear canal. Small bits of Gelfoam moistened with saline or an antibiotic ear drop are used as packing. Eventually a thin layer of skin or squamous epithelium grows across the outer surface of the fascia, and mucous membrane from the middle ear side grows across its inner surface. The final results are good in most instances. The new graft forms an eardrum to protect the middle ear cavity from contamination from the outside, and in many instances the hearing is improved.

Other types of tympanoplasty (classified as types II through V) do more than merely patch a perforation in the eardrum. For example, in type III, the eardrum or graft replacing the eardrum is made to touch the head of the stapes. The normal route of sound transmission across the middle ear (eardrum to malleus to incus to stapes) has been disrupted by disease, and the new arrangement permits sound to pass directly from eardrum to stapes, often with excellent hearing as a result. A few otologic surgeons are using an intact tympanic membrane with one or two of the ossicles attached (taken from a cadaver). This composite graft is then used in place of fascia. It is also necessary to use fascia to supplement this graft. The results generally have been good but the technique is still new and one cannot yet make a definite statement about the eventual success of this technique.

Although in *theory* hearing loss from defects of the middle ear can always be restored, in *practice* the situation is sometimes different. Because of postoperative infection, bad technique, or rejection of grafts and prosthetic devices, results often are less satisfactory than expected.

Small tympanic perforations with apparently clean middle ear mucosa and no evidence of cholesteatoma can sometimes be closed successfully by office treatments. The margins of the perforation are cauterized with a tiny applicator moistened with trichloroacetic acid. This destroys the margin of squamous epithelium that often grows about the edges of the perforation and thus prevents healing. A patch of cigarette paper or other material is then placed across the perforation and the ear wet with Cortisporin or other ear drops. The epithelium grows across the paper, or starts to grow across, and the paper is extruded spontaneously or removed by the doctor. Then the process is repeated. When this technique is successful, it works very well indeed. The trouble is that in many cases a number of visits are required, even as many as ten or twenty, and sometimes there is no response at all. Because of the simplicity of the method, however, it is worth a trial in suitable patients.

Postoperative nursing care. After tympanoplasty the patient is hospitalized for three or four days. The inner dressing in the ear canal is left undisturbed; but if it becomes saturated with blood or drainage, the external dressing may changed. The patient should be instructed to avoid wetting the ear when bathing and to avoid blowing his nose because of danger of forcing a strong stream of air up the eustachian tube into the middle ear, which might dislodge the graft. Once healing is complete, most patients may swim and travel by air without restriction.

As with any operative procedure on the middle ear, patients with tympanoplasty are sometimes dizzy for a day or two postoperatively. The nurse may need to assist the patient when he first tries to walk. Some patients who are quite dizzy will exhibit nystagmus—a jerking movement of both eyes resulting from labyrinthine stimulation. The vertigo and accompanying nausea may be relieved by antimotion drugs and sedatives such as dimenhydrinate (Dramamine), diazepam (Valium), or chlorpromazine (Thorazine).

CHAPTER THIRTY-TWO

Otosclerosis and stapedectomy

OTOSCLEROSIS

Otosclerosis is a disease causing a gradually *progressive* hearing loss for which there is no medical treatment but an excellent operation—stapedectomy.

Otosclerosis produces loss of hearing by fixing or immobilizing the footplate of the stapes in the oval window. The cause of otosclerosis is unknown, but it has nothing to do with previous ear infections. The disorder tends to run in families, and it is more common in women than in men. It is rare in the Negro. Characteristically the hearing loss starts during the teens, but it is so gradual that patients seldom realize their disability for several years. It gradually worsens over the next ten to twenty or more years. As a rule, both ears are affected, although often not equally.

The new growth of bone about the stapes blocks its movement so that it is no longer free to vibrate effectively in response to sound pressure. At first there is little interference. In time, however, as the process advances, the stapes becomes so firmly fixed that it cannot move at all. You might think such a patient would be totally deaf since his stapes is useless. Actually he can still hear very well any sounds brought to his inner ear by "bone conduction." In short, although he hears poorly by the usual route, he hears clearly if a tuning fork, for example, is applied to his skull. Distinguishing between the patient's ability to hear by air and by bone conduction is important in diagnosing otosclerosis. When a patient with a *normal eardrum* and a history of *slowly progressive* hearing loss hears as well *by bone conduction as by air conduction,* or hears better, he almost certainly has otosclerosis.

STAPEDECTOMY

Stapedectomy is almost a hundred years old. Early attempts to restore hearing by this procedure were largely unsuccessful because of lack of antibiotics, adequate illumination, and magnification. Accordingly the operation was abandoned, and the fenestration ("window") operation, devised in Sweden and perfected by Julius Lempert, became a standard procedure to use in patients with otosclerosis. This operation worked well, but because of its disadvantages, when stapedectomy was revived and perfected during the 1950's, the fenestration operation was discarded. Now otologic surgeons rarely, if ever, do the fenestration operation.

The technique of fenestration included a preliminary mastoidectomy to gain working room, drilling an opening into the horizontal semicircular canal (a part of the inner ear), and sealing the opening with a skin graft. No effort was made to remove the immobilized stapes bone; it was left in place and bypassed. Now sound could enter the new window ("fenestra") in the inner ear, and the patient could again hear serviceably. This operation worked well, but it had the disadvantages of being a major surgical procedure, of leaving a mastoid cavity that required cleaning for the rest of the patient's life, and of not restoring all of the hearing because of loss of use of the eardrum and auditory ossicles (which were bypassed by the surgical procedure).

Stapedectomy, while still not altogether standardized, has become perfected to the point where the patient has about a 90% chance of a successful result. Minor alterations in techniques are still being suggested.

Figs. 32-1 to 32-7 indicate some of the more important aspects of tests for hearing. *Study the captions.* Keep in mind that diseases of the external ear and middle ear produce one type of hearing loss ("conductive"), whereas diseases of the inner ear cause a "sensorineural," or "perceptive," hearing loss. It is important to distinguish between the two.

In otosclerosis the surgical problem is largely a mechanical one. With

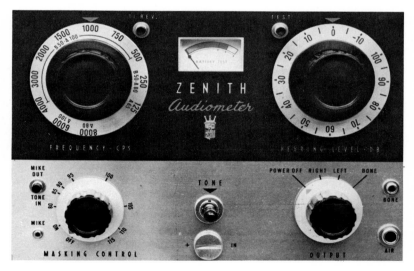

Fig. 32-1. Electric audiometer. Upper left-hand dial varies the frequency of the sound emitted through the earphone from very low to very high tones. Upper right-hand dial increases the intensity of the stimulus until the patient responds and indicates that he hears the signal. Lower left-hand dial presents a masking noise to the ear *not under the test* to make certain it is excluded from the test.

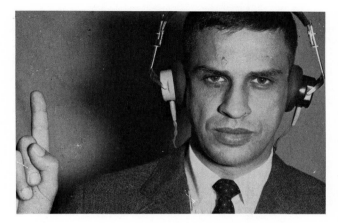

Fig. 32-2. Audiometry. Test sound is delivered through one earphone; the other earphone is used to present a masking noise. Patient signals if he hears the test sound.

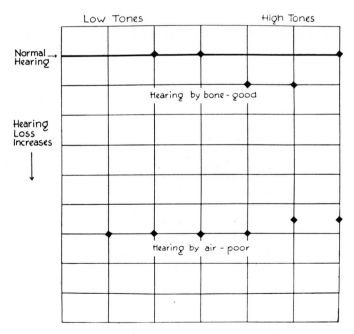

Fig. 32-3. Typical audiogram (shown without usual decibel and frequency scales) indicates good hearing by bone conduction and poor hearing by air conduction. This is the case in otosclerosis and other conditions in which the hearing loss is caused by a defect in the external or middle ear. When the inner ear is diseased, bone conduction measurements are no better than air conduction measurements.

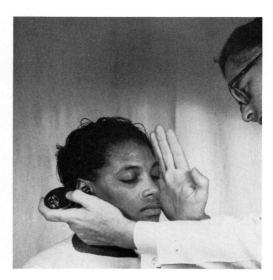

Fig. 32-4. Barany noise box (one of several methods) used to mask the ear *not* under test. *Failure to mask one ear is a common error in testing hearing.* Also note the examiner's hand shielding the patient's eyes so that she cannot read his lips as he delivers the numbers, words, and test phrases.

the stapes fixed in the oval window the surgeon must either break it loose so that it can move again or remove it completely and replace it with an artificial "bone." Until recently, medical opinion held that it was best simply to break the stapes loose and leave the middle ear as normal as possible. Now, however, most authorities agree that only to loosen the stapes (the "stapes mobilization" operation) is not enough; they think it is better in most cases to remove the entire bone. Stapedectomy (removing the stapes) is generally preferred to the stapes mobilization operation because, although the mobilization operation restores hearing for a time, the otosclerotic process continues and eventually refixes many of the "mobilized" stapes. Patients with good hearing immediately after the mobilization operation are disappointed when their hearing later drops back to what it had been. We will not discuss the mobilization operation here. You can better understand otosclerosis and its surgical treatment by learning about the stapedectomy procedure.

To enter the middle ear for *stapedectomy* the surgeon must turn or reflect the eardrum. With the patient under local anesthesia the surgeon makes a curved incision deep in the ear canal close to the rim of the eardrum. He does not cut the eardrum itself. The back half of the eardrum, freed from its attachment to the bone of the ear canal, is folded forward on itself like an omelette. As he works through the ear canal, the surgeon uses an operating microscope, which provides binocular vision, excellent illumination, and magnification. The tiny middle ear bones appear large and clear.

In otosclerosis the footplate of the stapes is solidly attached to the mar-

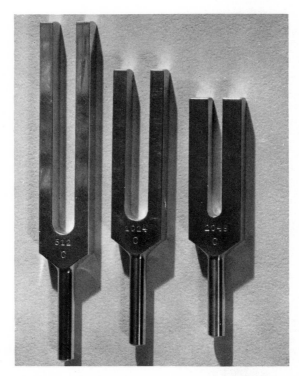

Fig. 32-5. Tuning forks used in testing hearing. The 512 fork (on the left) corresponds to middle C, and the others (1024 and 2048 double vibrations per second) are one and two octaves higher. This range represents the heart of the speech frequencies.

gins of the oval window. Pulling on the head of the stapes usually does not remove the entire bone; instead, the legs break off at the footplate. Head, neck, and both legs (the "superstructure") lift out, but the footplate remains fast. So, to dislodge and remove the footplate, sometimes in one piece and sometimes in several, the surgeon uses various picks or needles and sometimes an electric drill. Once the footplate is removed, the surgeon must seal the open oval window and then connect the oval window with the incus to restore the normal pathway of sound conduction. Several methods are in common usage. In one method a preformed prosthesis of wire with Gelfoam fixed to one end is introduced into the ear. The Gelfoam, which seals the window, is absorbed after a week or two. The wire to which it is attached is looped over the incus and the loop crimped to fix it in place. Sound pressure is transmitted from incus to wire and finally reaches the liquids of the inner ear where hearing takes place. Mucous membrane replaces the Gelfoam after a few weeks (Fig. 32-8, right upper figure).

Another method uses a small piece of vein from the back of the hand or fascia from the temporalis area. The vein or fascia is stretched across the open oval window, and then any one of several prostheses is used to bridge the gap between incus and vein. The original method (Shea) was a plastic tube cut on a bevel at one end and straight across at the other. The lower beveled end was placed on the vein graft and one end of the incus dropped into the upper end of the prosthesis (Fig. 32-9, *B*). This method has been replaced largely by other prostheses, some of which are seen in Fig. 32-8. As soon as the connection is made with the incus, the patient's hearing is improved. When the eardrum is returned, he hears even better.

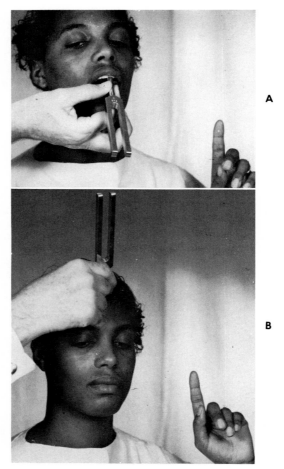

Fig. 32-6. A, Weber test. A ringing tuning fork on the midline of the skull or upper incisor teeth is *normally* heard with equal loudness in both ears. In *conductive* hearing loss (caused by diseases of the external or middle ear) bone-conducted sound lateralizes to the *poorer* ear. In *nerve* or *perceptive* hearing loss (caused by disease of the inner ear or central nervous system pathways) the fork is heard louder in the *better* ear. **B,** Weber test—alternate placement of fork.

Later that day blood forms in the middle ear and in the ear canal so that the hearing is usually reduced again for a week or so until the blood clot dries and cracks open to again admit sound pressure through the external auditory canal.

After stapedectomy, hearing improves permanently in the great majority of patients. This is not to say that completely normal hearing is restored, although often it is, or that in a few instances hearing may not become even worse. *Stapedectomy is done on only one ear at a time—the poorer ear.*

The patient's course after operation is ordinarily smooth, but an occasional patient may experience vertigo for a few days. If vertigo does occur postoperatively, patients should be cautioned against rapid turning. They

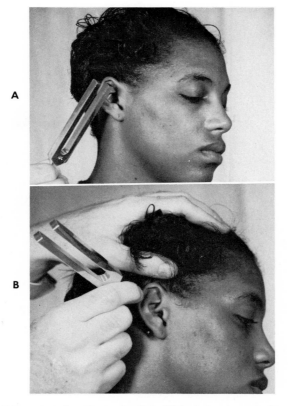

Fig. 32-7. A, Rinne test for air conduction. This test compares bone conduction with air conduction—alternately. In the *normal* patient the fork is heard about twice as long by air as by bone conduction. In *conductive* hearing loss (external or middle ear) the ratio alters in favor of bone conduction, and in severe conductive loss the ratio may be 2:1 in favor of bone conduction. In *nerve* or *perceptive* hearing loss the ratio of 2:1 remains about the same, but *both* air and bone conduction are reduced. **B,** Rinne test for bone conduction.

should be given assistance when walking or getting in and out of bed. The usual hospital stay is two or three days.

Nursing care

The patient is told not to blow his nose for a week so that he will not force air up the eustachian tube and loosen his eardrum. The surgeon may leave instructions for the patient to maintain a particular head position

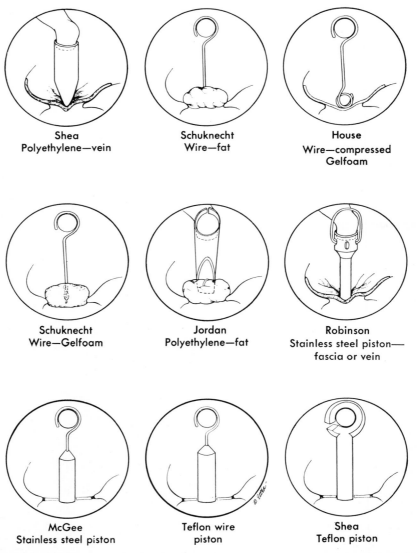

Shea
Polyethylene—vein

Schuknecht
Wire—fat

House
Wire—compressed
Gelfoam

Schuknecht
Wire—Gelfoam

Jordan
Polyethylene—fat

Robinson
Stainless steel piston—
fascia or vein

McGee
Stainless steel piston

Teflon wire
piston

Shea
Teflon piston

Fig. 32-8. The more commonly used prostheses shown immediately after being positioned. Later the various grafts thin out and become contiguous with the adjacent mucoperiosteum.

so that there is less likelihood of the plastic strut slipping. Blood usually forms in the ear canal, and cotton in the meatus is changed by the nurse as required. Pain is present for a few hours after operation, and one or two injections of meperidine, 100 mg., may be necessary. If the patient becomes vertiginous, the physician must be notified at once. Antibiotics are given to prevent postoperative infection.

The surgical nurse

During stapedectomy the nurse in surgery can be of inestimable value if she knows intimately the instruments required and if, between procedures, she keeps all instruments in working order. The fine hooks, needles, and forceps used in stapedectomy are, without a doubt, the most delicate and finest used in any type of surgical procedure. Many of the instruments have points or working ends measuring no more than 0.3 to 0.5 mm. Special needles used for suction are of the size of a No. 20- to 27-gauge hypodermic needle and become readily clogged with blood unless irrigated after each use. Furthermore, the operation is usually performed in semidarkness, with only the operating microscope for light. This means that there is no chance to look at instruments during the operation, since many are too small to identify even in a well-lighted room. Most surgeons have special trays in which each instrument is kept in a numbered slot.

HEARING AIDS

The hearing of persons with otosclerosis and many other patients can also be assisted by means of a hearing aid. Hearing aids are instruments

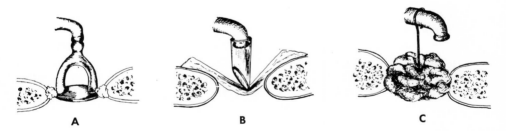

A   **B**   **C**

Fig. 32-9. **A,** Stapes fixed or immobilized by otosclerotic focus at each end of footplate. **B,** An early type of stapedectomy. The stapes bone which originally fitted in the oval window has been removed. Plastic tube or "strut" fits over lenticular process of incus and presses on vein graft which now lies across the oval window. With the otosclerotic obstruction removed sound can be conducted again from the eardrum→malleus→incus→ plastic strut→vein graft→fluids of inner ear→organ of Corti with its hair cells→acoustic nerve→brain. The particular arrangement is somewhat insecure and is not widely used at the present time. **C,** Another early method of stapedectomy. Alternate method of stapedectomy. Stainless steel wire is tied around small plug of fat from the ear lobe and the other end of the wire is crimped over the incus. The fat fits loosely in the oval window from which the obstructive stapedial footplate has been removed. Sound pressure is transmitted from the incus to the fat plug. **B** and **C** illustrate two *early* methods, neither of which are used commonly today.

like radios, which make sound more intense when a dial is turned. *They do nothing to improve* hearing but simply make sound louder. Therefore the person with middle ear disease generally uses a hearing aid well, because all that is needed to make him hear and to make him understand what he hears is to amplify the sound. When amplified sound reaches his normal inner ear, he responds as would a normal person. In contrast, when inner ear disease causes hearing loss, the person may still fail to understand speech even though it is amplified by a hearing aid. Such patients often complain that hearing aids do nothing to make speech more distinct. Consequently *patients with middle ear hearing loss generally make better users of hearing aids than do patients with inner ear hearing loss.* Sometimes, to determine whether a patient should be advised to buy an aid, it may be necessary to test the patient with and without an aid. Many times the gain is borderline. In such a case, if the patient buys an aid, he may later put it away because he finds it a nuisance rather than a help.

The following are answers to common questions about hearing loss:

1. *Will I ever go totally deaf?* Regardless of cause, most patients who can still hear when they ask this question never lose all their hearing. Total deafness is rare. Usually it results from a prenatal condition or a childhood illness or from some other condition that attacks the ears rather suddenly and leaves the individual without hearing. It is seldom the result of a hearing loss than increases gradually, year by year.

2. *Can I hear without an eardrum?* Yes, of course. Loss of the eardrum, or part of it, is one of the causes of middle ear hearing loss, and like all middle ear disorders, loss of the eardrum causes only partial deafness. Such hearing loss may be corrected, at least in some cases, by surgical treatment.

3. *Will a hearing aid help me?* A ready answer to this question is sometimes not possible, and special testing or a trial with an aid may required to make certain. However, in general, if a patient hears as well, or even better, by bone conduction as by air conduction, a middle ear defect and a normal inner ear are indicated, and therefore the patient should be a good user of a hearing aid. (Remember, too, that such a patient may do even better by having his hearing restored by surgery.)

If the patient has trouble hearing when there is a background of noise, or when several persons are talking at once, or if he knows he has a nerve loss, he will do less well with an aid. *But even these patients often profit from an aid,* and they are in the majority of patients with hearing loss.

4. *What percentage loss have I?* A percentage expression of hearing loss is inexact because hearing losses are usually different at different frequencies. Furthermore, loss of reception for pure tone signals (the usual test) may not correlate well with ability to understand speech.

5. *Which hearing aid is best?* Actually, few significant differences exist among the hearing aids produced by various manufacturers. The chief differences are in service. Most hearing aid dealers have little training in matters related to hearing; their training is in salesmanship. The dealer should know that his hearing aid serves only to make sound louder and that it

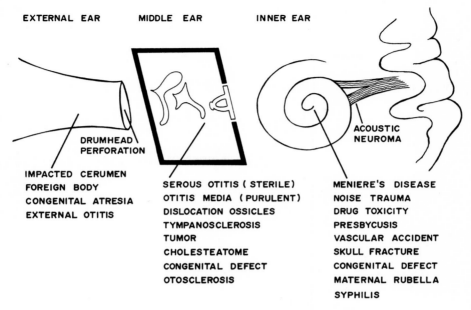

EXTERNAL EAR   MIDDLE EAR   INNER EAR

DRUMHEAD
PERFORATION

ACOUSTIC
NEUROMA

IMPACTED CERUMEN
FOREIGN BODY
CONGENITAL ATRESIA
EXTERNAL OTITIS

SEROUS OTITIS (STERILE)
OTITIS MEDIA (PURULENT)
DISLOCATION OSSICLES
TYMPANOSCLEROSIS
TUMOR
CHOLESTEATOME
CONGENITAL DEFECT
OTOSCLEROSIS

MENIERE'S DISEASE
NOISE TRAUMA
DRUG TOXICITY
PRESBYCUSIS
VASCULAR ACCIDENT
SKULL FRACTURE
CONGENITAL DEFECT
MATERNAL RUBELLA
SYPHILIS

Fig. 32-10. Causes of hearing loss in the three parts of the ear.

varies from another aid chiefly in price or appearance. The patient should be careful to choose a dealer he trusts and one who is expected to be in business next year. He must be wary of high-pressure salesmen.

Consultation with an otologist before purchasing an aid would save trouble and money for many patients. Then either the otologist or his audiologist can advise the patient concerning the need for an aid, which ear to fit, and other pertinent information.

6. *If I don't wear a hearing aid, will lack of use of the ear make my hearing get worse?* No. The ear, even though partially deafened, is stimulated constantly by loud sounds, and even if it were not, loss of hearing is not analogous to the wasting of muscular tissue that occurs from disuse.

For easy reference, Fig. 32-10 lists conditions causing hearing loss according to site of pathologic process. Those in the external ear and middle ear are generally correctable; those in the inner ear and central nervous system are not. (See also Chapters 33 and 34.)

SUGGESTED READING

DeLaney, R. E.: Stapedectomy, American
  Journal of Nursing **69:**2406, Nov., 1969.

CHAPTER THIRTY-THREE

Sensorineural hearing loss; functional hearing loss; tinnitus

Until now we have discussed what happens to hearing in diseases of the external and middle ears. The third part of the ear, the inner ear, serves as both the organ of hearing and the organ of balance. It is made of delicate nerve tissue, which, once damaged, does not recover. Therefore, for protection the inner ear is situated deep in the head in the petrous bone, the hardest part of the temporal bone. There are only three important symptoms caused by disease of the inner ear and its central nervous system pathways in the brain: *hearing loss, vertigo* (dizziness), and *tinnitus* (ear ringing). Pain and loss of consciousness are *not expected;* if these symptoms are present, they point toward disease of the central nervous system.

SENSORINEURAL HEARING LOSS

When we discussed hearing loss resulting from external and middle ear disease, we said that the difficulty was mechanical and that sound waves, for one reason or another, were impeded in the course of their passage toward the inner ear. As examples, we cited a perforation in the eardrum, preventing proper collection of sound; absence of one of the middle ear bones, preventing normal transmission of sound from the eardrum to the inner ear; and otosclerosis, in which there is a fixation of the stapes, preventing its normal vibration in the oval window. We learned that, at least in theory, all defects of the external and middle ear that produce hearing loss are remediable.

The special nerve tissue of the inner ear that forms the sensory organ for hearing will not regenerate after injury. Therefore, once neural tissue is damaged and hearing loss occurs, there are no medical or surgical measures that can be expected to restore hearing.

Sometimes inner ear hearing loss results from prenatal disease affecting the mother—one example is German measles during early pregnancy; the child is born hard of hearing or deaf, and no treatment will restore the hearing. More commonly, however, conditions arising after birth are responsible. Some of the more important causes include infections, especially viral infections such as mumps; drugs toxic to the inner ear; head injury; intense noise, especially when prolonged; and the aging process.

Among the *drugs severely toxic to the inner ear* are kanamycin, neomycin, dihydrostreptomycin, and gentamicin. These drugs should never be given by injection if equally effective drugs can be substituted. Neomycin can be given by mouth in relatively large doses, since it is not well absorbed from the gastrointestinal tract. It can cause ototoxicity if used as a wet dressing on raw surfaces of open wounds, or as an irrigant. Another drug, streptomycin, while not producing hearing loss, is toxic to the vestibular apparatus of the inner ear. Salicylates, including aspirin, quinine, and quinidine, are also recognized as ototoxic drugs. Tinnitus, for example, is a common symptom of overdosage with aspirin. For the most part, however, these drugs do not cause the severe ototoxicity with profound permanent hearing loss caused by the antibiotic group of ototoxic drugs.

It is unfortunate to have a hearing loss for which there is no medical or surgical treatment, but, as if to add insult to injury, still other factors make inner ear hearing loss especially difficult for a patient. One of these difficulties is the problem that the patient has in *understanding* what he hears. Sound may reach his inner ear with sufficient intensity to cause hearing, yet he may fail to interpret that sound as meaningful words. In contrast, to hear perfectly the patient with middle ear disease and a *normal inner ear* needs only to have the speaker raise his voice. But the patient with inner ear disease often fails to understand at least part of what he hears, *regardless of the intensity* of the speaker's voice because part of the function of the inner ear is to distinguish among words that sound alike. In a test to demonstrate this problem, if the words *sin, thin,* and *fin* are said loudly enough to a patient with middle ear hearing loss (or to a person with normal hearing), he should be able to repeat the words correctly. The patient with inner ear hearing loss, on the other hand, often fails when he tries to repeat the words because he does not hear the fine differences among them. He hears *in* but he guesses at the *s, th,* and *f.* As a result of his poor auditory discrimination, he may repeat the same word three times. The confusion is compounded when he listens against a background of noise or when several persons talk at the same time.

Noise-induced hearing loss

Hearing loss caused by loud noise is the most common and the most important type of occupational hearing loss. Exposure to industrial noise levels greater than 85 to 90 decibels for months or years causes cochlear damage. In the early stage there is a loss of hearing at or near the frequency of 4,000 cycles per second. Later the damage extends to both the higher and lower tones. The lowest tones are affected least.

If it is necessary for a person to continue working in the area of high noise level, he can use ear protectors, or plugs, as they are often called. These plugs are inserted into the external auditory canal, and in some persons they reduce the noise reaching the middle ear by 10 to 30 decibels. Earplugs are usually made of rubber or malleable plastic and come in several sizes to fit different auditory canals. Some protectors are custom-made; they are molded to the individual ear canal by impression techniques. They offer a better seal but are more expensive. In most industries the standard plugs are used.

In industries with extremely high noise levels, such as jet engine factories, simple earplugs do not afford enough protection. In such factories, where the sound level may reach 140 decibels, workmen wear earplugs, muffs over the ears, and, finally, a large shield over the entire head.

Similarly, hearing loss associated with firearms such as the M-16 rifle, but also with guns used in sports, can readily occur. The loss tends to be substantially greater in the left than in the right ear for a right-handed person shooting from the shoulder. With revolvers, the hearing loss is equal in both ears. Patients should be warned that, if firing guns causes tinnitus, a sensation of fullness in the ears, or temporary hearing loss, they probably should not fire or else should wear suitable ear protectors.

Also of interest is the observation that high-intensity music, such as rock music, is quite capable of producing hearing loss. Typical readings of 110-decibel sound-pressure levels at 30 feet from the loudspeaker will produce a severe temporary threshold shift in about 16% of young listeners.

Sudden deafness

Sudden deafness, unilateral and sensorineural, and usually profound, may appear instantaneously in a person who just previously had no apparent hearing loss. Some patients say they hear a "click" in one ear and then realize they are deaf in that ear. Others go to bed hearing normally but wake up deaf in one ear and thus are not certain just when their deafness commenced. Subsequently, over a period of days or weeks this profound loss may lessen, at least a little, and in some cases there is complete recovery. Vertigo as an associated symptom is inconstant. Some patients become sick and vomit and are incapacitated for several days. Others have only a transient and mild vertigo lasting for a few hours. Many have no vertigo.

The clinical entity of sudden, profound, sensorineural, unilateral hearing loss was long considered as a vascular accident until rather recently, when viral factors began to be recognized as causative.

Treatment of idiopathic sudden deafness has been with a great variety of drugs, including vasodilators and steroids, but it is not at all certain whether any of them have been helpful. The only alternative to treatment, however, is to do nothing, and most physicians will want to hospitalize these patients and offer therapy with either steroids or vasodilators, or both.

Presbycusis

Presbycusis is the term given to hearing loss associated with the aging process. It is probably the result of atrophy of the ganglion cells in the cochlea. The degenerative changes producing this type of hearing loss parallel those that occur in other tissues of the body as senility approaches. Presbycusis is characterized by bilateral gradual loss of hearing. Beginning with a loss of the high tones, it slowly progresses to involve the middle and lower tones.

Acoustic neuroma

Acoustic neuroma as a cause of hearing loss is rather rare but it deserves special attention because of its great importance. Usually the first symptom is tinnitus; the onset of hearing loss may be delayed months or years. In late stages there will be vertigo of a constant, usually mild, type, and finally facial paralysis as the seventh and eighth cranial nerves are compressed in the internal auditory canal.

Treatment is by surgical removal. Small and medium-sized tumors can be resected through a middle cranial fossa or translabyrinthine approach, whereas large tumors are best approached through the posterior cranial fossa by neurosurgical techniques.

FUNCTIONAL HEARING LOSS

One other general type of hearing loss is called *functional,* or hysterical. The condition is seldom understood by the patient, and the diagnosis is resented by relatives. *Patients with functional hearing loss have no ear disease.* In fact, they have no physical or "organic" abnormality at all; they have a psychologic condition that somehow prevents them from responding normally to sound. They are not malingerers. *Malingerers* are persons who intentionally feign hearing loss for secondary gains. They hope to derive some benefit, usually financial, as from an insurance company after an accident or to avoid certain duties, such as serving in the Armed Forces when drafted. Rather, these patients find their supposed hearing loss a convenient crutch or psychologic device to help them through life.

The recognition of functional hearing loss is of great importance since if overlooked and ascribed to an organic cause (sensorineural loss), the patient might needlessly be fitted with a hearing aid, or told that there is no help for his hearing loss, or (in the case of a malingerer) assisted in his unscrupulous design.

TINNITUS (EAR RINGING)

Tinnitus is the medical term for ringing in the ears, a very common condition. It may be unilateral or bilateral, or the patient may be unable to say just where the noise seems to localize and refers to it as head noise. Almost anyone with normal hearing, upon entering a quiet room and listening carefully, experiences a little tinnitus. Apparently this much is normal, or physiologic. At the other extreme are patients whose ringing is so great that they can think of nothing else but the terrible noise in their heads and what they can do to get rid of it. Some even threaten suicide. Heroic measures such as cutting the auditory nerve have been tried, but as often as not tinnitus persists. This persistence would indicate that not all head noise arises from the ear but that it results sometimes from disease of the central nervous system. Between these two extremes are the great majority of persons with tinnitus who have head noise and wish they did not but who can forget it most of the time. Their tinnitus bothers them most in quiet surroundings, for example, in their bedrooms when they are trying to fall asleep. They also become disturbed when they have an introspective turn and start to worry about themselves.

The character of the sound that patients hear varies greatly. Many liken their head noise to escaping air. Others say, variously, that they hear a sizzling or frying sound, crickets chirping, the hum of a telephone wire, running water, or just a loud noise which they say they cannot describe. One woman reported that her tinnitus sounded like a train running through her head. Sometimes a person can identify the approximate pitch of his ringing, and if he listens to several tuning forks presented to his good ear, he may be able to pick out a tone that matches his ringing. Others, however, have great difficulty making up their minds as to pitch, probably because their tinnitus is a mixture of sounds in which no one tone predominates.

Undoubtedly the loudness of tinnitus depends a great deal upon the patient's frame of mind. When all goes well, tinnitus is likely to be less annoying and less noticeable than when everything seems to be wrong. There is no accurate way to measure the loudness of a patient's tinnitus, because no one else can hear it and his statement as to loudness is the physician's only measure. An approximation of loudness can be made by placing a sound of known intensity in his good ear and asking him to compare the loudness of that sound with the loudness of his tinnitus. By knowing how other patients have matched the loudness of their tinnitus, the physician gets an idea of the patient's distress.

Causes of tinnitus

Many different conditions may produce tinnitus. Those related to the external or middle ear are well understood and are often correctible because they are accessible. A plug of wax in the ear canal, for example, may cause tinnitus. Another remedial cause is perforation of the eardrum, although of course, not all perforations produce ringing. If the coexistent hearing loss is not great (and often with a small perforation it is not), patients may complain more of the ringing than of the hearing loss. Many perforations heal spontaneously, but for those that do not, surgical repair may close the hole and relieve the tinnitus. Sometimes, however, it is not certain whether it is the perforation that causes the patient's tinnitus or whether coexistent disease of the inner ear is responsible.

Another rather common middle ear cause of tinnitus is the disorder called *otosclerosis*. In this condition the stapes, the innermost of the three tiny middle ear bones, gradually becomes fixed to the margins of the oval window. Normally the stapes vibrates in the oval window to transmit sound pressure to the inner ear. Patients with otosclerosis complain more of hearing loss than of tinnitus, but if asked, most will say that they have a noise in one or both ears. Often they volunteer that if the ringing would just stop, they could hear better. After a stapedectomy, the operation devised to improve hearing in these patients, ringing is often relieved.

The eustachian tube connects the middle ear with the back of the nose or upper part of the pharynx. When the tube fails to function properly (it should open during yawning and swallowing to admit air to the middle ear), there may be tinnitus. Minor degrees of tubal malfunction are common. Prolonged tubal closure may result in the collection of blood serum in the middle ear space; with the tube blocked, the little air that remains in the middle ear is absorbed into the bloodstream until a partial vacuum develops; then serum is pulled from the blood vessels into the middle ear by negative pressure. Since this disorder is usually self-limited, treatment for a newly blocked eustachian tube may not be necessary. The physician may prescribe medication such as the antihistimines to open the tube or he may blow air into the tube via a cannula inserted through the nose. The treatment is a good one when indicated. Unfortunately it is possible that more harm than good has been done by these manipulations, because many persons who have had repeated treatments for tinnitus or hearing loss never had tubal obstruction in the first place. If these patients had really been afflicted with tubal difficulty, one or two treatments should have cleared their tubes, but because their tinnitus usually comes from disease of the inner ear, no amount of treatment to the middle ear or eustachian tube does any good.

An unusual cause of tinnitus is dislocation of the middle ear bones. After a slap on the ear the incus may become dislodged from the stapes; tinnitus and hearing loss result. The bones can be replaced by a fairly simple operation. For example, one patient whose friend boxed him on the ear had severe hearing loss as well as a loud roaring in the ear. When the incus was repositioned and made to touch the stapes, tinnitus disappeared and hearing was restored.

Except for disorders such as the foregoing, which affect the external and middle ear, *most conditions that produce tinnitus affect the inner ear or its pathways in the brain.* These areas are hidden from direct observation so that information gained about them must come by testing their functions. Roentgenographic examinations do not help much. Even if it were possible to remove the inner ear in order to work on it, not much added information could be gained. Its parts are microscopic and complex, with thousands of delicate hearing elements called hair cells. Contrasted to the relatively large and accessible middle ear structures, these parts are almost unapproachable. Consequently treatment of tinnitus resulting from a disturbance of the inner ear or its central connections is definitely not a surgical matter. Alterations in function rather than gross changes in structure account for most examples of inner ear tinnitus.

A classic cause of tinnitus, common enough to deserve special mention, is Meniere's disease (see Chapter 36). This disorder also causes partial hearing loss in one ear and severe vertigo. Although vertigo may stop eventually, the hearing loss and ringing remain. Usually such patients have a noise in one ear all the time. During a crisis the ringing gets worse. The patient with Meniere's disease, however, tends to minimize his tinnitus because he is more concerned with vertigo.

Acoustic neuroma, a tumor arising in the internal auditory canal from the sheath of the eighth cranial or acoustic nerve, often causes tinnitus. Although rare, acoustic neuroma is an important cause of tinnitus because in such a patient it may be the earliest symptom, coming on before hearing loss, and long before the late symptoms of vertigo and facial paralysis.

Salicylate toxicity is another cause of tinnitus. Usually the symptom clears when the drug is stopped or the dosage reduced.

The role of noise in the production of tinnitus deserves special mention. Many persons, when exposed to an intense noise even for a short time, such as the report of a high-powered rifle, experience ringing for hours afterward. More prolonged exposure may cause ringing for days, weeks, or even permanently. There is a variation in the susceptibility of ears to injury by noise; noise that makes one man's ears ring all day may have no effect on someone else's. When tinnitus occurs after noise exposure, hearing loss, temporary or permanent, may also occur. As a matter of fact, many times hearing tests show a sharp dip near the frequency at which the patient complains of tinnitus. This writer tells patients that ringing produced by noise is a warning: It means that if they do not get away from the noise, they may lose their hearing.

The hearing test is an important part of the examination of the patient with tinnitus. Many patients, especially those who have had tinnitus for some time, are found to have hearing loss. Sometimes the hearing loss is a part of a clinical entity such as Meniere's disease or otosclerosis. A sharp dip in hearing in the higher frequencies is typical of an ear injured by noise. It is important to learn whether hearing loss is caused by middle ear or by inner ear disease; middle car disorders are often correctable, but inner ear disease is not.

Treatment

Were a physician to devise an effective surgical technique for the relief of tinnitus, he would be unable to care for the patients who would flock to his door. As you might guess, a number of operations have been tried. Some of them, when originally reported, seemed to be useful, but when other surgeons reported failure, the procedures were abandoned.

What of medical treatment? It, too, is unrewarding. On the assumption that many instances of tinnitus are caused by spasm of blood vessels that supply the inner ear, physicians may prescribe drugs to dilate cerebral vessels. Many physicians tell patients who have had tinnitus for a long time that there is no likelihood that any therapy, medical or surgical, is going to improve their head noise and that if they will just wait, the noise may decrease or stop altogether. This advice, of course, is given after a painstaking examination to exclude any remediable causes. Generally the patient accepts the explanation and appreciates the fact that he is not asked to return for a series of injections or office treatments. Nicotinic acid, a commonly prescribed medication, probably is of no value for patients with tinnitus.

In Meniere's disease medical treatment may improve all three symptoms, but usually the tinnitus and hearing loss persist even though the vertigo comes under control. Occasionally a patient with severe and frequent attacks of vertigo fails to respond to medical management. If the affected ear has poor hearing, and it usually does, an operation can abolish the attacks of vertigo permanently, but the operation destroys all function in one ear. Moreover, it does not always abolish the ringing.

CHAPTER THIRTY-FOUR ## Hearing impairment

Ernest R. Nilo, Ph.D.*

The intent of this chapter is to consider certain aspects of hearing impairment, with emphasis on some of the communicative problems which result and the therapeutic measures undertaken. The sense of hearing is critical to normal development and maintenance of speech. Through hearing the infant receives the speech patterns of others to emulate. Important to this developmental process is the infant's ability to monitor his own attempts at speech. Hearing is also critical to this monitoring function, which eventually guides him to the formulation of adequate speech skills.

The important relationship of hearing to speech is a continuing one; it extends from the developmental processes of speech through the maintenance of established speech skills used in everyday communication. When hearing is defective, a break results in this critical relationship.

NORMAL HEARING

General consideration of certain aspects of the normal hearing process is helpful to understanding the impairment of hearing and the ensuing problems of communication. From a physical standpoint, sound is a form of energy generated by a vibrating source. Simple sound waves may be called pure tones; an example are those generated by a tuning fork. Others are complex, like the sounds produced by the human voice. Two parameters of sound which are important in measuring hearing are "intensity" and "frequency."

Intensity refers to the pressure exerted by a sound, and the unit used to express intensity is the decibel (dB). "Loudness" is not quite the same as intensity, but rather refers to the sensation experienced by a person to the intensity of sound. The loudness of a sound of a given intensity is

---

*Director of Audiological Services, Department of Otolaryngology, The Ohio State University Hospital, Columbus, Ohio.

reduced for a person with impaired hearing compared to a person with normal hearing. The loud sound of a rivet hammer nearby has an intensity of about 100 dB; a low whisper at 5 feet is approximately 10 dB. Speech that is comfortably loud ranges in intensity from approximately 40 to 65 dB (Fig. 34-1).

Frequency refers to the number of vibratory cycles per second of sound and is expressed in Hertz (Hz), formerly expressed in cycles per second (cps). "Pitch" relates to frequency and, like loudness, does not describe a physical measurement but a sensation. A sound with a frequency of 125 Hz is perceived as a tone low in pitch, whereas one of 8,000 Hz is heard as a high-pitched tone. Generally a child or young adult can hear fre-

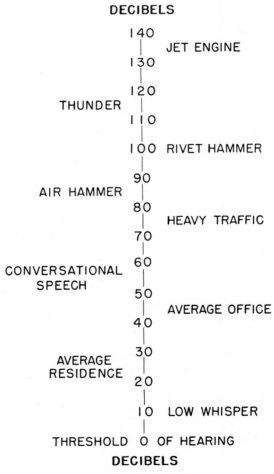

Fig. 34-1. Intensity range of human hearing—intensity levels of various environmental sounds and situations.

quencies from about 20 to 20,000 Hz. Hearing is most sensitive in the frequencies from 500 to 4,000 Hz, the range in which the important speech sounds occur.

Sound follows basically two pathways in reaching the inner ear, where its initial transformation in the processing to meaningful sensation takes place (Fig. 34-2). The more sensitive of the two pathways is through the ear canal and across the ossicular chain to the inner ear. This is commonly referred to as "air conduction hearing" in clinical measurement of hearing. The second pathway of sound transmission to the inner ear is through the bones of the skull, "bone conduction hearing." However, the inner ear is stimulated, whether by air or bone conduction, sound energy that has been a mechanical force begins its transformation in the inner ear into neural energy. As this neural energy continues on its way to the brain via the auditory nerve and pathways, it is somehow "decoded," and upon reaching the brain it is interpreted as meaningful speech.

IMPAIRED HEARING
Symptoms

Hearing loss is not always recognized by the patient. In the adult a sudden loss of hearing is usually noticed at once, but when the loss is gradual (as in ostosclerosis), many years may lapse before the patient is aware of

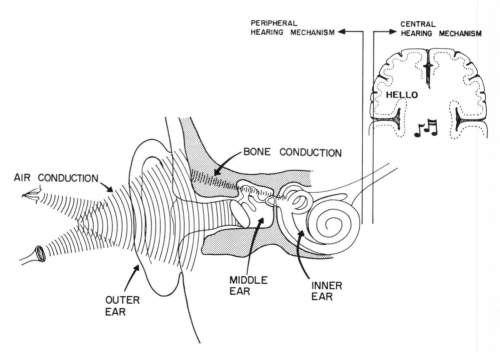

Fig. 34-2. This schematic drawing depicts the functions of the hearing mechanism as it translates sound waves into meaningful sensations.

hearing loss. With children the parents and teachers often are the first to suspect a hearing problem. In the young child total hearing loss may be more easily detected than partial loss, as the symptoms are usually more dramatic. However, a child with a severe *unilateral* hearing impairment may go undetected for years. The following are common clues that suggest hearing impairment in a school child:

1. Asking to have things repeated frequently
2. Irrelevant answers
3. Inattention and daydreaming
4. Scholastic performance below level of apparent ability
5. Hearing much better when watching the speaker's face
6. Tendency to withdraw from activities necessitating conversation
7. Deviations in speech-sound articulation

In the preschool child:

1. Absence or little babbling from the infant; also a failure of the infant to produce true syllables in which consonants are distinct (e.g., ba-ba, ma-ma, ga-ga, etc.). At the age of 9 months a baby should produce two- to three-syllable babbling.
2. Delayed speech and language development. A normal 2½-year-old child may have a vocabulary of 300 to 400 words with beginning skills in verbal communication.
3. More response to vibration and touch than to speech and surrounding environmental sounds; also, undue alertness to movement and other visual clues. For example, when sleeping, the child may need to be awakened by touching him, since verbal stimuli go unheeded.
4. Child makes his wants known more through the use of gestures and vocalizations than through speech attempts.
5. Behavior suggestive of emotional immaturity such as being demanding, fearful, having tantrums, etc.

Early detection of the hearing-impaired child is important from both a medical and an educational standpoint. Medically it offers both an opportunity for early treatment and an early information source of causal factors of hearing problems. From an educational standpoint it provides the opportunity to apply measures of habilitation and rehabilitation during the most critical remedial years for the child.

Testing

Two measurements of hearing commonly made are "sensitivity" and "speech discrimination." By "sensitivity" is meant one's ability to hear signals; by "speech discrimination" is meant how clearly one distinguishes different speech sounds.

The basic instrument used for measurement of hearing is called an audiometer (Fig. 34-3), an electrically calibrated instrument that affords careful control of test stimuli. Two different types of stimuli are presented: pure tones and specially selected words. Most audiometers generate the following pure tone frequencies: 125, 250, 500, 750, 1,000, 1,500, 2,000, 3,000,

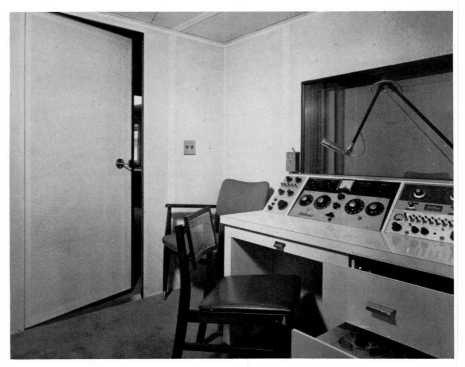

Fig. 34-3. An audiometric console in a prefabricated, sound-treated two-room test suite. The console-controlled presentation of pure tones and speech signals in a variety of ways permits the administration of many different diagnostic tests. The patient can be tested either in the same room with the examiner or in an adjacent chamber and seen through an observation window. A quiet area necessary for testing is provided by the sound-treated rooms. (Courtesy Industrial Acoustics Co., Inc., New York, N. Y., and Beltone Electronics, Inc., Chicago, Ill.)

4,000, 6,000, and 8,000 Hz. Each tone can be presented at different intensity levels, ranging from those that are barely audible to those that are uncomfortably loud. In the presentation of speech material, either the tester's own voice (live speech) or recordings of word lists are used. Pure tones and speech are normally presented through earphones; however, they can be presented through a loudspeaker. In either way the test signals reach the inner ear following the air conduction pathway. By placing a vibrator behind the ear on the mastoid process, measurement of bone conduction hearing for certain tones is also made. A comparison of how efficiently tones are heard by air and bone conduction is important in determining the site of hearing defects.

Information gained by pure tone audiometry indicates the reduction in hearing sensitivity and also points out the specific frequencies affected. It shows the extent to which difficulty exists in hearing barely audible sounds in the low, medium, and high frequencies, and it determines whether sound is heard better by air or bone conduction (Fig. 34-4). The primary importance of such information is the help it gives in differential diagnosis of the causes of hearing loss. It helps the physician decide whether the disease causing the loss is in the middle or inner ear.

To evaluate and determine sensitivity for speech, thresholds for specially selected words are determined. (Threshold means the lowest level of intensity at which the words are heard correctly at least 50% of the time.) A typical complaint voiced by patients with reduced sensitivity for speech is: "Everyone talks too softly. When they raise their voices, I can understand."

Also important to meaningful reception of speech is discrimination—a measure of how distinctly everyday speech is heard. To test discrimination, patients listen to specially selected lists of common one-syllabic words at an optimal intensity level, that is, at a level just where the patient wants it. Those who have difficulty in discrimination are likely to complain: "Words are loud enough but they're just not clear. I can't understand speech; words seem to run together."

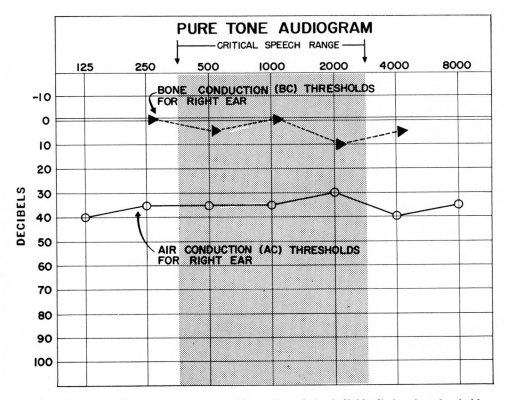

Fig. 34-4. An audiogram presents a graphic outline of the individual's hearing threshold sensitivity as measured by pure tones. Thresholds for the different tones as heard by air and bone conduction are plotted on the graph. The information is important in the diagnosis of the type of hearing loss. Also, by testing through the critical speech range, one can predict how much difficulty there may be in hearing and understanding speech.

Screening tests are used as rapid methods of separating persons who may have defective hearing (who will then need further testing) from those whose hearing is within acceptable limits. There are many different screening techniques. All should be simple, rapid, and capable of accurately detecting individuals with defective hearing.

An integral part of hearing conservation programs, screening testing is done in schools (Fig. 34-5), in industry, and in the Armed Forces. Importance of the early detection of hearing impairment is evident in the use of screening testing with preschool children and infants (Fig. 34-6).

Tests in children. Measuring the hearing of young children requires somewhat different techniques from those used in adults (Fig. 34-7). After 5 or 6 years of age conventional test procedures can be used satisfactorily. Below this age, however, lack of motivation, attention span, and coordination necessitate modifications of conventional test procedures. New techniques for testing young children are being developed regularly. The differentiation of hearing impairment from other disorders such as brain injury, mental retardation, and emotional disturbance is also important. The behavior manifested with these disorders may be mistaken for that of impaired hearing.

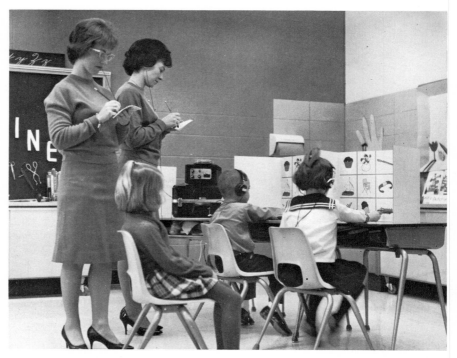

Fig. 34-5. Hearing screening of school children. Recorded words identifying the pictured objects are presented at a predetermined intensity level through earphones worn by the children. Incorrect picture selections warrant a detailed individualized test of the child's hearing. (Courtesy Zenith Radio Corp., Chicago. Ill.)

CLASSIFICATION OF HEARING LOSS

1. *Conductive hearing loss:* A conductive hearing loss results from dysfunction of the outer ear, middle ear, or both. Consequently conduction of sound to the inner ear is reduced, decreasing primarily the sensitivity and not the clarity dimension of sound. Since the inner ear is not affected, its function to "clearly" analyze the weakened sound it receives remains normal. Sounds that normally are comfortably loud are fainter to one with a conductive hearing impairment; how much fainter depends on the degree of the impairment. However, if the deficit in sensitivity is overcome, the

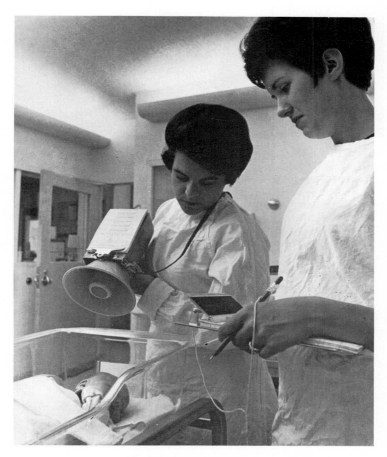

Fig. 34-6. Experimental behavioral hearing screening of the newborn. The girl on the left presents warbled signals of selected intensities with an infant audiometer. Responses elicited (auropalpebral, Moro's reflex, cessation or arousal of activity, etc.) are observed and recorded by the girl on the right. As yet no satisfactory technique for mass behavioral screening of the newborn is established. However what is advocated is a basic minimum screening program of the newborn with "high risk" factors, historical and physical, for hearing impairment. The great majority of deaf infants are implicated by a very small number of high risk factors. (Courtesy Tracor, Inc., Austin, Texas.)

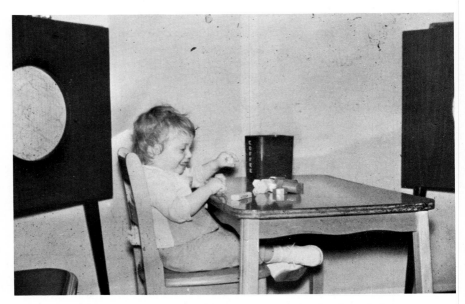

Fig. 34-7. Varied procedures are helpful in measuring the hearing of the very young. Conditioned play audiometry, a common approach, is being used to measure the little girl's hearing. Through conditioning the child is learning to perform a playlike activity (dropping the objects in the box) in response to selected sounds coming from the speakers. The next stage is to get the child to accept the wearing of earphones through which the sounds are presented and more definitive hearing information obtained. Factors of motivation, attention span, and motor coordination are important considerations in the hearing measurement of children. (Courtesy Hearing and Speech Center of Columbus and Central Ohio, Columbus, Ohio.)

loudness of sound is reestablished. For instance, speech heard over the radio as comfortably loud and clear by normal hearing listeners will sound distant and faint but still relatively clear to a listener with a conductive hearing impairment. By turning up the volume of the radio the reduced sensitivity is compensated for and the loudness dimension of the speech returns to a comfortable level.

As a rule, individuals with conductive hearing impairment make good users of hearing aids. All they need to hear adequately is greater amplification of sound, which the hearing aid provides.

2. *Sensorineural loss:* Sensorineural hearing impairment applies primarily to dysfunction of the inner ear mechanism. With outer and middle ear functions being normal, efficient conduction of sound to the inner ear is provided. Because of inner ear dysfunction, the sound it receives is not analyzed properly. Both sensitivity and discrimination of sound may suffer. Difficulty in discrimination compounds with that of reduced sensitivity produces a frustrating handicap. For those with problems in discrimination, speech sounds are distorted regardless of their volume. To make matters

worse, some of these hearing-impaired people have an intolerance for loud sounds in general. This creates an ironic situation—they want the speaker to "speak up"; yet when someone does, he is chastised with "Really now, you don't have to shout!" Intolerance for loud sounds tends to make these people poor candidates for hearing aids. The need for audiological consultation regarding hearing aid use is greater for persons with sensorineural than those with conductive hearing impairment, as the listening problems of the former tend to be more complex. This does not imply, however, that persons with sensorineural loss cannot be helped with an aid; many of them can. The purpose of consultation before buying a hearing aid is to determine through more objective measures whether or not use of an aid will be beneficial and to counsel accordingly.

3. *Mixed hearing loss:* A mixed hearing loss has both conductive and sensorineural components. It is common.

4. *Central hearing loss:* Central hearing loss refers to impairments that have their underlying difficulty in the central nervous system. In these cases the hearing difficulty cannot be explained adequately on either a conductive or sensorineural basis.

5. *Psychogenic hearing loss:* Psychogenic hearing loss is explained more on a psychological basis than in terms of any structural change in the hearing mechanism. Other terms used for this difficulty are "nonorganic" and "functional." Psychogenic hearing losses are not intentional and should not be confused with malingering, in which individuals knowingly fabricate or pretend a hearing problem. Hysterical, or conversion, deafness is the most common type of psychogenic deafness. The hearing loss, often total, is a manifestation of emotional conflicts.

The educational and rehabilitative needs of a hearing-impaired person vary, depending on the time of onset and the nature of the hearing loss and their effect on speech and language development. Classification systems which include these factors are helpful in the selection of proper training programs for those with impaired hearing.

In England the following classification with three grades for children with hearing impairment makes distinctions on the basis of the acquisition of speech:

Grade I—Children with defective hearing (usually those who are amenable to medical treatment) who do not need hearing aids or special educational treatment.
Grade II—Children with some naturally acquired speech but who need special educational treatment. Many of these children need hearing aids.
Grade III—Deaf children without naturally acquired speech when admitted to school. Many of these children are not totally deaf and can be helped in learning to speak by use of hearing aids.

The Conference of Executives of American Schools for the Deaf proposed the following system, which is based primarily on two factors: (1) time of onset of hearing loss and (2) functional status of hearing:

1. The deaf—those in whom the sense of hearing is nonfunctional for the ordinary purposes of life. This general group is made up of two distinct classes:
   (a) The congenitally deaf

(b) The adventitiously deaf—those born with normal hearing in whom the sense of hearing became nonfunctional through illness or accident.

2. The hard of hearing—those in whom hearing, although defective, is serviceable with or without a hearing aid.

These systems of classification have merit in providing the bases for differentiating the educational and rehabilitative needs of hearing-impaired persons.

AURAL REHABILITATION

The concern of aural rehabilitation is in restoring and maintaining efficiency in oral communication. This is done through the use of amplification, application of residual hearing, and increased reliance on other sensory modalities.

A distinction should be made regarding the purposes of training in speech and language skills for the hard of hearing and the deaf. With the hard of hearing, the purpose is rehabilitative—to correct, restore, complement, and maintain normally acquired skills in oral communication. For the deaf it is habilitative; language and speech skills have to be taught by special methods from the start, since conditions are lacking for their normal development.

The following approaches are commonly used for both habilitative and rehabilitative purposes:

1. Hearing aids—amplifiers of sound used to compensate for reduced hearing sensitivity

2. Auditory training—improvement of listening skills and use of residual hearing

3. Speech reading—use of many visual clues such as facial expressions, gestures, body movements, situational circumstances, as well as lip movements, for more effective communication

4. Speech training—either "speech conservation," the prevention of possible deterioration of speech skills relating to impaired hearing, or "speech therapy," the correction of defective speech skills caused by impaired hearing.

Hearing aids

Hearing aids are instruments through which sounds are amplified in a controlled manner. Generally an aid consists of a microphone to receive and convert speech and other sounds into electrical signals, an amplifier to increase their strength, and a receiver to reconvert the electrical signals back into sounds of greater magnitude.

The chief benefit derived from a hearing aid is amplification. Therefore a hearing aid is most helpful when the basic hearing problem is reduced sensitivity and when there is difficulty with the loudness dimension of sounds. When the difficulty is reduced speech discrimination, that is, words sound distorted and are not heard clearly, benefit from the use of an aid is more restricted.

A variety of hearing aids is available (Figs. 34-8 and 34-9). Basically they are grouped into those worn about the head and those worn on the torso. The headborne type may be built into temples of eyeglasses or worn as individual units behind the ear or in the ear canal.

The following are some points to consider in evaluating a person's performance with a hearing aid:

1. How much improvement is there in sensitivity for speech sounds?
2. Is discrimination for speech sounds maintained?
3. In which ear should the aid be worn? Should aids be worn in both ears?
4. What type of aid is indicated—body type or headborne? If the latter, hearing-aid glasses or a behind-the-ear model?
5. How does the person react to the use of an aid?

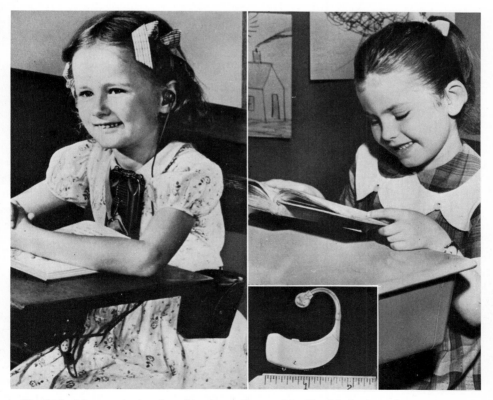

Fig. 34-8. Advances in hearing aids. An earlier model aid with its large battery, transmitter, receiver, and wires is worn by the girl on the left. In contrast the girl on the right is wearing a modern headborne aid. The basic components are contained in a single housing, shaped and sized as shown in the inset to lie behind the ear. (Courtesy Zenith Radio Corp., Chicago, Ill.)

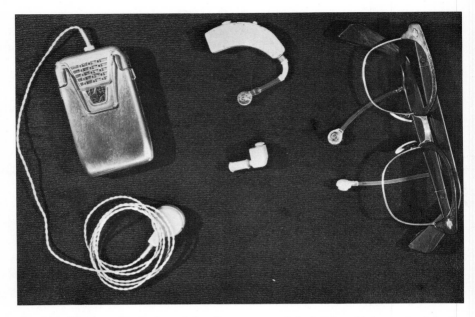

Fig. 34-9. Hearing aids, body and headborne types. A body-type aid is on the left. Its button receiver is coupled to the ear with an insert, and its component housing is either clipped to one's clothing or worn on the body in a harnessed cloth pouch. Remaining are different types of headborne hearing aids. Top center is a behind-the-ear aid, at the right is an eyeglass aid, and in the center is an in-the-ear aid. (Courtesy Audiology Division, Department of Otolaryngology, The Ohio State University, Columbus, Ohio.)

Auditory training

Auditory training teaches those who are hard of hearing to use their residual hearing more effectively and is accomplished by developing listening skills. Basically the training seeks to enhance the patient's ability in discrimination, a function already described as the ability to distinguish among similar speech sounds.

Techniques in auditory training vary, depending on when hearing impairment developed. In children auditory training is designed to follow the lines of normal development of auditory discrimination. These stages of development are as follows:

1. Awareness of sounds—recognizing the presence and meaningfulness of sounds
2. Gross discriminations—discriminating between highly dissimilar environmental sounds
3. Discriminations for speech—training beginning with broad discriminations for simple speech patterns and leading to the more precise discriminations of normal speech

In adults auditory training counteracts the effects of hearing impairment on established discrimination ability. This is done by (1) establishing an attitude of critical listening, (2) developing an awareness of the listening errors that are more likely to be made in view of the nature of the hearing impairment, (3) compensating for these errors by using other speech clues that are still heard accurately, and (4) generally improving listening habits and skills.

In either approach assistance in the adjustment and use of hearing aids is important.

Speech reading

Speech reading concerns greater use of visual clues to maintain effective oral communication. A more commonplace term is lipreading. However, lipreading tends to be misleading by implying that the lips are the only source of visual clues, whereas actually the entire body and circumstances pertinent to the speech situation also provide visual clues. Facial expressions, gestures, body movement, and the immediate physical setting are examples of visual clues that supplement the hearing function in oral communication.

Objectives important in speech reading training are as follows:

1. Understanding of how visual and auditory clues can combine to serve in speech communication
2. Development of skills in the perception of visible aspects of speech
3. Improvement of general observation ability

Speech training

It was pointed out earlier that hearing is important not only for the development of speech but also for its maintenance. Normal hearing permits a person to hear his own voice and so constitutes a monitoring function for regulating it. Occasionally the monitoring function is brought to light in a startling manner. For example, a speaker using a loud voice in order to be heard in a noisy situation may be caught off guard when the noise is unexpectedly reduced; he finds himself shouting momentarily before he can adjust the loudness of his voice.

Attributes of speech maintained by this monitoring function are loudness, clearness, pitch inflection, quality, and rate. Hearing impairment reduces the reliability of the monitoring function, and in turn these attributes may be adversely affected, causing speech to deteriorate.

Speech training with hearing-impaired persons may take two forms: (1) conservation and (2) correction. The former is undertaken when there is little or no evidence of speech deterioration with the goal of conserving speech skills. If speech deterioration has already occurred, corrective procedures are undertaken.

SERVICE PROGRAMS

Service programs for those with impaired hearing vary in terms of sponsorship and scope. Universities sponsor many of the programs, and there they are commonly identified as audiology or hearing and speech programs. In hospitals these programs are frequently associated with departments of otolaryngology. Community programs may be privately sponsored or sponsored in part by organizations such as the Junior League or the various united appeals. Other programs are under the auspices of state and local departments of health and education. The Veterans Administration maintains several audiology and speech facilities throughout the country. Specific services are as follows:

1. Screening of hearing for early detection of hearing losses
2. Complete evaluation of hearing losses for diagnosis and rehabilitation
3. Evaluation of hearing aid use
4. Training in speech reading, auditory training, speech conservation, speech correction, and language development

SUGGESTED READINGS AND FILM
Readings

Characteristics of persons with impaired hearing, Public Health Service Publication No. 1000, Series 10, No. 35, April, 1967.

Davis, Hallowell, and Silverman, S. Richard: Hearing and deafness, ed. 3, New York, 1970, Holt, Rinehart & Winston, Inc.

Hearing sensitivity and related medical findings among children, United States, HEW Publication No. 72 1046, Series II, No. 14, March, 1972.

Newby, H. A.: Audiology, ed. 3, New York, 1970, Appleton-Century-Crofts.

Film

The Deafness Research Foundation and Churchill Films: Silent world, muffled world, U. S. Department of Health, Education and Welfare, Public Health Service, Audiovisual Facility, Atlanta, Ga. 30333.

CHAPTER THIRTY-FIVE Hearing impairment—the nurse's role

Not only must the nurse understand the pathophysiology of hearing impairment, but she must have some understanding of the psychologic impact that a hearing loss or deafness has for the individual who has learned speech normally. Changes in personality are not necessarily proportionate to the degree of hearing loss. Often those with mild hearing impairment tend to have more changes of behavior than those with a more severe hearing impairment. The problems of the congenitally deaf are very different. Their lack of aural stimulation and consequent development of speech and conceptual ability imposes a severe handicap to both personality and intellectual development. The lack of sensory gratification in the newborn can have a severe effect on the health and life of the infant. What happens to the individual when impairment and distortion of hearing occur?

In the previous chapters the nurse's role in the care of patients with specific diseases of the ear and corrective surgery was presented. In this chapter aspects of the psychologic problems of the aurally handicapped are presented. Means of improving communication with those who have a hearing loss are also discussed. The *detection* of persons with hearing impairment and the *prevention* of hearing loss are important nursing responsibilities.

MEANING OF SOUND

To better understand the person who has a hearing deficit one must examine the importance of sound as well as speech in our daily lives. We hear environmental sounds that we cannot see such as rain on the roof or footsteps approaching from behind. It is hard for the hearing person to imagine and nearly impossible to experience a world in which he does not perceive sound. As you read this you are perceiving sound—some unconsciously and some of which you are aware, such as background noises, a fan, the ticking of a clock, the shuffling of feet, or the radio. As you concentrate these environmental sounds are shut out, or on the unconscious level. These vague background sounds associate us with the world around us; we feel a part of the activity or related to the movements about us. Our mind is constantly

403

reacting to these sounds on the unconscious level, and it is not until a sound is interpreted as a *signal* that we will consciously hear it and, depending upon our interpretation, change what we are doing. The bell signaling the end of a class period or the sound of a bee will cause us to take action. This unconscious level of hearing, called the *primitive level* by one author, is what hard-of-hearing persons no longer perceive and consequently refer to the "world as being dead" about them. Not only is the deaf person isolated from the interchange of conversation of family and friends but he no longer experiences the sounds of his environment. Because some of the sound was on an unconscious level, the person is unable to identify exactly what is lost or lacking but a feeling of sadness and insecurity is expressed.*

Not only is sound perceived as signals and as background sound, it is also used for *symbols* or speech. Speech, whether an interchange between oneself and a friend or the bus driver or just listening to radio, television, and others conversing, is essential to our relatedness to others and also to the world about us. Not only do words or symbols communicate experiences, feeling tone is also communicated such as friendliness, acceptance, and anger. Our thoughts are organized and clarified, and social and moral codes are learned through these symbols.

Sound also provides us with aesthetic experiences such as the sounds of nature and music. Individuals vary as to their enjoyment and/or need for the auditory aesthetic experience. The need for visual experience may be more developed in some individuals, whereas others rely on auditory experience for satisfaction such as listening to a concert or jazz or the sound of wind in the trees. Auditory and visual aesthetic experience is of little importance to others. The person who has developed a need for auditory aesthetic experience will find it more difficult to adjust to a soundless world.

The one word that would best describe the plight of the person who is hard of hearing or deaf would be *isolation*. The lack of background noise, the signals no longer or poorly heard, the lack of verbal communication, and the loss of aesthetic auditory experiences all influence the individual's confidence, self-concept, and feeling of well-being. Thus the individual must alter his means of equilibrium. Depending on his personality he may react to this stress or threat by withdrawal, by becoming suspicious as others omit him from the conversation, by depression, and by aggressiveness and cynicism.

Another factor to consider in understanding the problems of the person with limited hearing is that this handicap is not readily recognized by others. One readily identifies the person with limited vision or who is blind by the way he moves, by his white cane, and by his general appearance. The immediate and usual reaction to the blind is compassion and sympathy. This is usually not true of the aurally handicapped, as the per-

---

*Ramsdell, D. A.: The psychology of the hard-of-hearing and the deafened adult. In Davis, Hallowell, and Silverman, S. Richard: Hearing and deafness, ed. 3, New York, 1970, Holt, Rinehart & Winston, Inc.

son may appear quite normal and move about as any other person. When one speaks to the person with hearing impairment, he may not respond to our greeting, may completely ignore us, or may respond inappropriately. Because he appears physically able, he is viewed as slow or odd, and consequently the speaker may withdraw or avoid further contact. The aurally handicapped person may interpret such action as rejection. Not only is he isolated by the lack of perceived sound but as others respond to him, cues are picked up that cause further isolation and withdrawal.

Perhaps another factor that further enhances the gap between hearing and nonhearing persons today is the increasing use of auditory stimulation such as television, radio, telephone, records, and audiotapes. Of note is the increased use of background music during work hours to improve the morale of workers. As stated before, sound comes from all sides; it is heard around corners, behind us, over us, and in the dark. We cannot close it out by shutting an ear lid. The person who is unable to hear must depend upon visual clues such as lip or speech reading and only "hears" when the speaker (sound) is directly in front of him and in the light. He must become adept at using other visual clues to understand part of what is said.

Thus the person with an aural handicap will experience varying degrees of stress and behavior change depending upon his personality, the extent and type of hearing loss, and the age at which this occurred, whether congenital or acquired. Reaction of family and friends to this loss will also play an important role in the adjustment of the individual.

VARIOUS GROUPS WITH HEARING IMPAIRMENT

Incidence. It was estimated by the National Health Survey of 1961* that 7 million persons have various degrees of hearing impairment. Males are twice as frequently affected as females. Of interest to the nurse is the fact that nearly one half or 3,500,000 persons with hearing impairment are 65 years of age and over. A more recent estimate, however, indicates 10 million or more persons have hearing impairment.†

The person with slight hearing loss. The person with decreased hearing may at first be unaware of it and, as the impairment progresses, tries to minimize or hide the defect. Consequently he will strain to listen; further frustration is caused by embarrassing situations that develop throughout the day. Irritation and exhaustion occur, and social contacts are avoided. If communication is essential in his employment, difficulties arise; he may resign or be passed over when promotions are made, and further isolation occurs. Others find communication difficult at home and minor irritations and disputes occur. Perhaps the most important factor in helping this group is the recognition of defective hearing by the individual in order that corrective or rehabilitative steps can be taken. Once others who are impor-

---

*Statistical Bulletin, Metropolitan Life Insurance 47:3-5, Sept., 1966.

†Mindel, Eugene D., and McCay, Vernon: Out of the shadows and the silence, Journal of the American Medical Association **220**:1127-1128, May 22, 1972.

tant to the person are aware of the impediment, means for more effective communication can be established.

The older person with hearing impairment. Because of the increase in our aging population and resulting increase in incidence of presbycusis in this age group, this group of persons requires special consideration. Between the ages of 65 to 74 years, inclusive, it is estimated that 129 per 1,000 persons have a hearing handicap.* Of course some of this group will have experienced conductive hearing loss in earlier years; the sensorineural loss compounds the problem. Typically the person has decreased ability to hear or discern the higher sounds such as those produced by the consonants "f" and "s," and increasing the loudness of the voice only increases the distress of the individual. Fortunately these sounds can be perceived visually fairly well, and lip reading would be of some help. With this age group the individuals themselves and their family and friends tend to accept decreased hearing ability as part of the aging process and think little can be done. The older person who is well aware of his declining physiologic functioning interprets his confusion in comprehending what others are saying as caused by mental deterioration and is fearful of seeking help. Isolation because of loss of contemporaries and other health problems causes further social withdrawal. There are a few in this group who no longer care to hear any more and are content to be in a silent world, but this is not the usual reaction.

The person with severe hearing loss. Because of the problems the person with severe hearing loss has, he seeks help and is more likely to use facilities available if these are known. This person is unable to hear signals essential to his safety and functioning, such as the automobile horn, the whistle of the train, or the telephone and doorbell. Because he no longer hears himself speak, his speech may be slurred or too loud. Should the hearing loss be sudden, as occurs with an accident, although rare, the individual will experience much confusion, fear, and even panic to be suddenly thrust into a soundless, moving world. If the person experiences sudden hearing loss in one ear, there will be difficulty in locating the source of sound that he cannot associate with visual clues. As one woman aptly described the experience of suddenly not hearing in one ear when she awoke one morning, "I felt I was half gone." She immediately sought medical help.

The congenitally deaf person. The child who has little or no hearing is severely limited in his psychologic and mental development without the ability of hear words and associate them with things, ideas, and feelings. It is known that the child without hearing has disturbed visual perception. Profound deafness from infancy alters the perceptual processes and the individual's awareness of self. Deaf children perceive their body differently when compared to other children. Emotional and social immaturity are noted on tests. The congenitally blind child is more dependent than the deaf child; however, both groups score higher in dependency than the av-

---

*Statistical Bulletin, Metropolitan Life Insurance 47:3-5, Sept., 1966.

erage child in the same age group. Perhaps the most significant feature of the deaf child when compared to other children of the same school age is his inability to use the written word and to read well. By test the deaf child reaches a plateau in language development of 11 years of age, with little progress beyond. Today more emphasis and research are being directed toward the learning abilities of the deaf child and how best to help him learn. It is essential that such a child be found early and corrective measures be taken prior to school age, and more specifically before the child is a year old, as speech is most effectively learned between the ages of 2 and 5 years. Parents can do much if the nature of the handicap is understood. The John Tracy Clinic correspondence course is especially prepared to assist parents with preschool children who are deaf and are in the home.

COMMUNICATING WITH THE PERSON WITH DECREASED HEARING

It is essential that the nurse be aware of the specific problems and note any behavior of the person that may indicate withdrawal and/or confusion. A great deal of patience and ingenuity is required. If the deaf or hard-of-hearing person is hospitalized, a new environment and unfamiliar faces may accentuate isolation and loneliness. Increased anxiety and apprehension also make hearing more difficult. The following are specific points to facilitate speech reading* and/or hearing:

1. Draw attention by raising an arm or hand; do not touch first, as this may unduly startle the person.
2. Stand with the light on your face; do not stand in the window.
3. Look directly at the person (see Fig. 35-1).
4. Speak normally—slowly and distinctly.
5. Move closer to the person—toward the better ear if he does not hear you. Often the person will turn his better ear toward the sound.
6. Do not shout; this overemphasizes normal speaking movements and may cause distortion and be too loud for the person with sensorineural damage.
7. Rephrase if the person is not comprehending; white, red, and green appear the same.
8. Write out proper names, as these are difficult to speech read.
9. Avoid mannerisms that block the sight of your face and lips. Smoking, chewing gum, and eating interfere and should be avoided.
10. Inattention may indicate tiredness and/or lack of understanding.
11. Avoid one-word answers unless "yes" or "no." Phrases are used to comprehend meaning rather than single words.
12. Do not show annoyance by careless facial expressions. Hard-of-hearing persons depend more on visual clues for acceptance.

---

*Speech reading is a term used to denote lip reading but also includes observing the whole face and body to comprehend what is being said. Thus the hard-of-hearing or deaf person observes more than just the lips to comprehend.

13. If in a group, repeat important statements and avoid asides to others in the group.
14. Allow the person time to assimilate all clues and understand what is being said.

If the person has a *hearing aid,* he should be encouraged to use it. In speaking to a person with an aid, allow him to adjust the distance; moving closer or directing your voice toward the aid may increase his discomfort. Remember that the aid *amplifies,* and shouting is unnecessary. Should the the patient not have his hearing aid or if he cannot hear, amplification can be accomplished by speaking into the diaphragm of a stethoscope with ear pieces in the patient's ears. A rolled paper or magazine will also amplify the speaker's voice.

If the individual is learning to use an aid, it is well to remember that it may take as long as six months to become accustomed to an aid. Periodic discouragement occurs; motivation and perseverance are necessary. Conversation directed toward areas of interest will be more stimulating. The hearing-aid wearer should follow the directions provided by the company in caring for the aid. He should know how to obtain batteries and have extra batteries on hand. Often it is advisable to remove the battery to conserve its life when not in use. The aid should be stored in a dry place

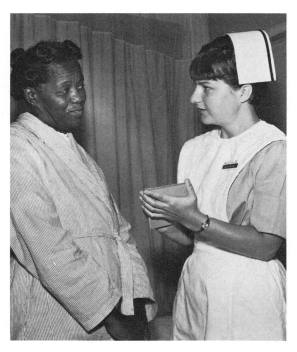

Fig. 35-1. Student nurse communicating with a patient who is deaf and has only a small amount of hearing in the right ear. Note that the patient is intently watching the nurse's face to speech read. The nurse is using a pad and paper to write key words.

when not in use. Sharp blows should be avoided, as the aid can be damaged. If an ear mold is used, special instructions are provided for cleaning the mold, and they should be followed. Cerumen may accumulate in the ear canal when a mold is worn; temporary difficulty in hearing may result until the impacted cerumen is removed.

The intercommunication system used in many hospitals to communicate with patients from the nurse's station may be poorly understood and distorted for one who has impaired hearing. Since the hard-of-hearing person depends upon *visual* clues to pick up changes in the environment, it is wise to place this patient in a bed where he can observe activities and anticipate others approaching him. Should he be in the corner behind partially pulled screens, he can be startled easily as people suddenly enter his unit because he will not hear their approach. A deaf person will scan the environment periodically to check for changes that a hearing person can identify by sound alone. Special effort must be made to communicate to him the hospital routine and to prepare him for special tests and treatments.

Anyone who is hard of hearing will also depend upon the *tactile* sense to gain information about the environment. The nurse should be mindful of the use of touch in relating to the patient. Many patients will feel less isolated if the nurse places her hand on his arm after his attention is gained. At times, instead of arousing a patient with loud shouts, a hand placed on his hand or shoulder may be a less frightening awakening. Of course, each patient will vary in the approach most beneficial for communication. Once the specific approach and means of implementing effective communications are identified, it is essential that a plan of care be made and shared with others caring for the patient.

Another point worth noting is that muscular movement can compensate for the involuntary shifts of muscle tension that resulted from background sound heard on the unconscious level. Purposeful activity such as knitting, sewing, playing cards, and other hobbies are rewarding and satisfying. The nurse can assist in finding activities that involve others yet require little communication such as putting a jigsaw puzzle together, playing cards, or viewing television.

To further assist the deaf person at home an amplifier can be placed on doorbells and telephones. A flashing light can be used to various parts of the house to signal the ringing of the doorbell and telephone or the crying of a child in another room. Special headphones may allow the enjoyment of radio, records, and television.

PREVENTION AND DETECTION OF HEARING LOSS

The nurse can do much to help in the prevention of hearing loss. By an understanding of the causative factors of hearing impairment *early prenatal care* will be taught and encouraged. Any person in the first trimester of pregnancy who has not had measles (rubella) should be cautioned regarding exposure to the disease and to seek immediate medical advice if contact occurs. Should the pregnant woman experience any viral disease such as measles, influenza, or mumps, medical supervision should be sought. Medical supervision is imperative in the first several months of pregnancy if congenital defects are to be avoided. Vaccination for measles should be given to all children and especially to any young girl who has not had measles.

There is increased incidence of hearing impairment in the premature infant, the jaundiced (related to Rh incompatibility) infant, and the infant who experiences anoxia in the postnatal period. The nurse who sees these infants in the nursery and later in the home should observe their ability to hear and their speech development. Infants can be tested for hearing as early as 3 months of age, or earlier if indicated (Fig. 34-6), and other diagnostic and rehabilitation resources can be made available to the parents and child. A rehabilitation program will be prescribed to meet the individual needs of the child. The parents can do much to help in the rehabilitation program once they are aware of the diagnosis and are helped to understand their role.

Children who have frequent upper respiratory infections with tonsillitis and/or earache should have medical supervision. Often the school nurse or public health nurse may be the first to recognize the child who already has some hearing loss by his behavior, such as inattentiveness, difficulty with speech, and other related symptoms. The child who has a discharge from the ears or who is a mouth breather should be examined medically and receive appropriate therapy.

Any patient receiving *ototoxic* drugs, which cause damage to the eighth cranial nerve, need to be questioned regarding subjective symptoms that relate to dizziness, decreased hearing acuity, and tinnitus. The patient may credit these symptoms to his illness and fail to report them to the medical staff. Observation regarding the patient's equilibrium, including nystagmus, should be made. Any of these untoward effects should be reported and the next dose of medication withheld until the patient is examined by a physician. Oxotoxic drugs include streptomycin, dihydrostreptomycin, neomycin, kanamycin, gentamicin, viomycin, the salicylates including aspirin, and quinine. As new drugs are marketed, the nurse should be aware of similar side effects.

In various contacts with the public the nurse may be asked for advice regarding hearing problems. She may also identify persons whose behavior may indicate difficulty in hearing. She should recognize that some people may be unaware of or may fail to accept a hearing loss; skillful use of interviewing techniques may assist in identifying and accepting their problems. Certainly the nurse can help members of the family in understanding how to communicate better with the patient. The availability of resources and the places where further information can be obtained that would help the individual and his family should be known. The nurse should be aware of the various adult age groups that would be affected with specific types of hearing loss. For example, a young woman who complains of head noises and has some hearing impairment may have otosclerosis, which is amenable to surgical treatment by stapedectomy. The older patient who has difficulty distinguishing words probably has presbycusis and should be encouraged to seek evaluation by an audiologist and/or an otolaryngologist. Often the older person buys one or more hearing aids from one or more dealers without benefit of an audiogram and specific diagnosis.

Acoustic trauma. An area of national and international concern is the problem of *noise prevention.* It is estimated that city noise is increasing 1 dB per year. Presently the average community has noise levels of 70 dB or more, which has been designated as a minimum level for potential hearing loss. Not only is the noise level increasing in the city, but noise levels are increasing within the home. Use of more powerful appliances such as dishwashers, mixers, and disposals has increased the noise level to higher and more irritating levels. Individuals vary in their susceptibility to noise. For some a noisy environment causes nervous irritability and fatigue.

Historically, occupations of boilermaking and weaving were known to produce hearing loss and deafness resulting from acoustic trauma. Beginning in 1948 federal and state laws have established compensation for hearing loss, although no wages were lost during employment. More interest has been shown in the evaluation of damaging noise, and regulations have been established in many industries. Other occupations known to produce deafness are aircraft maintenance and manufacturing, riveting, blasting, machine manufacturing, gun firing, metal working, drop forging, and other occupations using high pressure steam, large presses, wood and metal saws, and heavy hammering operations. The following are noise conditions that cause hearing loss:

1. Short, high-intensity exposure to noise (160 dB) can rupture the eardrum and drive the stapes through the oval window. Temporary hearing loss can also occur because of intense noise. Usually hearing is recovered the following day. This is called auditory fatigue, or temporary threshold shift. No damage is done unless continued exposure occurs.

2. Prolonged exposure to intense noise is difficult to evaluate. It is known that such exposure to noise damages the hair cells of the organ of Corti. There is decreased ability to hear at the 4,000 Hz (the higher pitched tones of normal speech) as measured by audiometric tests. The individual is usually unaware of this loss. With continued exposure to noise, further damage occurs, and the loss involves the 3,000 to 4,000 Hz range. The loss will measure 40 to 50 dB.* In other words, the individual will have difficulty hearing speech in the higher frequencies (the consonants) of normal conversation, which mainly will be reflected as an inability to understand what is being said. This is sensorineural hearing loss similar to that caused by presbycusis, but can be differentiated by thorough and periodic testing and other diagnostic means.

If the individual is identified who is experiencing a beginning hearing loss due to noise exposure and is removed or protected from the noise en-

---

*Sataloff, Joseph: Hearing loss, Philadelphia, 1966, J. B. Lippincott Co., pp. 175-177.

vironment, progression of the hearing loss does not occur. The person with presbycusis, however, will demonstrate slow progression of sensorineural hearing loss although removed from the noise.

Factors requiring consideration in evaluating industrial noise are overall noise level of the environment, composition, duration, and distribution of the noise daily and throughout the working life of the individual. The individual's own sensitivity, age, and aural pathology are also factors that influence his susceptibility to industrial noise.

The use of protective devices is recommended in many industries. The protective ability and acceptance of this protection vary. These devices include earplugs that fit only the meatus or actually insert into the ear canal, earmuffs, and helmets. The workers wearing protective devices should be able to hear each other. The industrial nurse, as part of the hearing conservation program of the industry, should be able to assist and encourage the worker in wearing protective devices and to evaluate their effectiveness. In some areas of industry, perspiration may decrease the effectiveness of protective devices. Any hearing conservation program should include the measurement of noise in each area of work, preemployment audiometric test, and education regarding the use of protective devices. As more research is done in the area of noise and industry, better ways of protecting the individual in industry will be found. The Subcommittee on Noise of the Committee on Conservation of Hearing of the American Academy of Ophthalmology and Otolaryngology has established a research center that devotes full time to the study of noise in industry.

ORGANIZATIONS CONCERNED WITH HEARING AND SPEECH PROBLEMS

Many organizations are devoted to the problems of the deaf and hard of hearing. Several organizations have been in existence for fifty or more years, indicating the courage, thinking, and dedication of the pioneers in this field such as Alexander Graham Bell and Rev. Thomas Gallaudet. Gallaudet College, Washington, D. C., named for Rev. Gallaudet and his two sons, provides education, including higher education, exclusively for the deaf and is over 100 years old. Many other organizations have developed, reflecting the increased interest in the prevention of hearing loss as well as research and rehabilitation of the deaf and hard of hearing. The following are professional organizations specifically concerned with the education of the deaf child:

1. Convention of American Instructors of the Deaf. Membership is limited to those who teach the deaf in the United States and Canada. The convention is one of the few educational organizations that has been in existence for over a century. The official publication, *American Annals of the Deaf,* is the oldest educational publication in the United States.

2. Conference of Executives of American Schools for the Deaf. Membership is limited to administrative heads of schools for the deaf in the United States and Canada. This group is concerned with the management of schools for the deaf and certifies teachers of the deaf. *American Annals of the Deaf* includes this organization's proceedings, also; a listing of schools and classes for the deaf and hard of hearing is included annually.

National organizations for and concerning the deaf and hard of hearing are many. A list of the major organizations follows. Brief information regarding their purpose is provided; however, more complete information can be obtained by writing directly to the organization.

1. Alexander Graham Bell Association for the Deaf, Inc., Headquarters: Volta Bureau, 1535 35th St., N. W., Washington, D. C. 20007. Membership includes parents of deaf children, educators, scientists, physicians, and others. Many adults with hearing impairment are members. The Volta Bureau, which is owned by the association, contains the largest collection of books on deafness in America. The *Volta Review,* published monthly, is the official journal of this organization and contains articles specifically written for parents, teachers, and professional persons. Reprints are available at a low cost.

2. American Hearing Society, 919 18th St., N. W., Washington, D. C. 20006. Membership in this society is open to all who have a hearing problem. The purposes of this organization are multiple and include prevention of hearing loss and rehabilitation of the deaf and hard of hearing. Assistance with hearing aids and classes for speech reading are provided by local chapters. *Hearing News,* a bimonthly periodical for members, contains articles related to the problems of deafness, hearing aids, speech reading, and rehabilitation. Pamphlets are also available.

3. American Speech and Hearing Association (ASHA), 9030 Old Georgetown Road, Washington, D. C. 20014. This is a scientific and professional organization with approximately 15,000 members. Members must have a Master's degree or equivalent in the field of human communication. The purposes of the organization are to encourage basic scientific study of the processes of human communication, with special reference to speech, hearing, and language, to promote investigation of disorders of human communication, and to foster improvement of clinical procedures with such disorders. Official communications include: *The Journal of Speech and Hearing Disorders* and *The Journal of Speech and Hearing Research. The Annual Directory,* published yearly, lists all members and their qualifications, and recognized state associations.

ASHA and *Language, Speech and Hearing Services in Schools* are monthly publications; *ASHA Monographs* and *ASHA Reports* are others.

The American Speech and Hearing Association and Gallaudet College founded *Deafness Speech and Hearing Publications, Inc.,* which publishes *dsh Abstracts.*

The American Speech and Hearing Foundation is a charitable trust established by the American Speech and Hearing Association. The purpose of the foundation is to advance scientific and educational endeavors in speech pathology. Funds are awarded to qualified applicants as training and research grants in the fields of speech pathology and audiology.

4. American Academy of Ophthalmology and Otolaryngology of the American Medical Association is the chief organization of otolaryngologists. Several significant committees are the Committee on Conservation of Hearing and its Subcommittee on Noise and the Subcommittee on Hearing in Children. Research in specific areas of deafness and hearing is being conducted, and information is published for the public as well as for members of the health professions.

5. The Deafness Research Foundation, 366 Madison Ave., New York, N. Y. 10017. In order to study causes of deafness, Temporal Bone Banks have been established in leading medical centers and universities. Persons with hearing loss can bequeath their temporal bone for scientific study. The Temporal Bone Banks are cosponsored by the Academy of Ophthalmology and Otolaryngology (Fig. 35-2).

6. The John Tracy Clinic, 806 West Adams Blvd., Los Angeles, Calif. 90007. A private, non-profit organization offers a free home course by correspondence for parents of young children who are deaf or have a severe hearing loss. The course is prepared in English and Spanish and is adapted to individual and special needs of both child and parents through exchange of correspondence and reports.

7. Perkins-Tracy Home Study, Perkins School for the Blind, Watertown, Mass. 02172.

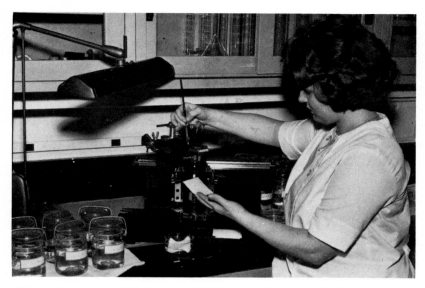

Fig. 35-2. Section of decalcified temporal bone is being prepared for mounting on a slide. Jars at the left contain temporal bones in a decalcifying solution. After six months in various solutions the bones can be used to study causes of hearing loss. The temporal bone contains the middle and inner ear. The inner ear cannot be examined during life.

The John Tracy Clinic with the Perkins School for the Blind provides a home study program for parents of deaf-blind children. The purpose is to provide parents with basic information, guidance, and encouragement to begin the training of a child who can neither see nor hear.

8. The National Association for the Deaf, 2025 Eye Street, N. W., Suite 321, Washington, D. C. 20006. Over eighty years ago the first meeting of this organization was held and since then this organization has done much to eliminate unjust traffic and liability laws and to promote the welfare of the deaf in education, legislation, and employment. The *Silent Worker* is the official monthly publication.

9. The National Fraternal Society for the Deaf, 6701 W. North Ave., Oak Park, Ill. 60302. This society was organized by young deaf men in 1901 to reduce discrimination against the deaf, especially by social orders and insurance companies. Life and automobile insurance can be obtained through this organization.

10. The American Public Health Association, 1790 Broadway, New York, N. Y. 10019. This is a professional society for those involved in the field of public health that concerns itself with the development and publications of standards. Surveys are made of various agencies and services.

11. The National Easter Seal Society for Crippled Children and Adults, Inc., 2023 W. Ogden Ave., Chicago, Ill. 60612. Information can be obtained regarding each state's chapter and the various services that are offered for the hearing handicapped.

Other organizations that make contributions regarding the problem of hearing and deafness include the Acoustical Society of America, the American Federation for the Physically Handicapped, the Council for Exceptional Children, the National Rehabilitation Association, Junior Leagues of America, and Sertoma International.

Government agencies have also been active in the problem of hearing and deafness. In the Department of Health, Education and Welfare, Washington, D. C. 20201, specific agencies that are interested in the aurally handicapped include the following:

1. National Institutes of Neurological Disease and Blindness, National Institutes of Health, Bethesda, Md. 20014. Funds are provided for basic and applied research and training purposes.
2. The Office of Vocational Rehabilitation, Section of the Deaf and Hard of Hearing. This agency promotes and upgrades the employability of those with severe hearing loss.
3. The Children's Bureau. This agency is concerned about the acoustically handicapped child.
4. United States Office of Education. Statistics regarding the handicapped child are reported by this agency. Studies have been made concerning teachers of the deaf.

Since World War II, the Veterans Administration has conducted specific programs and clinics for those whose hearing loss was incurred while in the service. Hearing aids are provided as well as specific training. The regional Veterans Administration Office should be consulted for further information.

SUGGESTED READINGS

Bell, Alan: Noise; an occupational hazard and public nuisance, Geneva, 1966, World Health Organization.

Bender, Ruth E.: Communicating with the deaf, American Journal of Nursing **66:** 757-760, April, 1966.

Canfield, Norton: Hearing; a handbook for laymen, Garden City, N. Y., 1959, Doubleday & Co., Inc.

Conover, Mary, and Cober, Joyce: Understanding and caring for the hearing-impaired, Nursing Clinics of North America 5:497-506, Sept., 1970.

Davis, Hallowell, and Silverman, S. Richard: Hearing and deafness, ed. 3, New York, 1970, Holt, Rinehart & Winston, Inc.

Grested, Naomi L.: The role of the occupational health nurse in noise control and hearing conservation, Occupational Health Nursing 20:17-18, Jan., 1972.

Hearing Aids, Consumer's Reports **31:**30-39, Jan., 1966, and **36:**310-320, May, 1971.

Henriksen, Heide L.: The nurse's role in an industrial hearing conservation program, American Association of Industrial Nurses Journal 12:14-16, Dec., 1964.

Linnell, Craig, Long, Sister Victorine, and Proehl, Janet: The hearing-impaired infant, Nursing Clinics of North America **5:**507-515, Sept., 1970.

Miller, James D.: Effects of noise on people, Washington, D. C., 1971, U. S. Environmental Protection Agency, Office of Noise Abatement and Control.

Moore, Mary Virginia: Diagnosis: deafness, American Journal of Nursing **69:**297-300, Feb., 1969.

Myklebust, Helmer R., editor: The psychology of deafness, ed. 2, New York, 1964, Grune & Stratton, Inc.

Neuschutz, Louise M.: If your patient is deaf, American Journal of Nursing **52:** 578, May, 1952.

Payne, Peter D., and Payne, Regina L.: Behavior manifestations of children with hearing loss, American Journal of Nursing **70:**1718-1719, Aug., 1970.

Riley, Edward C., and others: Focus on hearing, American Journal of Nursing 63:80-93, May, 1963.

Sataloff, Joseph: Hearing loss, Philadelphia, 1966, J. B. Lippincott Co.

Stone, Virginia: Hearing problems for our older population, Nursing Outlook 12:54-55, Nov., 1964.

U. S. Department of Health, Education, and Welfare: Hearing loss; hope through research, Public Health Service Publication No. 207, Washington, D. C., 1964, National Institute of Neurological Diseases and Blindness.

CHAPTER THIRTY-SIX

Inner ear—dizziness and vertigo; Meniere's disease

DIZZINESS AND VERTIGO

Dizziness and *vertigo* are terms sometimes used synonymously. When referring to dizziness, otolaryngologists generally mean a milder degree of unsteadiness than when they refer to vertigo, which implies a severe whirling sensation in which either the patient or his environment seems to spin. True vertigo occurs if one turns around and around rapidly and then tries to stand still.

Disorders of different bodily systems may produce vertigo. The otolaryngologist tries to diagnose and treat those conditions that arise from diseases of the ear. Vertigo may be produced by disturbances of the ocular system, the proprioceptive (muscular reflex) system, the vestibular system, and the central nervous system.

A person is able to walk reasonably steadily if he retains *two of the three* basic mechanisms for the maintenance of equilibrium: vision, proprioceptive reflexes from muscles, and labyrinthine function. For example, a blind man who has no other disease is able to walk without staggering, and a man with a reduced or absent labyrinthine function can walk as long as he can see. The latter, however, has great trouble at night or in a dark room, and both would be incapacitated if they had a disease of the spinal cord and could not receive proprioceptive reflexes from leg muscles to help in establishing their positions.

In taking the *history* it is important to establish whether the patient actually has true vertigo or whether he has another symptom he erroneously calls vertigo. If he has vertigo, the room should spin about him or he should feel as if he is whirling in space. Patients often mistakenly report as vertigo a momentary lightheadedness or even what may turn out to be a brief loss of consciousness. These entirely different states must be clearly distinguished, because both treatment and prognosis are different. Questions should be asked concerning loss of consciousness, head pain, hearing loss, and tinnitus. Great emphasis must be placed on the severity, duration, and mode of onset of the vertigo. It should be noted that when a patient has vertigo that is the result of inner ear disease as, for example,

Meniere's disease, there *never is expected to be loss of consciousness or pain*. The simultaneous presence of pain or unconsciousness and vertigo points away from disease of the inner ear and toward brain disease. Vertigo lasting for several days or months also leads the diagnosis away from disease of the inner ear and toward disease of the central nervous system.

As a rule, vertigo associated with disease of the inner ear (Meniere's disease is a good example) comes on suddenly and is severe. It lasts for a moderate length of time, minutes or hours, but not for seconds or for days or months. When disease of the inner ear causes vertigo, there often is an associated loss of hearing in one ear.

In *physical examination* of the vertiginous patient the ears are usually found to be normal, and this is always the case when it is the inner ear that causes vertigo. Occasionally, when disease of the middle ear produces vertigo, there are changes in the tympanic membrane that give a clue to diagnosis. If disease of the central nervous system is causing vertigo, the ears will be normal but there may be changes in the ocular fundi or the patient may exhibit abnormal behavior. Patients who feel dizzy momentarily upon standing suddenly from a sitting or stooping position have no ear disease but aging blood vessels that leave them with brief cerebral ischemia before arterial tension adjusts itself.

Functional examination of the inner ear is done by testing the hearing (audiometry) and by testing function of the semicircular canals. When vertigo and dizziness result from disease of systems other than the ear, ordinarily there is no associated loss of hearing, whereas vertigo resulting from disease of the ear is frequently associated with a unilateral loss of hearing.

There are two common methods of testing the labyrinth: (1) turning the patient in a chair and (2) douching cold water into one ear (caloric examination). In the *caloric examination* (Fig. 36-1) tap water is douched into the external auditory canal to stimulate the labyrinth. Stimulation is caused because the cold water cools the inner ear and sets up a current in the endolymph that stimulates the vestibular endorgan. Ice water is used ordinarily, but sometimes water at 86° F. is used for a longer period. The examiner must perform his tests in exactly the same way on every patient if he wants to compare results accurately. After cool water runs into the external auditory canal for twenty-five seconds (ten seconds for ice water), the patient starts to become dizzy. If stimulation is excessive, some patients even vomit. Besides dizziness and nausea, there is nystagmus (see following paragraph) with the quick component toward the opposite ear and falling toward the douched ear (when the patient stands and closes his eyes). Both ears are tested in exactly the same fashion. A five-minute waiting period is advisable between testing of the two ears to ensure that reaction from the first labyrinth has subsided completely.

Electronystagmography (ENG) (Fig. 36-2) is a test that records the position and movement of the eyeball by recording the changes in the electrical field around the eye when there is a change in position of the eye. Thus a

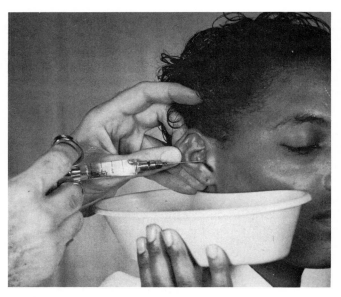

Fig. 36-1. Caloric test. Ice water is used to cool the tympanic membrane and middle ear and, in turn, the semicircular canals of the inner ear. Note the Luer-Lok syringe—an important point, since the needle must not come off the syringe.

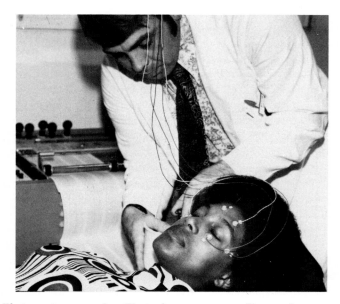

Fig. 36-2. Electronystagmography. Electrodes near eyes will record nystagmus on the recording sheet when physician irrigates ear with cold or warm water.

permanent record is made on prepared graph paper, allowing later study and actual mathematical calculations of amplitude, direction, and speed of nystagmus. Obviously it can be used to record either spontaneous nystagmus or induced nystagmus (the caloric test).

Nystagmus is an abnormal rhythmic, jerking movement of the eyes with a quick and a slow component. The direction of nystagmus is named according to the quick component and is said to be toward the right if the quick component carries the eyes toward the right, with the slow component returning them to the left. With the head upright nystagmus is rotary; that is, the eyes do not jerk directly laterally but have a slight rotary component. With the head tilted back 30 degrees, nystagmus is exactly horizontal. Vertical nystagmus is abnormal. It and other abnormal forms of nystagmus occur particularly in disease of the central nervous system.

Nystagmus occurs in normal persons only after stimulation of the vestibular labyrinth with cold or warm water or after rapid turning. Both methods of labyrinthine stimulation produce nystagmus by initiating a current in the semicircular canals of the inner ear. This movement of endolymph stimulates receptor cells and provides a clinical means for testing function of the vestibular components of the inner ear.

The caloric test is done to learn something about the functional state of the vestibular labyrinth. In patients with no labyrinthine function there is no reaction. In those with partial function the test may show hypoactivity. The most important observation comes in comparing one ear with the other. The physician must not overemphasize results of the caloric test; it is not a very precise test, and there may be variations in responses even among normal patients. The caloric test is confirmatory but seldom absolutely diagnostic.

The nurse should anticipate the possibility of the patient's vomiting during the caloric test and be on hand with emesis basin and towel. Most patients, however, do not get such a severe reaction. After douching, the ear canal is dried with a loose wisp of cotton. The caloric test may be done with the patient in either the sitting or reclining position.

The nurse may assess the patient's stability for walking and assist him as needed. A wheelchair may be required to take the patient to another location where he can rest more comfortably. Even with a severe reaction, however, complete recovery is expected after a brief rest and the patient can drive himself home.

MENIERE'S DISEASE

Meniere's disease causes a triad of symptoms: vertigo, unilateral hearing loss, and tinnitus. But other diseases or combinations of diseases may cause similar symptoms, and one must know how to differentiate among them. The cause of Meniere's disease is unknown, but it seems to be related to dysfunction of the autonomic nervous system, producing a temporary constriction of blood vessels supplying the inner ear. *Vertigo,* the outstanding symptom, comes in attacks or crises at irregular intervals of days, months, or years. The onset of an attack of vertigo is sudden and without warning.

Patients with Meniere's disease have true vertigo. During an attack or crisis, most of them are so completely disoriented in space that their surroundings whirl wildly about them. Usually they must lie down or they fall down. In a crisis the patient staggers when attempting to walk.

The duration of vertigo in a crisis of Meniere's disease is also characteristic and very important in differential diagnosis. In a crisis the patient remains vertiginous for several hours or all day. On the other hand, patients with intracranial disease are often dizzy for several weeks or months but never experience true vertigo. Other patients, for example, those who had cerebral arteriosclerosis or postural hypotension, may have transient episodes of dizziness or lightheadedness but do not remain dizzy for any length of time.

Between attacks the patient with Meniere's disease is not vertiginous. He is able to work normally and has no complaint except tinnitus or deafness. Some patients seem to have occasional tipping sensations, feelings of lateral pulsion, or dizziness, but for the most part they have normal equilibrium except during an attack. Most patients with Meniere's disease have several attacks each year. After many years the attacks become less frequent or cease altogether. The disease in itself is never fatal.

In Meniere's disease, hearing loss is always of the sensorineural type. Symptomatically it is unilateral, although a lesser degree of hearing loss in the opposite ear is not uncommon. The hearing loss varies from mild to severe but is rarely, if ever, total. The hearing loss generally appears months or years before the vertigo, but because the hearing loss appears very gradually, the patient often does not notice it. Even at the time of the first vertiginous crisis, hearing loss may not be great. Because the hearing loss often fluctuates, patients say they hear better one day than another. Patients with Meniere's disease often complain of a sensation of fullness in one ear, and some think that their ears have water in them. Because hearing in the good ear is usually normal, the loss of hearing associated with Meniere's disease is not incapacitating. Although the hearing loss does improve from time to time, the general trend is downward. After Meniere's disease has been present for several years, often not much serviceable hearing remains in the affected ear.

Tinnitus or ringing is present in one ear most of the time. There is no particular characteristic of this tinnitus. Like the hearing loss it may worsen during a crisis, but usually it is present all the time.

Except during a crisis, which lasts several hours, there are no symptoms between attacks except for hearing loss and tinnitus. There are also no abnormal physical findings in Meniere's disease. The eardrums are normal because this is a disorder of the inner ear, not the middle ear. Meniere's disease is *not* expected to be associated with *pain or loss of consciousness,* and if a vertiginous patient also has these symptoms, one should suspect disease of the central nervous system.

There is no medical treatment for Meniere's disease that has proved entirely successful. Many have been suggested, and most of them seem to work some of the time. But the very fact that there exists such a variety of treatment is evidence that no one medical treatment is always effective. In one regimen patients are given a salt-free diet and ammonium chloride tablets, 0.5 Gm., six tablets with each meal (eighteen tablets daily). They use these pills three days on and two days off. Other patients are treated with nicotinic acid, 100 mg., three times a day before meals. These medications and many others are given in an effort to prevent attacks. To treat a patient *during an attack or crisis,* atropine, 1/100 grain, should be given intramuscularly or intravenously. Atropine acts by abolishing impulses from the autonomic nervous system that, according to some authorities, may have precipitated the attack.

There are several surgical treatments for patients with Meniere's disease. The most effective and certain is ablation or destruction of the inner ear or membranous labyrinth, but it also destroys all hearing in the ear operated upon and therefore is reserved for patients with severe attacks who already have nonserviceable hearing in one ear. The eardrum is reflected, the stapes avulsed from the oval window, and the contents of the vestibular labyrinth aspirated. To seal the inner ear from infection the stapes may be replaced or Gelfoam used to close the oval window.

Postoperatively nursing care is of importance, since these patients are likely to be very dizzy and often vomit for a day or two. Careful notation of intake and output is important, and antibiotics are given to avoid infection of the inner ear. Medications designed to reduce nausea may be useful but may have to be given by injection if the patient is vomiting. After the initial severe reaction (which is not always present) there may be several days of relative unsteadiness during which the nurse may need to support the patient or provide him with a walker.

This procedure abolishes vertigo, but it also leaves the patient with a deaf ear. However, since the operation is reserved for patients whose hearing in one ear is already below the serviceable level, it makes no appreciable change in hearing. If there is a suspicion that Meniere's disease is present in both ears, this operation is not done even on one ear.

In addition, there are other surgical treatments, some new and others old, that have their proponents. Generally we may say that the best technique is not yet agreed upon and that certain methods now in use will be abandoned and others tried before there is consensus.

Therapy using ultrasonic vibrations is also used. This requires a mastoidectomy to give access to the horizontal semicircular canal of the inner ear. The pencil-sized probe or applicator of the ultrasound generator is then applied directly to the bone of the horizontal canal, and energy is directed into the labyrinth in this fashion. Advocates of this treatment point out that vertigo can be abolished and yet the hearing preserved. Therefore this treatment may be useful in patients who have symptoms of vertigo but who still have worthwhile hearing that should be preserved.

Similarly, there are advocates of the use of cryogenic (freezing) therapy, which is performed similarly to the ultrasonic therapy except that it can be done through the ear canal without mastoidectomy.

Meniere's disease is never fatal in itself, although a patient might have an accident if he fell from a ladder or was caught in moving machinery. Because there is no medical treatment that works for all patients, many continue to have crises at irregular intervals over a period of years. Eventually, although the vertigo tends to burn itself out, a patient may be left with poor hearing and tinnitus in the affected ear.

DIFFERENTIAL DIAGNOSIS

Of course, many other conditions besides Meniere's disease may cause vertigo, and other bodily systems besides the ear may be responsible.

Diseases of the central nervous system. In disease of the *central nervous system* dizziness is likely to be much less severe but to last longer than in Meniere's disease. A patient with a brain tumor, for example, may be a little unsteady for months yet never experience the severe whirling vertigo associated with a crisis of Meniere's disease. Also, there are expected to be other signs and symptoms that clinch the diagnosis: papilledema, cranial nerve palsy, headache, and episodes of unconsciousness, none of which is present in the patient with Meniere's disease. Furthermore, except in acoustic neuroma, hearing should be unaffected in most patients with disease of the central nervous system.

Acoustic neuroma. Acoustic neuroma, a tumor affecting the auditory division of the eighth cranial nerve, is another condition that must be differentiated from Meniere's disease. This is a slow-growing tumor that may cause a gradual loss of hearing over a period of several years before the patient begins to notice a mild instability or staggering. There may also be a tinnitus or ear noise just as there is in Meniere's disease. In addition, because a large neuroma compresses the brain, there may be headache, papilledema, and other symptoms suggestive of an expanding intracranial tumor. The protein level in the cerebrospinal fluid is usually elevated. The vertigo in Meniere's disease is explosive, severe, and lasts only a few hours, whereas in acoustic neuroma the patient is likely to be a little dizzy all the time, but never experiencing vertiginous crises with clear intervals between attacks. Also, modern audiometric tests help distinguish between lesions of the inner ear (Meniere's disease) and lesions of the acoustic nerve (acoustic neuroma).

Treatment of a small acoustic neuroma is done by the otologist by means of a mastoidectomy approach in which the cochlear and vestibular labyrinth are drilled out (therefore destroyed) to gain access to the internal auditory canal just behind or deep to these structures. Great care is taken to spare the facial nerve in this location. Removal of the tumor removes the danger of further expansion of the growth; tinnitus may not be relieved; if vertigo was a symptom, it is relieved; the patient is permanently deaf in the affected ear.

Larger acoustic neuromas that have grown out of the internal auditory canal to press on the brain are better handled through a neurosurgical approach. In either case, postoperative nursing care is most important. The patient is partially deafened, is vertiginous, has head pain, and may develop meningitis.

Positional vertigo. The cause of positional vertigo is unknown, but the disorder is common. Ordinarily it is self-limited and disappears after several weeks or months. Testing for positional vertigo is done by tipping the patient backward from the sitting position and then turning his head first toward the left, then toward the right. These maneuvers sometimes produce nystagmus and a brief but severe vertigo. A patient who gives this abnormal response to positional testing will say that he often becomes dizzy when he turns his head suddenly in looking up to pull down a blind or when he gets into bed.

Postural hypotension is a common cause of momentary lightheadedness that may be called vertigo, although really it is not. When a person stoops to tie his shoe and then stands quickly, there may be temporary cerebral anoxia. This is a normal manifestation in most people over 40 years of age and means that the blood vessels leading to the brain are less elastic than they were earlier in life.

Epilepsy may be associated with vertigo occasionally. These patients have periods of dizziness and short periods of memory lapse in which they are not quite sure just what happened. Hearing is normal. An electroencephalogram may help in diagnosis and antiepileptic drugs in treatment.

Eustachian tube disorders. Occasionally, probably much less often than is generally believed, occlusion of the eustachian tube causes dizziness. Similarly middle ear disease such as serous otitis media or external ear disease such as impacted cerumen may cause dizziness. All of these disorders produce findings that are detectable by otologic physical examination.

The dizziness caused by tubal obstruction is not severe and is intermittent. Furthermore, the associated deafness is of the conductive or middle ear type. A diagnosis of occlusion of the eustachian tube is sometimes made erroneously when the patient actually has Meniere's disease.

A simple test for patency of the eustachian tube is to have the patient hold his nose and swallow. If he feels pressure in the ear, or if the examiner, looking with an otoscope, sees the drumhead move outward at the moment of the swallowing action, the tube is certainly patent and further tests are unnecessary.

The eustachian tube has been incriminated far too often as the cause of dizziness, tinnitus, or deafness. Too many patients have been subjected to repeated tubal inflations or bouginage for disorders in no way related to the eustachian tube.

Chronic mastoiditis may also cause vertigo. This is especially likely to occur when the patient has a cholesteatoma that has caused pressure erosion of the horizontal semicircular canal, producing a fistula leading into the inner ear. Then any increase in pressure at the external acoustic meatus will transmit pressure through the fistula to the inner ear, and the patient momentarily becomes very dizzy. The physician may test the patient for the presence of a fistula by compressing air in the ear canal and noting any eye movements or a falling reaction. Treatment here, of course, is mastoidectomy to remove the cholesteatoma.

Thrombosis of the internal auditory artery. Rather rarely, a patient is seen who has suffered a thrombosis of the internal auditory artery or one of its branches. Depending upon whether the entire artery is affected or just the vestibular or the cochlear branch, the patient may have severe vertigo or profound deafness, or both. Usually the patient has had no previous cochlear or vestibular complaints.

The vertigo, when present, comes on abruptly, and often there is nausea and vomiting. It is very severe and lasts several days or a week. Later the caloric reaction usually indicates a dead labyrinth. If the cochlea is involved, the hearing loss is usually total. The deafness is generally permanent, although the writer has seen some patients recover partial hearing.

Other conditions. There are, of course, other conditions to be included in the differential diagnosis besides the few described. Among them are anxiety reaction, apoplexy, carotid or vertebral artery insufficiency, postconcussion syndrome, carotid sinus syndrome, multiple sclerosis, and viral infections of the inner ear.

Before one treats the patient for Meniere's disease, consultation is arranged with the internist, neurologist, and sometimes the psychiatrist. Routine laboratory studies are performed and roentgenograms of the skull obtained. An electroencephalogram is made occasionally.

SUGGESTED READING

Wood, Charles D.: Medications for vertigo and motion sickness, American Journal of Nursing **66:**1764-1767, Aug., 1966.

References

American Speech and Hearing Association: 1973 Directory, Washington, D. C., 1973, ASHA.

Bauman, Mary K., and Yoder, Norman M.: Adjustment to blindness—reviewed, Springfield, Ill., 1966, Charles C Thomas, Publisher.

Beland, Irene L.: Clinical nursing, ed. 2, New York, 1970, The Macmillan Co.

Bluff, Leighton E., and Johnson, Joseph E.: Clinical concepts of infectious disease, Baltimore, 1972, The Williams & Wilkins Co.

Chodil, Judith, and Williams, B.: The concepts of sensory deprivation, Nursing Clinics of North America 5:453-465, Sept., 1970.

Cullin, Irene C.: Techniques for teaching patients with sensory defects, Nursing Clinics of North America 5:527-538, Sept., 1970.

DeWeese, David D., and Saunders, William H.: Textbook of otolaryngology, ed. 4, St. Louis, 1973, The C. V. Mosby Co.

Directory of Services for the Deaf in the United States, American Annals of the Deaf, 114, May, 1969.

Fuerst, Elinor V., and Wolff, LuVerne: Fundamentals of nursing, ed. 3, Philadelphia, 1964, J. B. Lippincott Co.

Glorig, Aram, and Gerwin, Kenneth S., editors: Otitis media, Proceedings of the National Conference Collier Hearing and Speech Center, Dallas, Texas, Springfield, Ill., 1972, Charles C Thomas, Publisher.

Gordon, D. M.: Disease of the eye, Ciba Clinical Symposia 14:Oct.-Dec., 1962.

Gragg, Shirley H., and Rees, Olive M.: Scientific principles in nursing, ed. 7, St. Louis, 1974, The C. V. Mosby Co.

Guiding principles and procedures for industrial nurses in care of eye injuries, American Journal of Nursing 61:86, Sept., 1961.

Hogan, Michael J., and Zimmerman, Lorenz, E., editors: Ophthalmic pathology, an atlas and textbook, ed. 2, Philadelphia, 1962, J. B. Lippincott Co.

Lowenfeld, Berthold: Our blind children, ed. 2, Springfield, Ill., 1964, Charles C Thomas, Publisher.

Meyers, David, Schlosser, Woodrow D., and Winchester, Richard A.: Otologic diagnosis and the treatment of deafness, Ciba Clinical Symposia 14:73, April-June, 1962.

Newell, Frank W., and Ernest, J. Terry: Ophthalmology—principles and concepts, ed. 2, St. Louis, 1974, The C. V. Mosby Co.

Reese, Algernon B.: Tumors of the eye, ed. 2, New York, 1963, Harper & Row, Publishers.

Shafer, Kathleen N., and others: Medical-surgical nursing, ed. 5, St. Louis, 1971, The C. V. Mosby Co.

Vaughan, Daniel, Cook, Robert, and Asbury, Taylor: General ophthalmology, ed. 4, Los Altos, Calif., 1965, Lange Medical Publications.

Worrell, Judith Deignan: Nursing implications in the care of patients experiencing sensory deprivation. In Kintzel, Kay Corman, editor: Advanced concepts in clinical nursing, Philadelphia, 1971, J. B. Lippincott Co.

GLOSSARY

Glossary of eye terms

Throughout the text the majority of common ophthalmologic terms have been described in more detail than is possible in a list of definitions. Reference to the index will locate these terms. This glossary is a supplement to the text and is not intended as a complete dictionary.

A

abducens nerve sixth cranial nerve, which innervates the lateral rectus muscle.

abduction rotation of an eye temporally.

abductor a muscle, such as the lateral rectus, which rotates the eye temporally.

abiotrophy synonym for degenerative change.

accommodation near focusing of the eye, accomplished by an increase in strength of the lens achieved by contraction of the ciliary muscle.

accommodation-convergence ratio relationship between accommodation and convergence of the two eyes, which determines (in part) whether they will be straight.

acetylcholine the chemical that transmits parasympathetic impulses to the muscle fiber (e.g., sphincter of iris) and transmits impulses across most nerve synapses.

achromatic corrected for chromatic distortion.

achromatopsia color blindness for all colors.

acne rosacea chronic dermatosis of unknown cause, which may result in corneal scarring.

acuity ability of the eye to see fine detail.

add additional lens strength of the bifocal part of an eyeglass.

adduction turning of an eye toward the nose.

adductor a muscle, such as the medial rectus, which turns the eye toward the nose.

Adie's syndrome slowness of the reflexes, including a tendency for one or both pupils to respond only slowly to light or dark.

adnexa adjacent structures of the eye; e.g., lids and extraocular muscles.

Adrenalin the chemical that transmits sympathetic impulses to the muscle fiber (e.g., dilator of iris).

advancement moving forward of an extraocular muscle for surgical correction of strabismus, with the intent of increasing its function.

afterimage visual sensation remaining even though the eye no longer looks at the object producing the afterimage (e.g., the bright sensation seen when the eyes are closed after looking at a light).

agnosia cerebral inability to recognize the meaning of details seen or otherwise perceived.

akinesia blocking of muscle movement (e.g., paralysis of orbicular muscle by anesthesia of the seventh nerve to prevent squeezing of eyelids during surgery).

albinism genetically determined deficiency of pigment, either localized or general throughout the body; if the retina is involved, vision is reduced.

alexia inability to read because of damage to the reading centers of the cerebral cortex.

amaurosis little-used synonym for blindness, frequently used to designate visual loss in a structurally normal eye (as from a pituitary tumor).

amblyopia reduced vision in an eye appearing normal to examination; this term is most commonly used as "suppression amblyopia," which refers to cerebral blocking of vision in an eye that is deviated or suffers from a refractive error more marked than that of the good eye.

amblyoscope a stereoscope-like instrument that can present different pictures to the two eyes at various angles of ocular deviation; such instruments are useful in orthoptic evaluation and treatment of patients with strabismus.

ametropia general term meaning the presence of refractive error of any type.

angioid streaks linear retinal change resembling a blood vessel, but representing a rupture of Bruch's membrane; this lesion appears in pseudoxanthoma elasticum, sickle cell anemia, Paget's disease, and senile elastosis.

angioscotoma extension of the normal blind spot caused by local blocking of vision by a large retinal vessel.

angle kappa angle between the direction of gaze and the apparent direction in which the eye points; this is normal but may cause errors in measurement of strabismus.

aniridia absence of the iris.

aniseikonia difference in size of the images received by the two eyes.

anisocoria difference in size of the two pupils.

anisometropia difference in refractive error of the two eyes.

ankyloblepharon abnormal adhesion between the margins of the upper and lower eyelids.

annulus of Zinn circular fibrous origin of the extraocular muscles in the back of the orbit.

anomaloscope research instrument for measuring color vision.

anomalous retinal correspondence (A.R.C.) an adaptation to strabismus whereby the deviating eye relearns directional orientation in terms of its abnormal position (e.g., the brain no longer interprets the macula as looking straight ahead).

anophthalmos total failure of the eye to develop.

antagonist the extraocular muscle exerting opposing pull (e.g., the medial rectus is the antagonist of the lateral rectus of the same eye).

anterior chamber aqueous-containing space between the cornea and the iris.

aphakia absence of the lens.

applanation tonometry measurement of intraocular pressure by an instrument that flattens a predetermined area of the cornea

aqueous clear fluid secreted by the ciliary processes, which fills the anterior and posterior chambers.

arcus senilis the gray ring commonly observed in the peripheral cornea of older persons; represents a benign lipoid infiltration of no local or general significance.

argyrosis dirty blue discoloration of conjunctiva caused by deposition of silver, usually after prolonged use of Argyrol.

aspheric lens a special lens corrected for peripheral distortions; such lenses give improved vision after cataract extraction.

asteroid hyalitis degenerative vitreous change causing numerous tiny white nodules to develop within the vitreous; rarely impairs vision.

asthenopia inability to use the eyes for a reasonable length of time without discomfort or fatigue.

astigmatism optical distortion usually caused by irregular corneal curvature, which prevents a clear focus of light at any point.

atropine a drug that blocks parasympathetic innervation (causes dilation of the pupil and paralysis of accommodation); used in treatment of intraocular inflammation and in refraction of the eyes of children.

axis direction in which astigmatism is oriented.

B

bedewing a delicate edema of the corneal epithelium, recognizable by biomicroscopy.

bifocal the double lens usually prescribed for older persons who can no longer accommodate; the lower portion focuses for near vision.

binocular vision normal simultaneous use of both eyes (which results in depth perception).

biomicroscope the clinical examining instrument (slit lamp) that combines a microscope with a very thin beam of light and permits observation of minute details within the transparent eye.

blepharitis inflammation of the eyelid.

blepharochalasis excess of the upper lid skin.

blepharospasm involuntary contraction of the orbicularis muscle.

blindness although the ophthalmologist usually considers blindness to mean inability to see, legal blindness is defined as vision (corrected by eyeglasses) of 20/200 or less, or less than 20 degrees of visual field, in the better eye.

bombé (of iris) forward displacement of iris caused by block of the pupil, which prevents forward flow of aqueous.

buphthalmos enlargement of the eye caused by secondary glaucoma at an early age.

butyn a topical anesthetic, little used because it is uncomfortable and frequently causes allergy.

C

campimeter synonym for tangent screen; a flat black surface used for evaluation of the central part of the visual field.

canal of Schlemm important aqueous drainage channel encircling the periphery of the anterior chamber.

canaliculus that portion of the lacrimal drainage apparatus between the punctum and the sac.

canthus the outer or inner angle between the eyelids.

carbachol a synthetic parasympathomimetic drug frequently used in treatment of glaucoma; a miotic.

caruncle the normal nodular elevation of the inner corner of the eye.

cataract any defect in transparency of the lens.

chalazion cystic dilation of a meibomian gland, usually caused by postinflammatory blockage of its duct.

ciliary body that portion of the uveal tract between the iris and the choroid which contains the muscles of accommodation and secretes aqueous.

cilium eyelash.

cocaine a narcotic that was the first anes-

thetic used topically in the eye; because of its corneal toxicity, cocaine is rarely used except as a diagnostic aid in Horner's syndrome.

collyrium synonym for eye drops.

coloboma any notchlike defect in the eye or lids.

color blindness inability to differentiate normally between colors; the most common type causes confusion between red and green.

comitant nonparalytic; a strabismus that does not change in amount with different positions of the eyes.

commotio retina edema of the retina after ocular contusion.

concave lens an incurved (center thinner than edges) lens that corrects nearsightedness.

cone retinal cell used for daylight vision.

conformer an oval shell fitted in the eye socket immediately following surgical removal of the eye in order to minimize contraction before fitting of the artificial eye (usually done one month postoperatively).

conjunctiva the mucous membrane lining the back of the lids (palpebral) and the front of the eye (bulbar) except for the cornea.

contact lens a very thin lens that fits directly upon the cornea under the eyelids.

conus a crescent-shaped degenerative area adjacent to the optic nerve; myopia is a common cause.

convergence turning of the two eyes toward each other.

convex lens an outcurved (center thicker than edges) lens that corrects farsightedness.

corectopia eccentric position of the pupil; normal in small amount.

cornea the normally transparent anterior surface of the eye.

couching primitive surgical practice of dislocating a cataract into the vitreous; visual improvement obtained in this way is transient, since lens-induced inflammation usually destroys the eye.

craniostenosis an inherited fault of the skull suture lines; of eye interest because of the frequency with which an abnormally shallow orbit develops and because bony constriction may damage the cranial nerves.

cross cylinder a lens made up of two astigmatic lenses at right angles to each other; this is used in refraction to measure astigmatism.

cross-eyes lay term for convergent strabismus.

cul-de-sac upper or lower conjunctival recess.

cyclitis inflammation of the ciliary body.

cyclodialysis antiglaucoma operation that separates the ciliary body from the sclera, thereby creating a new exit for the aqueous.

cyclodiathermy antiglaucoma operation that partially destroys the ciliary body, thereby reducing aqueous formation.

cyclophoria a tendency for the eye to become misaligned by rotating on an anteroposterior axis.

cyclopia developmental anomaly in which both eyes are joined together to form a single partially duplicated eye located in the central forehead.

cycloplegia paralysis of accommodation.

cylinder a lens for the correction of astigmatism.

D

dacryoadenitis inflammation of the lacrimal gland.

dacryocystectomy surgical removal of the tear sac.

dacryocystitis inflammation of the tear sac, usually caused by faulty drainage.

dacryocystorhinostomy surgical communication between a blocked tear sac and the nose.

decentration an eccentric positioning of a lens used to produce a prism effect.

deorsumvergence turning of both eyes downward.

descemetocele protrusion of Descemet's membrane, which occurs after the loss of corneal structure from disease or injury.

Descemet's membrane the elastic layer on the posterior corneal surface.

detachment separation of one layer of the eye from the adjacent one, a choroidal detachment is separated from the sclera; a retinal detachment, from the pigment layer; a vitreous detachment, from the retina.

deuteranomaly mild form of red-green color blindness, with reduced sensitivity to green.

deuteranopia type of red-green color blindness, with greatest loss of sensitivity for green.

deviating eye the eye that is not straight in strabismus as distinguished from the "fixing eye."

dextroversion simultaneous turning of both eyes to the right.

DFP diisopropylfluorophosphate; isofluorophate; a very long-acting cholinesterase inhibitor used in the therapy of glaucoma and accommodative esotropia; a miotic.

dictyoma a neoplasm originating from the neuroepithelium of the pars plana.

dionine an irritant causing vasodilation after topical application, used without success to "slow the growth" of cataract.

diopter the unit in which the refracting strength of a lens is designated (diopters are calculated as the reciprocal of the focal length of a lens measured in meters).

diplopia double vision, usually caused by faulty alignment of the two eyes.

discission technique of incising a cataract with a knife-needle in order to create an optical opening; this method is applicable to cataracts in children or to thin secondary membranes in adults but will not remove the nucleus of an adult cataract.

disk that portion of the optic nerve visible with an ophthalmoscope.

distichiasis reduplication of the eyelashes; the inner lashes originate behind the gray line and usually irritate the cornea.

divergence movement of the two eyes apart from each other.

drusen hyaline nodules of the lamina vitrea of the choroid, very commonly present but rarely disturbing vision.

dyscoria distorted pupil shape.

dystrophy inherited degenerative change; the cornea may be affected by a number of different types of dystrophy.

E

ectasia bulging forward of a weakened cornea; ectasia to be differentiated from staphyloma, which is a bulging area lined with uveal tissue.

ectropion abnormal outward displacement of the lid away from the eye.

eikonometer an instrument that measures the relative size of images seen by the two eyes.

electrooculogram recording of the electrical potential of the whole eye.

electroretinogram recording of the electrical potential of the retina.

elevator an extraocular muscle that rotates the eye upward.

embryotoxon developmental opacity of the posterior surface of the peripheral cornea.

emmetropia the refractive condition of an eye that is perfectly focused for distance without the aid of accommodation.

endophthalmitis infection of the interior of the eye.

enophthalmos abnormal displacement of the eye backward into the orbit, caused by atrophy of the orbital contents or their loss through a fracture.

entoptic phenomena sensations perceived because of mechanical reasons within the eye (e.g., the floaters and flashes caused by retinal detachment).

entropion abnormal inward displacement of the lid margin toward the eye.

enucleation surgical removal of the entire eye, including the sclera.

epiblepharon congenital redundant skin fold overlying the inner portion of the lower lid.

epicanthus congenital skin fold overlying the inner portion of the upper lid and the inner canthus; this simulates the appearance of esotropia.

epinephrine the chemical mediator at sympathetic nerve endings; useful as a vasoconstrictor in ophthalmic surgery and may be used in glaucoma therapy to reduce aqueous secretion.

epiphora tearing; caused by blockage of the lacrimal drainage apparatus or overproduction of tears.

episclera loose connective tissue on the scleral surface.

episcleritis an allergic response of the episclera; to be differentiated from other causes of red eye.

equator midportion of the eye, of significance in surgical or retinal localization.

erisophake small vacuum cup designed to hold a cataract during its removal.

eserine (physostigmine) an indirect-acting parasympathomimetic drug used in treatment of glaucoma; a miotic.

esophoria latent convergent deviation of the two eyes.

esotropia convergent strabismus.

euthyscope an instrument designed to treat excentric fixation by excessively illuminating the retina adjacent to the macula, thereby relatively enhancing macular vision.

evisceration removal of the contents of the eye with retention of the sclera.

exenteration removal of all soft tissues within the bony orbit.

exophoria latent divergent deviation of the two eyes.

exophthalmometer an instrument that measures the anteroposterior position of the eye within the orbit.

exophthalmos abnormal displacement of the eye forward out of the orbit caused by increase in volume of orbital contents or abnormally shallow orbital bony structure.

exotropia divergent strabismus.

extraocular pertaining to structures outside the sclerocorneal covering of the eye.

F

farsightedness the refractive error in which parallel light is focused behind the retina; accommodation is required in order to see clearly in the distance.

field of vision the entire area that can be seen by an eye.

fixing eye the nondeviating eye in strabismus.

floaters opacities within the vitreous space that cast moving shadows upon the retina.

fluorescein a harmless indicator stain useful in recognizing corneal epithelial abrasions and in verifying the fit of contact lenses.

focus to adjust a lens system to produce a sharp, clear picture.

folliculosis a chronic conjunctivitis that causes multiple tiny lymphatic nodules to become visible, especially in the inferior cul-de-sac.

footcandle unit of illumination; 1 footcandle is generated by 1 lumen upon a square foot of surface.

fornix conjunctival recess; cul-de-sac.

fovea centralis central portion of the retina with the highest visual acuity, ophthalmoscopically visible as a bright light reflection seen in healthy eyes.

fundus internal surface of the eye, including the optic disk, the retina, and the choroidal or scleral details visible through the retina.

fusion cerebral synthesis of the two ocular pictures into a single mental picture.

G

gerontoxon arcus senilis.

glare irregularly scattered light, which interferes with the focused retinal picture and reduces visual acuity.

glaucoma abnormally increased intraocular pressure, which causes irreversible death of the optic nerve fibers.

gonioprism (gonioscope) special type of contact lens that permits examination of the periphery of the anterior chamber; study of this portion of the eye is of importance in patients with glaucoma.

goniopuncture antiglaucoma operation that makes a tiny slit through the trabeculum and anterior sclera to permit aqueous to flow into the sub-Tenon's space.

gonioscopy study of the angle of the anterior chamber with the aid of a special contact lens (gonioscope).

goniosynechia tiny adhesions between the peripheral iris and the trabecular meshwork.

goniotomy antiglaucoma operation that cuts the abnormal tissue present in the anterior chamber angle of eyes with congenital glaucoma.

granulomatous uveitis inflammation of the iris, ciliary body, or choroid characterized by a chronic, destructive course, and supposedly caused by active bacterial infection (e.g., tuberculosis).

H

haploscope stereoscope-like instrument used in orthoptic training and diagnosis.

hemeralopia inability to see well in daylight illumination, with preservation of good night vision.

hemianopia loss of vision in approximately one half of the visual field.

heterochromia difference in color of the two irides or in parts of the same iris.

heteronymous indicates involvement of the temporal visual field in both eyes or of both nasal fields (to be distinguished from homonymous).

heterophoria tendency for the eyes to deviate from straightness.

heterotropia strabismus.

hippus rapidly alternating increase and decrease of pupil size associated with neurologic disturbances or occurring to a lesser degree physiologically.

homatropine a parasympatholytic drug with shorter action than atropine; useful in refraction.

homonymous indicates involvement of the same side of the two visual fields (e.g., right homonymous hemianopia).

hordeolum (sty) infection of a gland near the eyelid margin.

horopter the curved plane in space seen simultaneously by corresponding portions of the two retinas at a given position of the eyes; this concept is of value in theoretical considerations of binocular vision.

hue color.

hyalitis vitreous inflammation or degeneration.

hydrophthalmos congenital glaucoma.

hyperopia farsightedness; the refractive error in which light rays focus behind the retina.

hyperphoria latent upward deviation of an eye.

hypertelorism lateral displacement of the eyes because of an orbital anomaly.

hypertropia vertical strabismus.

hyphema blood in the anterior chamber.

hypopyon purulent discharge in the anterior chamber.

I

implant the rounded prosthesis buried in the orbit to replace partially the volume of an enucleated or eviscerated eye.

infraversion rotation downward of both eyes.

intorsion rotation of the eye on an anteroposterior axis so that the upper portion of the eye moves toward the nose.

intraocular within the eye.

iridectomy antiglaucoma operation that removes part of the iris.

iridencleisis antiglaucoma operation that uses a wick of iris to maintain a scleral opening through which aqueous drains to the sub-Tenon's space.

iridocyclitis inflammation of the iris and ciliary body.

iridodialysis tearing of the iris from the ciliary body, either traumatic or as part of an antiglaucoma procedure.

iridodonesis trembling of the iris with eye movement, indicating loss of lens support, as in aphakia or dislocated lens.

iridectomy prophylactic antiglaucoma procedure that makes a small cut through the peripheral iris.

iridoplegia paralysis of the iris.

iris colored portion of the eye surrounding the pupil.

isopter outer limit of the visual field as measured with a specific test object.

J

Jaeger type print of varying size used for measurement of near visual acuity.

jaw-winking a congenital anomalous connection between innervation to the levator and the pterygoid muscles of the jaw, resulting in elevation of the upper lid when the mandible is moved.

K

keratectomy excision of a superficial portion of the cornea.

keratic precipitate (K.P.) inflammatory deposits on the back surface of the cornea.

keratitis corneal inflammation.

keratoconus cone-shaped distortion of the central cornea resulting from degeneration of the stromal lamellae.

keratomalacia corneal breakdown resulting from vitamin A deficiency.

keratometer an instrument for measuring corneal curvature; useful in fitting contact lenses and in refraction.

keratoplasty corneal transplantation.

L

lacrimal pertaining to the structures that produce or drain the tears.

lacrimation excessive tearing.

lagophthalmos failure of the eyelids to close completely.

lamina vitrea inner layer of the choroid.

lens focusing structure immediately behind the iris with which accommodation is accomplished.

lensometer instrument that measures the strength of an eyeglass.

lenticonus inherited abnormal curvature of posterior or anterior lens surface.

leukocoria a white pupil caused by opaque tissue within the eye.

leukoma a dense scar of the cornea.

levator palpebrae the muscle raising the upper lid.

levoversion simultaneous rotation of both eyes to the left.

limbus junction of the cornea and sclera.

loupe binocular magnifier; useful in ophthalmic surgery.

lumen unit of light energy.

lysozyme an enzyme present in tears that can destroy some types of bacteria.

M

macula lutea central portion of the retina, several disk diameters in area.

madarosis loss of eyelashes.

Maddox rod a lens composed of a parallel series of very strong cylinders; when viewed through a Maddox rod, a point of light appears as a line; used to measure extraocular muscle balance (phoria).

magnification increase in size achieved by a lens system.

megalocornea an inherited abnormally large cornea; must be differentiated from the enlarged cornea resulting from congenital glaucoma.

meibomian glands sebaceous glands within the tarsal plates that open just behind the gray line of the lid margin.

melanin uveal pigment.

melanoma neoplasm arising from the uveal tract.

melanosis bulbi congenital hyperpigmentation of an eye.

metamorphopsia distortion of vision caused by retinal edema or damage.

microcornea an abnormally small cornea on an otherwise normal-sized eyeball.

micronystagmus very fine movements of the eyes normally present at all times.

microphthalmos abnormal smallness of the entire eyeball.

micropsia minification of vision caused by retinal edema.

migraine unilateral headache associated with premonitory visual disturbances; attributed to cerebral vasospasm.

minus lens a concave lens.

miotic a medication causing the pupil to become small.

monochromatopsia total color blindness.

monocular pertaining to one eye.

morgagnian cataract a hypermature, partially liquefied cataract, with a freely moveable central nucleus.

mucocele a mucus-filled distention of a sinus or the lacrimal sac.

muscae volitantes small floaters caused by minute opacities contained within the vitreous humor.

mydriatic a medication causing the pupil to become large.

myectomy surgical removal of part of a muscle; most often done to correct overaction of the inferior oblique muscle.

myokymia twitching of the orbicular muscle, usually because of fatigue.

myopia nearsightedness; the refractive error in which parallel light rays focus in front of the retina.

myotomy surgical transection of a muscle; most often done to correct overaction of the inferior oblique muscle.

N

nasolacrimal duct channel between the lacrimal sac and nasal cavity.

needling incision of the lens capsule with a tiny knife intended to remove a secondary membrane or to permit absorption of a cataract in a young person.

neuroepithelium rods and cones.

nevus localized hyperpigmentation of choroid, iris, or conjunctiva.

nicking compression of a vein by an arteriosclerotic arteriole at an arteriovenous crossing.

nictitation blinking of the lids.

noncomitant describes a strabismus varying in amount with the position of the eyes, thereby indicating the presence of a paralyzed muscle.

nyctalopia night blindness, with preservation of normal daylight vision.

nystagmus rhythmic involuntary oscillation of the eyes caused by abnormal innervation or by lifelong reduced vision.

O

occluder a cover for the eye; used in therapy of suppression amblyopia, to eliminate diplopia, for examination purposes, or to conceal deformity.

oculist a medically trained eye specialist.

oculomotor third cranial nerve.

O.D. oculus dexter; right eye.

ophthalmia ocular infection or inflammation.

ophthalmodynamometer instrument for clinical measurement of the blood pressure of the ophthalmic artery.

ophthalmologist a medically trained eye specialist.

ophthalmoplegia paralysis of ocular muscles.

ophthalmoscope instrument for clinical examination of the posterior portion of the eye.

opsin protein constituent of the visual pigment, rhodopsin.

optician the technician who prepares and dispenses eyeglasses.

optometrist a nonmedically trained refractionist.

ora serrata anterior boundary of the retina.

orbicularis oculi the muscle that closes the eyelids.

orbit bony eye socket.

orthophoria freedom from a latent tendency to ocular deviation.

orthoptics techniques used in diagnosis and treatment of strabismus or heterophoria.

O.S. oculus sinister; left eye.

O.U. oculi uterque; both eyes.

P

palpebral referring to the eyelids.

pannus a vascular corneal scar.

panophthalmitis generalized infection of the eye.

papilledema ophthalmoscopically visible swelling of the optic disk resulting from increased intracranial pressure or other cause of vascular stasis.

papillitis (optic neuritis) inflammatory swelling of the optic disk.

papilloma a benign ectodermal tumor that may arise from any surface part of the eye and its appendages (except the cornea).

paracentesis surgical drainage of the aqueous; very rarely indicated since the development of modern medical therapy.

parafoveal area retinal area adjacent to the fovea; usually the site of eccentric fixation in suppression amblyopia.

parallelepiped the corneal section illuminated by a slit lamp.

paresis incomplete paralysis.

P.C.B. punctum convergens basalis; near point of convergence plus the distance to the center of ocular rotation.

P.D. interpupillary distance.

perimeter instrument for clinical measurement of the visual field.

periorbita periosteum lining the inside of the orbit.

peripapillary surrounding the optic disk.

peritomy surgical separation of the conjunctiva from the limbus, performed as a preliminary step in various procedures.

phaco-anaphylaxis intraocular inflammation resulting from sensitivity to lens material.

phacolytic glaucoma increased intraocular pressure resulting from the toxic effect of liquefied lens cortex.

phakomatoses inherited neoplasms, all of which frequently affect the eye and the skin; include neurofibromatosis, encephalotrigeminal angiomatosis, tuberous sclerosis, and cerebelloretinal angiomatosis.

phlyctenule a localized conjunctival or corneal inflammatory nodule, supposedly caused by tuberculous hypersensitivity.

phoria latent tendency to ocular deviation.

phorometer instrument for clinical measurement of ocular muscle balance.

phoroptor instrument for clinical measurement of refractive error and ocular muscle balance.

phosphene sensation of light caused by mechanical or electrical stimulation of the retina or optic nerve.

photochemical light-sensitive visual pigments.

photocoagulation use of an intense, precisely focused light beam for sealing of retinal tears or for destruction of intraocular vascular anomalies or neoplasms.

photopic vision vision at daylight illumination.

photopsia flashing light sensations resulting from retinal disease.

photoreceptor rod or cone cell.

phthiriasis palpebrarum body louse infestation of the lids.

phthisis bulbi a mushy, soft atrophic destruction of the eye caused by very severe infection or injury.

physostigmine (eserine) an indirect-acting parasympathomimetic drug used in therapy of glaucoma; a miotic.

pilocarpine a direct-acting parasympathomimetic drug used in therapy of glaucoma.

pinguecula an inherited benign elastic nodule situated in the interpalpebral space several millimeters nasal or temporal to the cornea; long-continued irritation may cause transformation into pterygium.

pink eye acute bacterial conjunctivitis.

placidoscope an illuminated pattern of concentric rings that reveals abnormalities of corneal curvature when reflected from the corneal surface.

plano- a lens having no refractive strength.

pleoptics orthoptic method of treating eccentric fixation.

plica semilunaris remnant of the third eyelid situated in the inner canthus.

plus lens convex lens.

polycoria a congenital anomaly in which an eye has more than one pupil.

Pontocaine a topical anesthetic used for minor ocular surgery and tonometry.

presbyopia loss of accommodation because of age.

prism a wedge-shaped lens that displaces the position of objects viewed through it.

protanomaly mild form of red-green color blindness with reduced sensitivity to red.

protanopia type of red-green color blindness with greatest loss of sensitivity for red.

pseudoglaucoma optic atrophy and cupping resembling glaucoma but caused by vascular damage rather than by increased intraocular pressure.

pseudoneuritis physiologic variation in appearance of the optic disk that may be confused with the appearance of papillitis.

pseudopterygium a superficial vascularized corneal scar.

pterygium an elastic degenerative change that slowly proliferates from the conjunctiva upon the cornea; it originates from a pinguecula in response to irritation.

ptosis drooping of the upper eyelid resulting from deficient innervation or muscular strength.

pupil central opening encircled by the iris.

Q

quadrantopia loss of approximately one fourth of the visual field.

R

recession operation for strabismus in which the effect of a muscle is decreased by moving its insertion backward.

refraction clinical measurement of the error of focus in an eye.

resection operation for strabismus in which the effect of a muscle is increased by shortening its tendon.

retina innermost, light-sensitive layer of the eye.

retinoblastoma a malignant tumor of childhood originating from the retina.

retinopathy noninflammatory disease of the retina.

retinopexy operation for the correction of detached retina.

retinoscope instrument for the objective determination of refractive error.

retrobulbar behind the eye; the site of injection anesthesia for ocular surgery.

retroillumination valuable technique of examination of translucent tissues by light reflected from behind; useful in biomicroscopy and ophthalmoscopy.

retrolental fibroplasia destructive vascular and fibrous overgrowth of the retina occurring in premature children placed in high concentrations of oxygen.

rhodopsin light-sensitive pigment contained in the rods.

rod visual cell used when the eye is dark adapted.

rubeosis iridis neovascularization of the iris resulting from diabetes, occlusion of the central retinal vein, or some chronic inflammatory conditions.

S

sclera tough white outer layer of the eye.

sclerectomy antiglaucoma operation permitting aqueous to escape through a notch cut from the sclera.

scleromalacia perforans extreme thinning of the sclera usually associated with rheumatic uveitis.

scotoma area of loss of vision within the visual field.

scotopic vision night vision, performed by the rods.

siderosis bulbi iron deposits resulting from a retained intraocular foreign body; iron is toxic and causes extensive degenerative changes within the eye.

situs inversus a mirror reversal of the appearance of the optic disk in which the large vessels run predominantly nasalward from the disk; associated with myopia and uncorrectable visual loss and usually affects only one eye.

skew deviation vertical nonparalytic deviation of the eyes caused by cerebellar disease.

skiascope synonym for retinoscope.

slit lamp (biomicroscope) instrument for examining the eye under high magnification and in optical section obtained by a finely focused slit of light.

socket conjunctival sac remaining after enucleation into which an artificial eye fits.

spasmus nutans a syndrome including nystagmus and head nodding, occurring transiently in infants.

spectrum various wavelengths of light in orderly sequence.

spherophakia a small round lens found in patients with certain mesodermal anomalies (Marchesani's syndrome).

sphincter iridis constrictor muscle of the iris.

squint synonym for strabismus.

staphyloma a bulging defect of cornea or sclera that is lined with uveal tissue.

stenopaeic slit narrow aperture that excludes stray light and thereby enhances the focus of the retina image.

stereocampimeter instrument for measurement of the central visual field of each eye separately, although both eyes are used for fixation.

stereopsis binocular depth perception.

stereoscope instrument that permits different pictures to be positioned before each of the two eyes.

strabismus failure of straightness of the eyes; one eye (the fixing eye) looks directly at the object of attention, whereas the other eye (the deviating eye) does not.

sty (hordeolum) infection of a gland of the eyelid margin.

subluxation of lens partial displacement of the lens from its normal position.

suprachoroid outer layer of the choroid.

supraversion simultaneous rotation of the eyes upward.

suture junction of the ends of the lens fibers, which results in the formation of γ and stellate figures within the lens.

symblepharon adhesion of the lid to the eyeball.

sympathetic ophthalmia sensitization to the uveal pigment of an injured eye, which results in severe uveitis in the uninjured fellow eye.

synchysis scintillans a degenerative vitreous condition in which cholesterol crystals float freely within the liquefied vitreous cavity.

synechia adhesion of the iris to the lens or cornea.

synergists (yoke muscles) the two muscles, one in each eye, that move the eyes in the same direction (e.g., right lateral and left medial recti).

synoptophore stereoscope-like instrument used in orthoptic diagnosis and treatment.

T

tachistoscope instrument that projects a slide for only a fraction of a second; helpful in measuring speed of perception and possibly in some types of visual training.

tangent screen instrument for clinical measurement of the central visual field.

tarsorrhaphy partial fusion of the lids for the purpose of protecting the cornea from exposure.

tarsus fibrous plate that forms the lid contour and provides its strength.

tears lacrimal secretion.

Tenon's capsule connective tissue sheath encircling the eyeball posteriorly.

tenotomy severing all or part of a tendon; performed to decrease the function of a muscle in the surgical correction of strabismus.

tetartanopia a type of blue-yellow color blindness.

tonography measurement of the rate of aqueous outflow; this is clinically feasible and is a valuable method of evaluation of glaucoma.

tonometer instrument for measuring intraocular pressure; this is vitally important for the early detection of glaucoma.

trabeculum meshwork in the anterior chamber angle through which the aqueous flows to leave the eye.

trachoma a blinding virus infection of the cornea and conjunctiva; widely prevalent throughout the world and probably the most common cause of blindness.

transillumination method of determining with transmitted light whether a lesion is solid or cystic.

trephine antiglaucoma operation in which a small circular scleral opening is made to permit aqueous to escape to the sub-Tenon's space.

trichiasis aberrant lashes that turn against the cornea.

triplopia abnormal perception of three images corresponding to only one object.

tritanopia a type of blue-yellow color blindness.

trochlea fibrous pulley of the superior oblique tendon.

trochlear nerve fourth cranial nerve, which innervates the superior oblique muscle.

tucking folding of an extraocular muscle tendon in order to shorten it and increase its action to correct strabismus.

U

uvea vascular and pigmented layer of the eye, including the choroid, ciliary body, and iris.

V

vergence movement together (convergence) or apart (divergence) of the two eyes.

version similar movement of the two eyes in the same direction (e.g., dextroversion).

visuscope modified ophthalmoscope used to identify the fixation characteristics of an amblyopic eye.

vitreous the gel that fills the eye behind the lens.

X

xanthelasma yellowish lipoid plaques in the eyelids of patients with excessive cholesterol.

xerophthalmia dryness of the eyes.

Z

zonule fibers that suspend the lens.

zonulolysis dissolving of the zonules by a solution of alpha-chymotrypsin in order to facilitate cataract extraction.

Glossary of ear, nose, and throat terms

A

achalasia cardiospasm; failure of opening of the lower end of the esophagus.

adenoid pharyngeal tonsil.

adenotome instrument for removal of the adenoid.

aditus ad antrum communication between the mastoid antrum and epitympanum.

ala cartilaginous outer side of each nostril.

alaryngeal speech speech produced after a total laryngectomy.

allergic rhinitis reaction of nasal mucosa to an allergen.

angiofibroma rare nasopharyngeal tumor in young boys.

annulus fibrous peripheral ring of the eardrum.

anosmia loss of sense of smell.

anterior tonsillar pillar fold of mucosa and muscular tissue just anterior to the tonsil.

antrum largest of the mastoid air cells.

antrum of Highmore maxillary sinus.

aphonia loss of voice.

Aspergillus niger black fungal growth sometimes found in the ear canal.

atresia pathologic closure or congenital absence of a normal opening such as the esophagus.

atrophic rhinitis disease causing atrophy, crusting, and bleeding of nasal mucosa.

audiology study of hearing.

audiometer electrically calibrated apparatus used to test hearing.

aural referring to the ear.

auricle external ear exclusive of the ear canal.

B

Barany noisebox apparatus for producing a masking noise.

barotrauma injurious effect on the middle ear or sinuses caused by a sudden change of air pressure.

Bell's palsy idiopathic facial paralysis, usually unilateral.

biopsy removal of living tissue for examination.

blastomycosis a fungal disease.

bone conduction hearing hearing as transmitted through the skull—in contrast to air conduction hearing.

bouginage passage of an instrument through a tubular organ as the eustachian tube or esophagus as a means of increasing its caliber.

branchial referring to the embryonic apparatus that sometimes persists into adult life, causing cervical and cephalic fistulas and cysts.

bronchi air passages leading from the trachea to the lungs.

bronchography outlining the bronchi by instillation of radiopaque oil and making a roentgenogram.

bronchoscopy visual examination of the bronchi through a bronchoscope.

C

calculus salivary stone.

Caldwell-Luc an operation on the maxillary sinus.

caloric test douching the external auditory meatus with cool or warm water to stimulate the labyrinth.

440

carcinoma cancer; a malignant neoplasm of epithelial origin.

cardiospasm achalasia.

carina ridge formed by bifurcation of the trachea.

cauliflower ear contracted and deformed auricle after injury or infection.

cerumen earwax.

cervical referring to the neck.

choana one of the openings of the nose—two anterior and two posterior.

cholesteatoma ball of desquamated skin found in the mastoid and middle ear of some patients with chronic mastoiditis.

chondroma benign cartilaginous tumor.

chorda tympani nerve supplies taste to the anterior part of the tongue; crosses the middle ear space and may be injured during stapedectomy.

cilia hairlike processes on certain epithelial surfaces, especially those of the nose, trachea, and bronchi.

circumvallate papillae large taste buds on the posterior part of the tongue.

cocaine a topical anesthetic.

cochlea bony housing for the organ of hearing.

cold coryza; a viral infection.

concha nasal turbinates.

conductive hearing loss a defect in the external or middle ear, causing an impedance to sound; contrasts with nerve or perceptive hearing loss.

cone of light reflection from the eardrum.

contact ulcer laryngeal ulceration at the vocal processes.

conus elasticus fibroelastic tissue directly under the true vocal cords.

corniculate small, horn-shaped laryngeal cartilage.

cornu horn-shaped processes of thyroid cartilage or hyoid bone.

coronal incision incision made across the crown of the head in surgery.

Corti, organ of organ of hearing in the inner ear.

cribriform plate part of the ethmoid bone, containing perforations for the olfactory fibers.

cricoid ring of cartilage directly under the thyroid cartilage.

croup noisy breathing with hoarse, ringing cough caused by disease of the trachea or larynx.

cuneiform small, wedge-shaped laryngeal cartilage.

cystic hygroma cavernous lymphangioma of the neck.

D

deafness partial or total loss of hearing.

decibel commonly abbreviated db, a unit used to express the intensity level of a sound.

diplacusis hearing the same frequency as a different pitch in the two ears.

discrimination ability to distinguish correctly between words having a similar sound.

diverticulum pouch or sac, especially in the pharynx or esophagus.

drumhead eardrum or tympanic membrane.

dysphagia difficulty in swallowing.

dysphonia difficulty with speech.

dyspnea difficulty in breathing.

E

eardrum tympanic membrane.

endaural through the ear canal, as in endaural mastoidectomy.

endolymph liquid in the inner ear bathing the sensory organs of the acoustic nerve.

endoscopy visual examination of air or food passages using laryngoscope, bronchoscope, or esophagoscope.

ephedrine a drug causing vasoconstriction and used to shrink nasal mucosa.

epidemic parotitis mumps.

epiglottis lidlike cartilage about the larynx.

epistaxis nosebleed.

epitympanum the attic of middle ear, area above the drum membrane.

epulis fibrous tumor of the gingiva.

ethmoidectomy operation to exenterate ethmoid air cells.

eustachian tube channel connecting the middle ear and nasopharynx and through which air is admitted to the middle ear.

exostosis bony growth found in the ear canal or paranasal sinus.

external auditory meatus channel leading to the eardrum.

F

false vocal cord a fold of tissue directly above the true vocal cords.

fenestration operation effective but now seldom used operation to restore hearing in patients with otosclerosis.

filiform papillae one type of lingual papillae.

fistula abnormal communication between two body surfaces, e.g., skin and pharynx.

footplate that part of the stapes fitting in the oval window.

fossa of Rosenmüller a space above the torus tubarius in the nasopharynx.

frequency the number of sound waves per second determining the pitch of sound.

fungiform papillae one type of lingual papillae.

G

ganglion a point in a nerve at which fibers synapse or join other fibers.

geniculate ganglion ganglion associated with the facial nerve as it traverses the temporal bone.

geographic tongue migratory glossitis; an asymptomatic condition.

giant cell epulis a red gingival swelling containing characteristic giant cells.

gingiva gums.

glandular fever infectious mononucleosis; a viral disease.

globus hystericus sensation of a lump in the throat caused by functional disorder.

glossitis inflammation of the tongue.

glottis space between the vocal cords.

granular pharyngitis inflammation of lymphoid tissue on the posterior pharyngeal wall.

H

hairy tongue elongation of the filiform papillae.

hematemesis vomiting of blood.

hemoptysis expectoration of blood or blood-tinged sputum.

hemotympanum collection of blood in the middle ear.

hyperplastic mucosa that appears redundant or excessively thick.

hypoglossal nerve twelfth cranial nerve; controls movements of the tongue.

hypopharynx lower part of the throat; best seen with a laryngeal mirror.

hysterical aphonia loss of voice caused by functional disorder; more common in women than in men.

I

incus second or middle ossicle of the middle ear; articulates with the malleus and stapes.

infectious mononucleosis glandular fever; a disease of young people, probably viral.

inner ear that part of the ear containing the sensory structures for hearing and equilibrium.

intensity the magnitude of a sound relative to a reference standard.

intrinsic carcinoma, larynx malignancy arising on the true vocal cords.

J

juvenile laryngeal papillomatosis wartlike laryngeal growths in young children; often recurrent.

juvenile nasopharyngeal fibroma benign neoplasm of epipharynx found in young males.

K

keloid dense cutaneous scar tissue; most likely to form in the Negro.

keratin dead, superficial layer of squamous epithelium.

Kiesselbach's plexus formation of tiny blood vessels on the anterior part of the nasal septum.

L

labyrinth that part of the inner ear concerned with equilibrium.

laryngocele a dilated laryngeal ventricle; may present as a cervical tumor.

laryngoscope lighted instrument for direct examination of the larynx.

leukoplakia "white patch," premalignant change in mucous membrane, usually oral or laryngeal.

lichen planus dermatologic disease sometimes presenting oral lesions.

lingual thyroid thyroid tissue at the base of the tongue persistent from the embryologic state.

Lipiodol radiopaque oil used in bronchography.

lop ear outstanding auricle; caused by cartilaginous deformity of the external ear.

Ludwig's angina infection of the fascial spaces in the floor of the mouth.

lymphoepithelioma malignancy associated with lymphoid tissue of the nasopharynx or tonsillar region.

M

macroglossia large tongue.

malleus auditory ossicle attached to the eardrum and articulating with the incus.

manubrium handle of the malleus.

masking to introduce a noise in one ear so as to exclude that ear from the hearing test being given to the opposite ear.

mastoid part of the temporal bone.

maxilla upper jaw.

maxillary sinus large air space in the maxillary bone lined by mucosa and opening into the nose.

meatus opening or channel, such as the external auditory meatus.

Meniere's disease triad of symptoms—tinnitus, unilateral hearing loss, and vertigo —caused by a disorder of the inner ear.

metastasis spread of a malignant tumor by lymphatic or vascular channels.

microtia small external ear.

middle ear air-filled space behind the eardrum in communication with the mastoid air cells and, via the eustachian tube, with the nasopharynx.

modified radical mastoidectomy operation designed to remove disease from the temporal bone but to preserve hearing.

mucocele collection of mucous in one of the paranasal sinuses.

mulberry turbinates bluish, pitted posterior tips of the inferior turbinates.

mumps infectious parotitis; a viral disease.

myringitis inflammation of the tympanic membrane.

myringotomy incision of the tympanic membrane for drainage of pus from the middle ear.

N

nasofrontal duct drainage channel from the frontal sinus into the nose.

nasolacrimal duct drainage channel for tears; leads into the nose.

nasopharynx space above the soft palate and posterior to the nose—the epipharynx.

nicotine stomatitis inflammation of the mouth caused by smoking.

nystagmus jerking movement of the eyes that is sometimes the result of labyrinthine stimulation.

O

olfactory nerve first cranial nerve; associated with sense of smell.

organ of Corti sensory organ of the auditory nerve, located in the cochlea.

oroantral fistula abnormal communication between the mouth and maxillary sinus.

ossicles the three tiny bones of the middle ear—malleus, incus, and stapes.

ostium an opening (plural, **ostia**).

otitis inflammation of either the external or the middle ear.

otosclerosis a disease causing hearing loss by fixation of the stapes in the oval window.

ozena odor from the nose in patients with atrophic rhinitis.

P

papilloma irregular benign growth in the mouth or larynx.

paracentesis opening made in the eardrum for drainage of the middle ear.

parosmia perverted sense of smell.

parotitis inflammation of the parotid gland.

pars flaccida Shrapnell's membrane—a small part of the eardrum, superiorly, without a fibrous layer.

P-B words phonetically balanced words of one syllable used in speech audiometry, e.g., *eat*, *tree*, and *ice*.

perceptive hearing loss sensorineural, or nerve-type, hearing loss.

perichrondrium membrane covering cartilage.

perilymph liquid in the inner ear surrounding the membranous ducts that contain endolymph.

periodontoclasia pyorrhea.

periorbital abscess infection in the fatty tissue of the orbit.

peritonsillar abscess collection of pus just outside the tonsillar capsule.

PGSR psychogalvanometric skin resistance audiometry.

pharyngeal bands lymphoid tissue in the pharynx behind the posterior tonsillar pillars.

pillars (tonsillar) folds of mucosa and muscle just before and behind the palatine tonsils.

polypoid corditis edematous mucous membrane of the true vocal cords.

postcricoid carcinoma malignancy of the upper esophagus behind the cricoid cartilage.

presbycusis hearing loss caused by the aging process.

promontory basal whorl of the cochlea; forms the medial wall of the middle ear.

pulsion diverticulum Zenker's diverticulum of the lower pharynx.

pyocyaneus bacterial organism commonly causing external otitis and producing green pus.

pyorrhea disorder of the gingiva with infection and retraction of the gums.

pyriform fossa pear-shaped space opening into the esophagus posterior and lateral to the vocal cords.

pyriform recess space posterolateral to the arytenoid cartilages leading into the esophagus.

Q

quinsy peritonsillar abscess.

R

radical mastoidectomy operation on the temporal bone to remove disease from the mastoid and middle ear.

recruitment phenomenon of the inner ear in which there is an abnormally rapid increase in loudness.

Rendu-Osler-Weber disease hereditary hemorrhagic telangiectasia.

rhinophyma external nasal tumor caused by proliferation of sebaceous glands.

rhinoplasty reconstruction of the external nose done usually for cosmetic purposes.

rhinorrhea nasal discharge; sometimes specific as in cerebrospinal rhinorrhea.

Rinne test tuning fork test to compare air and bone conduction.

Rosenmüller's fossa a space above the torus tubarus in the nasopharynx.

S

saccule one of the parts of the inner ear concerned with static equilibrium.

Schwabach test tuning fork test that compares the examiner's hearing by bone conduction with that of the patient.

Schwartze sign a pink blush behind the eardrum seen in some patients with otosclerosis.

semicircular canals parts of the inner ear concerned with equilibrium—three membranous ducts filled with endolymph.

septum that part of the nose separating the two nasal chambers; composed of bone and cartilage.

sensorineural hearing loss damage to nerve tissue of the inner ear and/or sensory paths to the brain, resulting in inability to perceive all sounds. Called nerve or perceptive hearing loss also.

serous otitis media accumulation of blood serum in the middle ear.

sialography examination of the salivary glands by injection of radiopaque substance and by roentgenography.

singer's nodes small nodules on the vocal cords, producing hoarseness; speaker's nodules.

speech audiometry testing hearing by means of live or recorded speech as contrasted to pure tone signals.

spondee words bisyllabic words used in speech audiometry, e.g., *snowball, baseball,* and *doorway.*

Stensen's duct parotid duct.

stomatitis inflammation of the oral cavity.

stridor noisy, difficult breathing, usually inspiratory.

subcutaneous emphysema air in the subcutaneous tissue.

sublingual gland one of the major salivary glands.

submaxillary gland one of the major salivary glands.

sulcus furrow or groove, slight depression (ear gingiva).

T

thrush monilial infection of the oropharynx.

thyroglossal cyst swelling in a persistent remnant of the embryonic tract leading from the base of the tongue to the thyroid gland.

thyroid cartilage part of the larynx—the "Adam's apple."

tinnitus ear ringing or head noise.

torus palatinus overgrowth of bone in the midline of the hard palate.

trachea windpipe.

traction diverticulum outpocketing in the midesophagus; usually asymptomatic and small.

tragus cartilaginous, tonguelike projection in front of the external auditory meatus.

transillumination causing a light to shine through the paranasal sinuses.

trismus inability to open the mouth fully.

true vocal cord part of the larynx used in speech production, formed largely by the thyroarytenoid muscle.

tuning fork vibrating instrument used in testing hearing.

turbinates nasal conchae; internal bony parts of the nose along its lateral wall.

tympanic membrane eardrum.

tympanic sulcus bony groove that receives the margin of the tympanic membrane or annulus.

tympanoplasty reparative or reconstructive operation on the eardrum or middle ear.

tympanosclerosis deposit in the eardrum or middle ear in response to infection.

U

umbo a landmark of the eardrum.

utricle one of the parts of the inner ear related to static equilibrium.

uvula small, tonguelike structure hanging from the soft palate.

V

vallecula space between the epiglottis and base of the tongue, divided by the median glossoepiglottic fold.

varices dilated veins.

vasomotor rhinitis nonspecific congestion of the nasal mucosa.

ventricle a space between the true and false vocal cords formed by an invagination of mucous membrane.

vertigo a whirling dizziness, usually severe.

vestibule anterior part of the nares lined with skin.

vestibulitis inflammation of the skin of the nasal vestibule.

vibrissae hairs within the nasal vestibule.

Vincent's angina a specific infection of the mouth or pharynx.

vomer one of the bones forming the nasal septum.

W

Waldeyer's ring a collective name for all groups of lymphoid tissue found in the pharynx.

Weber test tuning fork test in which the fork is placed on the upper teeth or midline of the skull.

Wharton's duct duct of the submaxillary salivary gland.

X

Xylocaine an anesthetic for injection or topical use.

Z

Zenker's diverticulum outpocketing of mucosa at the hypopharyngeal level; also called pulsion diverticulum.

Appendix

Information and publications on blindness are available from the following organizations upon request.

American Foundation for the Blind, Inc. (founded 1921), 15 W. 16th St., New York, N. Y. 10011.

    A national research and service agency concerned with all aspects of work for the blind; serves as a clearinghouse on information about blindness. Publishes books, pamphlets, monographs, and reports of a professional nature, including the *Directory of Agencies Serving Blind Persons in the United States* and *The New Outlook for the Blind.* Sells special appliances for use by the blind.

American Printing House for the Blind, Inc. (founded 1858), 1839 Frankfort Ave., Louisville, Ky. 40206.

    Prints books and magazines in braille and manufactures talking books. Publishes *The Reader's Digest* in both braille and talking book editions and produces *Newsweek Magazine* in talking book form. Publishes books in large print, talking books, and recorded tapes for use in the education of visually handicapped children. Also conducts a department of educational research.

Braille Institute of America, Inc., 741 N. Vermont Ave., Los Angeles, Calif. 90029.

    Serves the United States through its printing plant. Produces books and magazines in braille and Moon type.

Eye-Bank Association of America, 3195 Maplewood Ave., Winston-Salem, N. C. 27103.

    A volunteer organization furnishing corneas, scleras, and vitreous to patients free of charge throughout the United States.

Fight for Sight, Inc., National Council to Combat Blindness, Inc., 41 W. 57th St., New York, N. Y. 10019.

    A national organization without geographical limitations, which concentrates on financing eye research. Grants are made to accredited medical colleges, hospitals, and eye centers. Disseminates information as to the need for, and potential of, increased eye research.

Hadley School for the Blind (founded 1922), 700 Elm St., Winnetka, Ill. 60093.

    A national school of tuition-free correspondence courses for the blind. The braille home-study courses include some elementary school subjects, a four-year high school program, some university courses, and selected vocational courses. Textbooks are available in braille and/or on records or tape.

Library of Congress; Division for the Blind and Physically Handicapped, Washington, D. C. 20540.

    Serves blind children and adults. Provides books in braille, talking book records, and reproducers for these records. Distributes, maintains, and replaces talking book machines through their thirty-four distributing libraries, which serve assigned geographical locales. Conducts a correspondence course in Standard English Braille to sighted volunteers who plan to become transcribers.

Local and/or state libraries

Supply books and magazines in large print, records, and games for the visually handicapped.

National Society for the Prevention of Blindness, Inc. (founded 1908), 79 Madison Ave., New York, N. Y. 10016.

Engages in a nationwide program to eliminate preventable blindness in both children and adults through field consultation, publications, statistical studies, and other means of public education. Publishes a quarterly periodical, *The Sight Saving Review*. Provides information on the education of partially seeing children.

Office of Education, Section for Exceptional Children and Youth, U. S. Department of Health, Education and Welfare, Washington, D. C. 20202.

The Office of Education provides consultative services to state, county, and city school systems as well as residential schools in the interest of all handicapped children. Conducts research and prepares publications to promote the development of educational programs to meet the needs of children requiring special provisions.

Recording for the Blind, Inc., 215 E. 58th St., New York, N. Y. 10022.

Provides free of charge records and tapes of textbooks and other educational material for any individual unable to read the printed word because of visual or other physical limitations. Will record books at the specific request of borrowers.

Rehabilitation Services Administration, Division of Services to the Blind, U. S. Department of Health, Education and Welfare, Washington, D. C. 20201.

Provides national leadership, technical and consultative assistance, and financial support to the federal-state programs of vocational rehabilitation. Each state administers its own program and provides complete rehabilitation services to eligible blind persons. Vocational guidance, training, placement, and follow-up are available. Information on local services can be obtained at individual state offices of vocational rehabilitation.

The Seeing Eye, Inc., P. O. Box 375, Morristown, N. J. 07960.

Serves the United States, Canada, and Puerto Rico. Qualified blind persons spend one month learning to use and control dog guides. Maintains a follow-up service for graduates. Conducts an extensive program of public education.

Veterans Administration, Washington, D. C. 20420.

The Department of Medicine and Surgery provides an intensive and comprehensive program of basic reorganization to blindness at the Blind Rehabilitation Center, Hines, Ill. Prosthetic and sensory aids are provided to help overcome the handicap of blindness for veterans who meet specific eligibility requirements. The Department of Veterans Benefits furnishes compensation and pension for disability and multiple vocational rehabilitation services.

Index